To Hasmi K
from William

02·11·17 LV

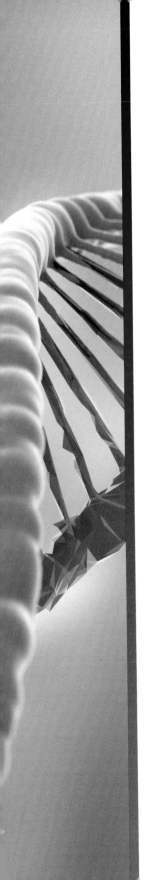

Dr William Amzallag

The Promise of Immortality
Telomeres, stem cells, nanomedicine.

Translated from **French** into **English** by *Zachary Weiss*
Edited by *Dr. Marian Baker*
Text and cover design by *Gregory Stark*

Varegus Publishing

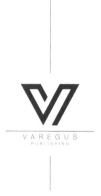

VAREGUS
PUBLISHING

Varegus Publishing

This book is above all a source of information, and is in no way a substitute for the advice of a medical professional. If you suspect you have a medical problem, we suggest you see your doctor. The author and publisher shall not be liable for any risk, personal or otherwise, resulting directly or indirectly from the use of the information found in this book.

Copyright

First edition : *October 2016*

w w w . j l i f e - s c i e n c e s . c o m

Contents

Content

Content

Foreword

« If you want to have good ideas you must have many ideas.
Most of them will be wrong, and what you have to
learn is which ones to throw away »

- Linus Pauling - Nobel Prize -

This book came about entirely unexpectedly: I had decided to compile my notes in a consistent form, in particular for my children. They had trouble keeping track of my various professional adventures and often asked me: « *Dad, what is it you do exactly?* ». It's true that I've pursued many different experiences and it is also true that I did not always follow all of them through to completion. In fact each one of them would have required a lifetime - so it's true, I am a bit of a « *mister incomplete* ». But nonetheless they have taught me lessons, about life which I would like to share with you.

I was born in 1941, I am a doctor, but above all. I am a humanist. Thirsty for knowledge I have spent most of my life, searching for rational explanations to things which most often had nothing to do with reason.

I began my career as an anesthesiologist and as such I had been educated in a strictly classical medical background - To my mind, treatment could only be administered through drugs or surgery, occasionally through psychology, and never through « *esoteric* » means - For me, medical techniques always had to be validated by serious clinical studies. For me, this was THE truth, and the proof was that, it worked! Thanks to this culture, this training, I was able to practice my craft. I was able to, prepare patients for surgical procedures, and lull them to sleep, protect them from the scalpel's assaults, and above all wake them up, all thanks to proven techniques.

Then one day, things changed. During a medical conference, one of my friends, a doctor, suggested that I attend a seminar on Chinese Medicine with him in Montpellier. Prof. J.A Lavier, who taught Chinese medicine, was a decidedly unique man, (and thanks to him), my fixed ideas about health and medicine started to be shaky and then to fall apart. Goodbye symptomatic medicine. Hello global, holistic medicine, welcome, metaphors, the eagle and the tortoise, vital energy, the five elements and the concept of yin and yang.

But what is even more surprising is that I managed to integrate all of these concepts without ever detecting any conflict or divergence from what I had learned. So with no problems I regularly attended this professor's classes for a few years. He was formerly in the US Marines corps, spoke twenty-seven Chinese dialects, and was so convincing!

Did I learn how to stick needles in people? Not exactly! But I discovered a brand new universe, the universe of Tao and of Chinese medicine as a whole. What struck me was the logic and the coherence of this philosophy. What did I hold on to? Two fundamental elements: first, the search for balance, what Taoists call « *the middle way* », second, the « *culture of paradox* », which afforded me real satisfaction in everyday life.

So here I am in 1975 practicing hard-line medicine every day with my desire for globality and my holistic visions: a first step into the universe of paradox!

In the early 80s, I decided to emigrate to the United States, in search of the American dream (paradox once more!).

My American adventure lasted seven years. A full cycle according to Aristotle. A cycle of trying, of stumbling, of falling, bouncing back and of starting over… I tried everything: retaking equivalency tests for my diploma, selling photocopy machines (a disaster) or sports apparel (a catastrophe) and finally returning to Health. My three kids were delighted, my wife much less so. An adventure of this kind cost a lot, my financial balance was starting to falter and even threatened to crumble. But it's always at that point that we bounce back: An old friend came to visit me in Boca Raton, Florida, where I lived, and made me an offer I couldn't refuse, on the condition that I come live in Paris.

And that's how the American dream ended!

Nevertheless, those seven years spent in the United States was one of the most rewarding periods of my life. In fact, I made two life-changing encounters which completely changed my perspective on health and medicine.

The first was in Los Angeles where I had the honor and privilege of meeting Dr. Linus Pauling, pioneer of Orthomolecular Medicine and of vitamin C megadosing. Twice winner of a Nobel Prize, Linus Pauling is the most complete, the most erudite, man I have ever met. He is, to my knowledge, the only scientist to ever have received (without sharing them) two Nobel Prizes in two very different areas (Nobel Prize in Chemistry in 1954 and Nobel Peace Prize in 1962).

The second encounter, which also changed things quite a bit, took place in Montreal, Canada. I had the chance to be able to follow closely the work of Prof. Hans Selye, the father of Stress, who, for the first time, explained and demonstrated the physicochemical and hormonal mechanisms which cause an excess or absence of stress known as « *general adaptation syndrome* ». Why was this so important? Because I suddenly realized that western medicine had just taken an important step forward by admitting what everyone recognizes today: the complex interrelation between the brain and the body.

Finally, after these 45 years of professional experience, I went from a hard and fast scientific mindset, to completely endorsing the concept of alternative medicine, to finally arrive at a reasonable compromise between Science and Traditional Medicine.

But this book is above all a mirror reflecting my personal experience and blindness when faced with a reality which was nevertheless obvious. For more than twenty years I suffered from rheumatoid arthritis which I self-medicated for with anti-inflammatory drugs. I put up with the joint pain more or less until the day the disease speeded up and became very aggressive. At this moment, everything changes: the drugs no longer work, the joint pain becomes debilitating, diabetes takes hold and a cancer forms. It is at this moment that I truly became aware of my mistake: I had quite simply gravely underestimated the ruthless efficiency of this inflammation, the cause (or result) of my polyarthritis. Thanks to this wake-up call I decided to undertake very extensive work on inflammatory phenomena and their harmful impact on our health. I decided to completely transform my lifestyle. Having regular, relatively intense physical activity, eating a healthy diet, eliminating « *toxic* » thoughts from my mind, managing bouts of stress in a positive manner, and taking dietary supplements which were adapted to my needs. After a few months, my polyarthritis was fully under control, I had lost 30 excess pounds as well as 4 inches around my waist, my diabetes vanished and there was no more news of my recent cancer. But even more surprising was that I felt as though rejuvenated: with more energy, better concentration, a « *youthful* » face, much stronger libido, and I could go on…

A few months before I had started writing this book, Laetitia, eleven years old, my wife's daughter, and very curious about life, asked me: « *Say Willy, will you be there with me when I get married and have kids. Will you hold my hand during the delivery like you did for all of your children?* ». I wanted very much to take part in all of my grandchildren's marriages and great grandchildren's births, but I wished with all my heart to be able to participate without having any disabilities, with the energy and mindset of a young man, so yes, in a way, writing this book was, at first, a somewhat egotistical way of finding a solution to live longer, but it is also a wonderful message of hope and optimism for all those willing to believe that aging is not inescapable. Science has made considerable progress in the past twenty years in understanding the phenomenon of aging, and consequently in learning how to slow it, and maybe even to reverse it. It is very likely that one of our great grandchildren will live… over two hundred years, or maybe more!!

William Amzallag
Doctor of Medicine.

Acknowledgments

This book is dedicated, above all, to my family:

To my wife, Julie, without whom it would never have existed;

To her children, Laetitia and Stephanie, whose curiosity compelled them to read along as it came together;

To my children, Kareen, Laetitia and Stefan, who have always followed in my footsteps as I chased paradox;

To my seven grandchildren, whom I don't see often enough;

And finally, to my dear Mother, to whom I owe my thirst for knowledge, and who always gave me her support.

My thanks as well :

To Wendy Lewis and Randy Ray, the co-founders of Jeunesse Global, who gave me their unconditional support for this undertaking and for its translation into English;

To Scott Lewis, Jeunesse Global Chief Visionary Officer, and to his wife Isabel, who have always supported me;

To Dr. Maurice Nahon, for his invaluable help in drafting certain chapters;

To Sylvie Le Bras for her help in editing and organizing this work;

To Gregory Stark for the quality of his layout work;

To Zachary Weiss for his patience in translating this book;

And finally, to Dr. Marian Baker, for her careful read-through.

But above all :

This book is dedicated to you, and the 60 trillion intelligent cells which make up your body and contribute to your well-being.

Introduction

*« Being born isn't a crime,
so why are we all sentenced to die? »*

4 th of August 1997: we are in France, in Arles, in the region of Bouches-du-Rhône, and Jeanne Calment, a French woman born on the 21st of February 1875 has just died. She has lived to be 122 years, 5 months and 14 days old: she has lived 44,724 days, and has since become the oldest living woman, having the longest lifespan on record. At the time, most specialists thought that we had reached, through Jeanne Calment the limits of the human lifespan.

Ten years later experts are proving the opposite. From now on we can already double the current lifespan. We can not only slow down aging but also turn things around, and rejuvenate, in the true sense of the word. We know how to rejuvenate cells, tissues and organs. What we do not yet know is if this can work for every single one of us!

How many times has the thought crossed our minds: *« ah, if only I were 25 years younger, with the experience I have now! »* That wish could be realizable today! Better yet, why not ten extra years? Ten years of good health, ten productive years, without cancer, without Alzheimer's! Or twenty more years to spend with our loved ones, enough time to accomplish all that we haven't been able to! What we want is not only a longer life, but a long life brimming with energy and creativity. Investing in our well-being today could prove to be profitable in the coming years. Technologies are advancing at an exponential pace, and the healthier we stay, the more we increase our chances of reaping the benefits of this progress.

Today, many experts consider aging a sickness whose death rate is, for now, 100%. We can survive certain severe illnesses, but not aging? Many of our fellow citizens do not accept the premise that we could live 'forever'. Many others, for various reasons, consider death to be a good thing; why these fixed ideas? Because, since our birth, we have been conditioned to accept death as inevitable, having no tools to fight it. And yet, if we look back, history shows us that our longevity has only grown over time, and there is no reason to believe that this will stop!

How long could we live? You might be disappointed to learn that at the moment we are not talking about « *eternity* » or « *immortality* ». Rather, the important thing is to eliminate the notion of a limit. Even if we do not wish to live forever, we do not want to die… today or even tomorrow… one day maybe, but not tomorrow: and that is the whole point! Because an answer to aging would place the choice in your hands; advancing years force our hand, suddenly we would like to live longer, to see our grandchildren grow up, or see through important projects, or for a million other reasons!

1 - Old Age: A Disease!

Natural death can no longer be considered a universal Law of Nature. Certain organisms like bacteria or perennial plants can overcome aging and thereby present a kind or immortality. Old age is therefore not an inescapable consequence of the deterioration of our vital functions since certain organisms can avoid it. Old age brings about most serious chronic diseases like diabetes, cardiovascular diseases, cancer, Alzheimer's disease or strokes. Certain preeminent scientists consider old age to be the illness, source of other illnesses rather than a foregone conclusion, and many research centers around the world are therefore working on possible treatments for the illness of old age. Certain research centers like that of Prof. Miroslav Radman (René-Descartes Medical Faculty, Paris, France) are attempting to explain the molecular basis of « *the robustness of life* ». Their first studies have mainly focused on molecular damage repair mechanisms, above all those concerning oxidative damage to DNA, which affects protein quality. Prof. Radman prefers to focus on ways to prevent damage to restorative molecules. Preserved, these will then be able to ensure quick and efficient maintenance. These protective molecules are present in nature, and exist in certain resilient species. These he believes could then protect non-robust species. It will be possible to extract these molecules and reuse them to protect our own cells.

2 - Aging: Three Different Forms!

We presume each living species to have a limited lifespan, which can vary widely depending on the species: a whale can live one hundred fifty years, a shrimp seven years, a crocodile over one hundred years, but a millipede only five years; a turtle one hundred eighty-eight years, a mouse three years. Man is no exception, he also has a limited lifespan, the all-time record (for now) being one hundred and twenty-two years. But he is the only one among all of the species which wants to change things. He already makes use of all means at its disposal: prostheses, transplants, medication, electronics, nuclear and nanotechnologies, everything which is able to neutralize his biological impairments and lengthen his lifespan.

According to Jean-David Ponci, aging takes three distinct forms in living beings:

1 - Those which experience « *gradual senescence* », such as man, which is due to the shortcomings of the organism's defenses when faced with its own deterioration. Man progressively loses vitality starting very early on, probably around 27-30 years old. Though he is still able to reproduce, his strength wanes. From a biological standpoint, it is accumulated damage which is therefore responsible for aging, whereas longevity depends on the efficiency and speed of the response to that damage. The more this response is efficient and expeditious, the more chances the individual has to be long lived.

2 - Those which deplete their organism for the purpose of reproduction. This strategy allows the species to ensure greater reproductive success. Many living beings go through very rapid

senescence once reproduction has been achieved. This is the case for, salmon; after a long migration and the effort expended for reproduction, the genitors are exhausted and let themselves be carried by the current towards calmer waters, where they remain for a few days, at which point they die. The study of all of the forms of accelerated senescence confirms that this process has no other objective than to optimize reproduction.

3 - Those whose longevity is not infinite but rather indefinite, such as certain plants; these living beings have the ability to regenerate their organism through certain specific cells. Their longevity is labeled as « *indefinite* » as it is unpredictable: they could live a single day or ten thousand years. Jean-David Ponci refers to this as « *overcoming senescence* » as the difference lies in that these organisms are able to perfectly repair the damage caused by aging or eliminate damaged elements by regenerating themselves. For example, when a part of the hydra's organism is amputated, the body regenerates it in 2 or 3 days. The hydra is therefore potentially immortal.

The fundamental issue is understanding what makes this or that organism enter one of these three categories rather than another. Jean-David Ponci thinks that the most likely hypothesis is to relate aging to the complete separation of reproductive functions from somatic functions within the organism. Germ/sex cells are responsible for reproduction, whereas somatic cells are responsible for all other functions. Living beings whose sexual and somatic functions are not differentiated could also use their reproductive function to ensure the integrity of their somatic cells; this is the case for bacteria, whose longevity is unlimited. Inversely, all beings in whom these two functions are separate (as is the case for human beings) would inevitably age. In plants, these two functions are not clearly separated. This is why it is always possible to cut off a piece of a plant and transplant it.

All three of these forms have one thing in common: the priority given to reproduction. This is the principle of primacy of the species over the individual. This principle is necessary because any species which invests too much energy into its individuals to the detriment of its reproductive success would inevitably become extinct. This leads to some questions which could bring about a metaphysical or religious debate: Man, who experiences this separation between maintaining somatic functions and reproduction, appears to only be a vehicle for immortal genes, which travel from one mortal body to another. So why isn't our genetic code assembled in such a way that we could live 300 or 600 or 6,000 years? How would these numbers hinder reproduction?

3 - Stem Cells

Stem cells have been discussed at length in the media, but there remains a lot of confusion in readers' minds, in particular as regards embryonic stem cells. Stem cells are, as their name implies, the source of all our cells. It all begins with the fusion of the winning sperm which found its way to the sought-after ovum and fertilizes it. This fusion will bear the first human cell, called a « *zygote* », which is also our first embryonic stem cell. This cell quickly duplicates and becomes a group of cells forming a « *blastocyst* », the origin of all our organs. This blastocyst plays a capital role, it will create the three fundamental tissues of which our body is composed: they are called: « *mesoderm, endoderm and ectoderm* ». The cells which constitute this blastocyst are called « *totipotent* » as they are capable of assembling these embryonic tissues at the root of human life.

After one week, once all three tissues are formed, each one will bear a new type of stem cell, called « *multipotent adult stem cells* ». These cells can take on the form and function of any specialized cell. They will therefore take an active part in the fetus's development.

The big difference between an embryonic and an adult stem cell lies in their potential: unlimited in the case of embryonic cells (cloning is possible) and more limited for the others. The term 'adult ' may cause confusion; in fact although adult these cells appear only seven days after conception. The difficulty in using embryonic cells is their extraction; as they come from human embryos, with all of the ethical consequences which that entails, but scientists have already solved this problem by converting adult stem cells into embryonic stem cells.

The use of adult stem cells has already revolutionized the medical world, from the moment we realized that we had stocks of these cells distributed throughout our bodies, certainly in the spinal cord… but also in abdominal fat! We had known for years how to use stem cells through spinal marrow transplants on leukemia patients but came up against two serious problems: that of the donor's tissue compatibility as well as anti-rejection treatment, which is very aggressive to all other cells.

Today these problems are mostly solved. We take autotransplants of the patient's own stem cells and reinject them into another part of the body. These « *autotransplants* » have drastically changed our prognoses for certain illnesses. We can also use our own adult stem cells to treat many illnesses: we have treated blindness by injecting these cells into the eyes of blind patients, we have managed to avoid certain heart transplants by injecting stem cells into the hearts of these transplant candidates. We regularly treat athletes by injecting their stem cells into their joints, greatly damaged by severe exertion, which allows them to perform for several more years in the professional arena. We have very promising experimental results for diabetes, Parkinson's disease, Alzheimer's disease, autism, inflammatory illnesses such as autoimmune diseases.... As such, the use of stem cells will gradually extend to all areas of medicine and surgery.

French researchers of the Institute of Functional Genomics of Montpellier have recently managed to reprogram senescent cells (that is, cells which have become incapable of duplicating as they have grown too old) into induced pluripotent stem cells (iPS cells), that is, 'blank' or 'general' cells, which can both duplicate very quickly and turn into any one of the organism's specialized cells (skin, brain, heart etc.) This work will obviously have significant applications; such a result suggests the possibility of one day healing old patients by regenerating their sick tissue thanks to cells taken from their own organism (for example skin or fat cells). Our stem cells could very well hold the formula for a fountain of youth which so many scientists have not stopped and will not stop searching for.

Unfortunately, these adult stem cells also undergo cellular aging. They also are not everlasting, at some point they become unable to play their part. But if scientists found a way to slow down or stop their aging, that would have a significant impact on our longevity and health.

4 - Telomeres and Telomerase

Telomeres, from the Greek « *telos* » (end) and « *meros* » (part) are the structures capping the end of the double-stranded DNA of our chromosomes, sort of like the crimp at the end of a shoe string. They are a repetitive DNA sequence, and these sequences are repeated hundreds of times, which means that even if, during every division, some DNA is lost at the end of the telomere, it has no immediate effect on the DNA's effectiveness, since the same sequence is found just before it... until we run out of these sequences, at which point cellular senescence begins... and we age!

These telomere sequences protect the genome from information loss caused by a gradual shortening of chromosomes during each cellular division. They also protect the natural extremities of chromosomes from end-to-end fusions and the recombination which could be brought about by DNA reparation systems. Many studies have shown that the length of telomeres present in human lymphocytes gradually shortens with the passing of time. The shortest telomeres are found in octogenarians (4,000 to 6,000 base pairs) whereas newborns have telomeres composed of 8,000 to 12,000 base pairs.

Other studies highlight a causal relationship between telomere loss, cellular aging, the reduction of cellular regeneration, and the loss of tissue function and structure. Epidemiological studies support this causal relationship by showing, in humans, that short telomeres are a risk factor for atherosclerosis, hypertension, cardiovascular disease, Alzheimer's, infection, diabetes, fibrosis, metabolic syndrome, cancer, and influence global mortality.

Telomere length has been analyzed in 150 people aged 60 or more. Those with the shortest telomeres were eight times as likely to die from infectious diseases and three times as likely to have a heart attack. For the authors of the study, these results may reflect the fact that immune cells have to replicate quickly in order to combat an infection. Telomere shortening could slow down replication, thereby increasing the risk of infection.

In 1985, Elisabeth Blackburn, Carol Greider and Jack Szostak identified telomerase. It is an enzyme of the reverse transcriptase family, capable of reversing this telomere degradation process. Their work was rewarded in 2009 with a Nobel Prize in physiology and medicine. Telomerase ensures the synthesis and growth of telomeres. It also has other functions, discovered more recently. In particular, it plays a part in protecting against apoptosis (programmed cell death), DNA differentiation and reparation.

In the scientific literature, the role of telomerase in cellular immortality is now well established. In laboratory tests, the insertion of telomerase into human cell cultures transforms cells which would up until now be mortal into immortal cells.

As a result of these discoveries, several small telomerase activating molecules have been developed to be used to treat cellular aging. Some are extracted from milkvetch (Astragalus membranaceus).

5 - The Promise of Genomics

Genetics is defined as the science of heredity. It studies the hereditary characteristics of individuals, their transmission over many generations, as well as their variations (mutations). The transmissible units responsible for the heredity of certain traits are called genes. Genes are our body's construction and operational blueprints. They give instructions on how to assemble the parts of the smallest unit of life: proteins

Our body contains around 60 trillion cells, each of which itself contains a nucleus with all of the genetic material necessary for the construction of our entire organism. This genetic material is spread over 23 pairs of chromosomes, one half of each pair coming from our father and the other from our mother. Each chromosome contains a DNA strand.

Genomics is the study of the composition of genetic material, DNA, our genes and our chromosomes. Nearly 99.8% of human DNA is identical in all of the human species, and our DNA differs from that of the chimpanzee by only 2%. And yet our differences are quite visible! Similarly, this 0.2% difference between each human is what makes us all different, unique, excepting homozygotic (identical) twins, who have exactly the same DNA.

Problems may arise during DNA duplication, which occurs billions of times during the production of all of the cells in our body, and alterations may crop up: They are called genetic polymorphisms. There are an estimated 10 million polymorphisms responsible for our biochemical personality. Some only involve a single nucleotide (A, T, C, or G). These are called single nucleotide polymorphisms (SNPs) and they are extremely common: each individual may carry up to one million SNPs. Predictive genomics attempts to identify the most important SNPs to determine if one might be predisposed to developing any particular disease in a specific environment. The consequences of this for our longevity could be capital. For example, a specific SNP has been found in the mitochondria of centenarians. Having this gene seems to multiply by four the chances of living past 100. If we could force such a beneficial mutation, we would thereby increase the chances of living past 100 for everyone.

6 - Active Nutritional Supplementation

Doctors, nutritionists and other scientists today have a better understanding of nutrition and biochemistry. Advances and discoveries in the past few years concerning illness and nutrition have underlined the essential role of vitamins, minerals, medicinal plants and other substances for our health. Furthermore, extensive evidence has shown that nutritional supplements can help prevent cardiovascular diseases, cancer, osteoporosis, as well as other chronic illnesses.

Just a few decades ago, clinical studies attempting to prove the effectiveness of dietary supplements were relatively rare, whereas today we are seeing a huge surge in these studies, thousands of researchers studying the role of certain plants on our health and longevity. Omega 3, resveratrol, telomerase activators and antioxidants - anti-aging supplements have benefited from tens of thousands of *in vitro* and *in vivo* clinical trials. There is ample evidence that this active supplementation, associated with a better lifestyle, will help to lengthen our lives, all while remaining in good health.

7 - The Influence of Lifestyle

Taking a nutritional supplement or taking advantage of the latest technological advances could change our lives, improve our performance, reduce the frequency of certain chronic illnesses and increase our longevity. The problem is that it can take some time for all of these health benefits to materialize. If we want to accelerate this process, we have to add an important ingredient: we have to significantly improve our lifestyle.

But what do we mean by lifestyle? As soon as weight management or anti-aging are brought up, words like lifestyle, way of life or quality of life come with it. But when we ask what exactly is meant by them, we're left with an awkward silence. At best, there will be talk of nutrition, physical activity or behavioral change.

In reality, most people think they already know what these words mean. But this assumption can be dangerous. We are going to focus on this well-worn word, lifestyle, and we'd be better off knowing exactly what it means before acting on it. First let's talk about what it isn't. It isn't dietary behavior, physical activity, positive thinking, or all three combined.

> *Quality of life is the interaction of our thoughts, our feelings, our attitudes, our goals, our values, our behavior, our nutrition, our physical activity as well as the interrelation between us and our environment.*

This balance is strongly influenced by biological and cultural factors. We must have a global and holistic approach. This is the only way that we can hope for long-term results.

8 - A Technological Tsunami : NBIC

Future-oriented, so-called convergent technologies, have been categorized as NBIC: *Nanotechnology, Biotechnology, Information technology* and *Cognitive science.*

Nanotechnology allows us to manipulate matter and build new structures at the nanometer scale (a millionth of a millimeter), the size of a few atoms or molecules. It paves the way not only for the conception of new materials, but also for biological, medical and pharmaceutical applications, in particular via artificial implants for the human body.

Nanorobots

Imagine a robot smaller than a micron with a DNA sensor which could in a few minutes or a few seconds detect a potential illness using a drop of saliva or blood. This is Prof. Lieber's goal at Harvard, who is developing nanowire sensors, almost as small as a molecule, and 1000 times more sensitive than the latest DNA tests. Thanks to this process, we will be able to detect for example, prostate cancer at its inception. Once the anomaly has been detected, some researchers have already developed nanorobots which can repair DNA. These machines are built to enter into the cell's nucleus, and are equipped with a nanocomputer containing genetic code and the machinery to produce the necessary amino acid strands. This nanocomputer could also block unwanted replication and instantly update our genetic code. The first trials have been carried out on 12 cystic fibrosis patients, who have an abnormal gene causing mucus to accumulate in the lungs.

Biotechnology aims to permit a detailed understanding of how genes and living cells function, as well as how illnesses and pathologies come about. With the help of computer science, it can model these biological processes. With the help of nanotechnology and microelectronics, it can lead to electronic sensors at the molecular level, or to applications which can provide diagnosis at the cellular level and to systems for dosage and administration of pharmaceutical molecules which are integrated into our organs and remotely controlled.

Information and Communication Technology (ICT) allow us to manage communication between microchips or nanochips and computer systems within their environment.

As for artificial intelligence, it is located at the limit of computer and cognitive science.

Cognitive science aims to better understand the mechanisms of perception. It interacts with neuroscience and disciplines within the social sciences, such as behavioral theories, and communication and representation theories. Along with ICT and nanotechnology, it aims to engineer sensorimotor or cognitive systems.

⬚ IN A NUTSHELL ⬚

DNA, stem cells, telomeres, nanorobots, biotechnology. Super longevity, Hyper longevity, Immortality? : Are these Superman-like fantasies? Dreams? Utopias? Not at all; this is reality.

This isn't the future, it is the present. Is that to say that we have the knowledge and technologies which would allow us to live eternally? Not yet! We can however, today, significantly slow down age-related illnesses as well as the aging process. Even if this is something which few people realize, even within the medical community.

The purpose of this book is precisely to show that it is possible to extend human life while remaining healthy. Today, we can see that human life regularly lengthens, by three months every year, but we don't know exactly why. Extending human life would therefore not be a discovery, as it is already happening. The only question is: can we understand this process and accelerate it?

This book is divided into five parts :

The first part will help you assimilate the information which we will refer to in the rest of the book, as part of a global and holistic approach to health. We will introduce the key players: Health, the dynamic balance essential for maintaining functional integrity, called « *homeostasis* », cellular physiology, and modern genetics. If you are already familiar with this scientific vocabulary, you can go straight to the second part.

The second part attempts to explain why and how aging takes place. There are many theories which try to explain the causes of aging. We will focus on those for which there is a consensus today: DNA damage, telomere shortening, and as a consequence of these two the accelerated aging of stem cells.

The third part takes the second to its logical conclusion: it poses the question how can we grow younger? It develops a response: by working collaboratively and simultaneously on the causes of DNA damage, by lengthening telomeres, and by protecting our stem cells.

The fourth part is dedicated to improvement of our lifestyle, an element indispensable not only in the prevention of diseases caused by aging but also in helping cellular regeneration

The fifth part, finally, will help you to put all this new knowledge into practice, thanks to its concrete solutions, with the J-Life longevity program.

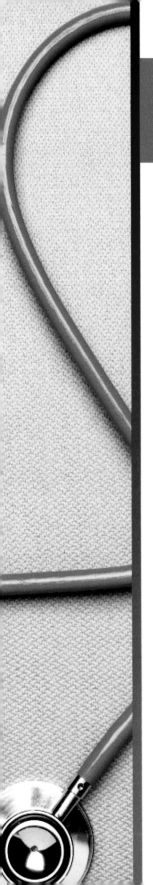

Part 1

HEALTH

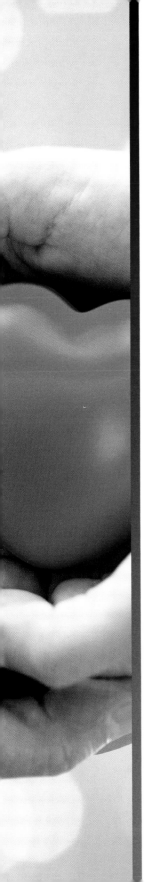

- Part 1 -

Chapter 1

Health

« The greatest wealth is health »

- Virgil -

1.1 - Health : What is it?

Health has always been the primary preoccupation of all societies. The ancient Greeks thought that health was the result of perfect physical equilibrium. For Indians, being in good health meant being in harmony with Nature. The ancient Chinese thought that health was a reflection of one's vital energy, which they called Chi. In the West, health proceeds from Darwin's theory on the evolution of species. This theory gave birth to the so-called « *Biomedical* » model, which describes human beings as having a biological identity stemming from nature. This approach has led medicine to essentially focus on illness and its treatment. Thanks to this approach, based on scientific rigor and experimentation, millions of lives have been saved and life expectancy has made a spectacular leap, going from 45 to 80 years within one century. This spectacular extension of lifespan, along with effective control over the great plagues and epidemics, has led our society towards a new way of thinking, no longer focused on the protection of life but on quality of life.

Most of our fellow citizens think that health means the absence of illness. « *I am not sick, therefore I am in good health* » : nothing could be further from the truth! All chronic illnesses take years to become detectable, and our genes, our potential weight problems, our nutritional habits, our physical, mental and emotional condition will positively or negatively influence the evolution of these silent problems. In 1946, the World Health Organization (WHO) was already introducing a positive (holistic) dimension to the definition of health: « *Health is a state of complete physical, mental and social well-being and not merely the absence of disease or infirmity* ».

There still remained one last step in defining health, however: how do we quantify it? What specific criteria could enable us to say: « *I am in good health* », « *I am in very good health* » or « *I am in perfect health* ». To define these criteria, scientists tackled this question in a new way: they studied the way in which our organism reacted when subjected to a change, constraint or stress. In particular, they took note of its capacity for resilience. They called this homeostasis.

1.2 - Homeostasis

> « *Homeostasis is defined as the organism's capacity to maintain the relative stability of the different components of its internal environment, and this despite constant environmental changes.* »

This is its scientific definition. But to properly understand this fundamental phenomenon, we'll have to put our imagination to work: suppose we are all born... on a steel wire stretched between two towers; our parents and their parents are all accomplished tightrope walkers and live permanently, twenty-four hours a day, on this wire. In order not to fall we will constantly need to acquire a dynamic balance which will require the involvement of hundreds of our muscles, our organs, our senses, our brain which will evaluate our strategic choices, our emotions which will have to be managed when danger lurks, and this... twenty-four hours a day, relentlessly. Not one second of relaxation! That is homeostasis!

Homeostasis is therefore not static, it is a constant search for equilibrium between activating and inhibiting forces. These variations should not exceed certain limits, however, beyond which cell survival is jeopardized. Homeostasis is stabilized when cellular needs are met. Yet the fulfillment of these needs is ensured by the synergistic work of all cells and therefore of tissue, organs, and all of the organism's systems.

Even if we cannot perceive it externally, our body's internal environment is the seat of countless and continuous changes which cause imbalances. And so, just as it is for the tightrope walker balancing himself on a wire, cells must react in order to adequately compensate these imbalances. So long as cells accomplish all of the needed compensatory actions, the organism remains in dynamic equilibrium, or homeostasis. If cells are not able to quickly restore internal balance by carrying out the appropriate compensatory actions, a major imbalance, called « *illness* », is unavoidable, just as f.a fall would be inevitable for the tightrope walker if he hesitated in the movements to recover his equilibrium.

The system's reorganization must be constant, mirroring its disorganization. All of this supposes precise mechanisms which take part in maintaining balance: this is called regulation. « *Regulation comprises all of the mechanisms ensuring the constancy of a chemical or physical characteristic of the internal environment* ». This is accomplished by error-correction systems. The correction mechanisms must be immediate and adequate: they process information through different receptors and work either by up- or down-regulating, or sometimes amplifying upward or downward trends when this proves to be necessary for our health.

☐ IN SUMMARY ☐

Health is defined today as our organism's adaptability to multiple and constant changes. This adaptability is effected through a coherent, complex and very efficient organizational system, which results in a permanent dynamic equilibrium which is constantly being put to the test. Homeostasis enables our functions to express themselves at peak efficiency. The gradual loss of this precarious balance is what brings about slowdowns in function and performance and thereby illness, including aging.

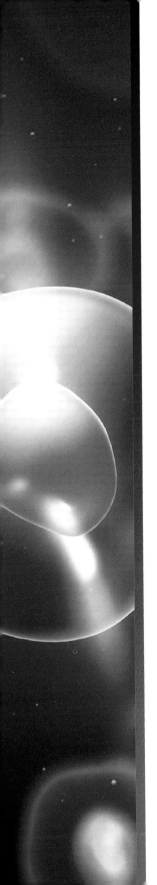

- Part 1 -

Chapter 2

The Cell

« Omnis cellula e cellula »
« All cells come from cells »

- Rudolf Virchow, 1858 -

2.1 - A Journey Inside the Cell

The cell is the unit on which all life on earth is based, from the humblest of bacteria, made of a single cell, all the way to the most complex organisms, like human beings, which contain more than 60 trillion of them. This small structure measuring 10 to 100 microns (10 to 100 thousandths of a millimeter) is one of nature's true masterpieces.

It is almost impossible to explain in a simple fashion the incredible complexity of what takes place every millisecond within a cell. When we know that this is also taking place at the same time in 60 trillion others, we can only humbly admire this technological marvel.

The Infinitely Big and Infinitely Small

Cells are a mirror of what takes place in microcosms as well as macrocosms, the infinitely small and infinitely big. A galaxy ten million light-years away from our planet looks eerily similar to a cell! The laws of nature are identical in both directions; at 10 microns we can see the inside of the cell; at 1 micron, the cell's nucleus. At 1000 angstroms we can see chromosomes, at 100 angstroms, DNA strands; at 10 picometers, electrons in an atom's field look strangely like a picture of the sky! Whether considering microcosms or macrocosms, basic structures seem identical and those of cells reflect this duality very well. The internal structure of the cell also mirrors the functional organization of the human body. This « *coherence* », in a biophysical sense, of the system, ensures the equilibrium necessary for our health.

2.2 - The Cell : A Spaceship!

Michael Denton, a biologist from Australia, describes the cell through the following analogy:

« To understand the reality of cellular function, let's enlarge the cell a million times until its diameter reaches 20 km and it looks like a spaceship the size of a large city. We would see a structure of unparalleled complexity and adaptability. There would be millions of openings on the spaceship's surface, the ship's portholes. If we entered through one of these openings, we would discover a world with astonishing technologies. »

Let's rework this analogy for our purposes: take the example of a molecule trying to enter into a cell to accomplish a specific action. It moves in the arteries' blood stream, until it reaches the exit leading it to the appropriate cell. When this substance nears the cell, it first searches for a door which will open as though reacting to a « *detector* ». The cell's doors function selectively: each molecule reaching a door is « *scanned* » to reveal any danger it may represent for the cell; the doors only open for useful molecules. If a harmful element, like a virus, tries to enter through one of these many entrances, it is immediately detected and the doors remain firmly closed.

The Cellular Membrane

This is the structure which controls the entrances. It surrounds the cell, is made of lipids and certain proteins and acts as a barrier made to contain all of the cell's activities within itself. It acts as a wall separating the internal and external environments. It contains a number of proteins called receptors which detect chemical signals present in the blood stream, transmitting coded messages to the cell and enabling it to react to environmental variations.

Having passed through the entrance, the molecule is immediately handled by specific proteins which execute the cell's functions. These proteins are called « *enzymes* ». If necessary, the enzymes will immediately use the molecule; if it is not immediately needed it will be stored in the cell's storage center, called the « *Golgi apparatus* ».

Bruce Lipton, in his research, has in particular analyzed « *the membrane's intelligence* ». He has demonstrated that a cell can survive without its genes for more than two months. When he removed nuclei from cells, he saw that they could sustain the coordinated operation of their physiological systems (respiration, digestion, excretion, motility, etc.). They could still communicate, protect themselves and grow appropriately, in response to the surrounding environment's stimuli. The reason they end up dying is that without DNA they can neither replicate nor replace weakened proteins. According to Lipton, the membrane receives information from the environment, decides what may enter the intracellular space, and regulates internal cell functions. « *Just like the nervous system, the cell membrane analyzes thousands of stimuli from the microenvironment* », (Lipton). This capacity for « *intelligent* » interaction with the environment is what makes the membrane the cell's true brain. When the membrane is destroyed, the cell dies. Without the receptor or executive proteins embedded in the membrane, « *they become comatose, similar to brain death.* »

The Golgi apparatus

The Golgi apparatus actively participates in the secretion process, that is, the process by which finished products are released out of the cell which produced them. Human cells produce all kinds of secretion proteins. But certain molecules like insulin, which transports sugars, are too big to pass through a standard door. The cell has a special entrance and exit system for these kinds of molecules. Once they have entered, enzymes retrieve the sugar carried by the insulin and bring it to the mitochondria, the cell's energy factories. Special ducts comprising the « *endoplasmic reticulum* » are in charge of logistics and transportation within the cell.

The Nucleus

The nucleus, a gigantic information processing center, is the cell's « *headquarters* ». Inside the nucleus we can find the chromosomes: 23 chromosome pairs, each one an enormous database. These chromosomes are comprised of entwined DNA strands. The detailed plan of all our body's functions are kept in store and coded into these strands. A DNA strand is similar in shape to a spiraling screw made of a sequential arrangement of 4 different molecules representing 4 different letters. Thanks to this sequential arrangement, an enormous amount of information, which would fill hundreds of encyclopedic volumes, is stored in our DNA. This coding system memorizes the detailed plans for thousands of enzymes and other proteins used within the cell. These 25 to 30,000 genes can produce more than 100,000 specific proteins.

DNA

In each cell, there are 23 pairs of long DNA strands which, if put end to end, would measure over 2 meters! The information coded into DNA is essential, and certain kinds of damage done to it can have deadly consequences for our organism. If we consider genes as coded blueprints (around 30 000 genes), DNA is a unique, extensive book indexing all of these blueprints. We then have 23 encyclopedias, each in 2 copies. These copies are so valuable that they cannot leave the central library (the nucleus). The information contained within each gene therefore is « copied » into a molecule called messenger RNA. Messenger RNA is taken out of the cell's nucleus and led to protein factories. In 1953, researchers Watson and Crick discovered the structure of DNA based on Wilkins' experimental work, a discovery which would earn all three of them the Nobel Prize in Physiology and Medicine in 1962. DNA lookslike a long spiraling ladder carrying all of this information; researchers call it a « double helix ». This information is written in an alphabet made up of four chemical letters called bases: adenine (A), thymine (T), guanine (G) and cytosine (C). A gene is therefore made up of a series of letters, looking something like ATGACACCGTGGA, whose pattern is unique for every gene, like a barcode. The interpretation of the information contained within DNA is achieved through a code: the genetic code, whose decryption is based on the fact that the four DNA bases must be enough to determine all of the twenty amino acids necessary for building proteins. Any spelling errors appearing in the DNA text are referred to as genetic mutations. Mutations can consist of letter inversions, deletions or insertions. Mutations can come from a reading error during DNA replication, through a viral infection or exposure to pollutants. They often lead to illness and occasionally to death.

Sequencing the human genome took about fifteen years. Three billion DNA letter combinations had to be transcribed and the very first sequencing cost one billion dollars. Today, an equivalent sequencing, of your DNA for example, would cost 100 dollars thanks to a microchip.

Mitochondrial DNA

Mitochondrial DNA is a circular DNA molecule found in mitochondria. This DNA molecule codes a portion of proteins and RNA specific to mitochondrial operations.

Mitochondrial DNA (or mtDNA) is very valuable for genetic analysis, as it only contains 37 genes in humans (compared to 30 000 in human DNA) and is generally better preserved, and obviously much faster to sequence. Also, and contrary to human DNA, which is a combination of half of the mother's genes and half of the father's genes (and therefore a quarter of each grandparent, an eighth of each great grandparent, and so on) making filiation extremely difficult to determine past a few generations, mitochondrial DNA is only transmitted through the mother, who herself took it from her mother, etc. This therefore simplifies the study of mother-child filiation and lineage dating immensely. Male mitochondrial DNA comes from the mother and is not passed on to the next generation. Recent studies have shown that all human mitochondria in the world have a common origin dating to around 150,000 years ago, in Africa. More recently, the remains of Tsar Nicholas II and of his family have been identified by comparing the mtDNA of the remains found in Ekaterinburg (Russia) with those of Prince Philip (whose maternal grandmother was the sister of Tsarina Alexandra). This identification is 99% certain.

Proteins

Proteins are the end product of nuclear DNA activity. These molecules carry out most operations necessary for cellular health: communication of messages, transportation and transformation of nutritional substances in order to produce energy.

The production of a protein molecule always starts with the identification of the gene holding the blueprint for the desired protein. An enzyme tasked exclusively with this mission opens up the DNA like one would a zipper; another group of enzymes divides the DNA strands into two. Another enzyme travels along the strands and quickly reads through the code; it will now copy the DNA. Once duplication is complete, this group of enzymes will reconnect the DNA and bring it back to its initial state. The copy made from the DNA is called « *messenger RNA* ». This messenger RNA contains the production blueprint for the protein which the cell requires at that exact moment.

There are two kinds of proteins: so-called « *structural* » proteins which constitute the structure for all of the body's tissues, and so-called « *functional* » proteins which ensure its proper operation. They can be regulatory proteins like insulin, defensive proteins like antibodies, or enzymes performing many different duties.

In order to synthesize all of these proteins, our body needs to obtain the building blocks with which to make them: amino acids. Food is our main source of amino acids.

Our cells are essentially an arrangement of protein blocks. Our body requires more than 100,000 different types of proteins in order to function properly. Each protein is a chain of amino acid molecules, similar to a string of interlocking plastic beads (Bruce Lipton). Each bead represents one of the twenty amino acid molecules used by cells. This structure is very flexible and can fold into a multitude of shapes. The flexible connections between the amino acids are called « *peptide bonds* » and can twist, flex, and even fold. This is due to the interaction of the electromagnetic charges of each amino acid: those with same-sign charges will repel each other and those with opposite-sign charges will attract each other! Certain proteins are so long that they need a special « *chaperone* » protein in order to fold. Proteins are constantly « *moving* » and their final form is a reflection of a stable state among all of their electromagnetic charges. If these charges are modified, however, the molecule will twist itself again until it reaches electromagnetic stability.

When a protein comes into contact with a molecule with a corresponding build, it will link to it, like a gear in a handmade watch. The cells take advantage of these protein gears' movement to ensure specific metabolic functions. This constant movement of proteins, changing shape thousands of times every second, is what animates every living thing.

Ribosomes

The copy of the genetic code is exported outside of the cell nucleus. It is then read by the cell's protein factories, the ribosomes. Ribosomes read the sentence (the copy of the gene) from beginning to end. And they will do so in three-letter packets. If a sentence is made, for example, of AUGGUGCACCUGACUCCUGAGGAGAAG, the ribosomes will read AUG, GUG, CAC, CUG, ACU, CCU, GAG, GAG, AAG.

You can find out how to build a specific protein within the copy of a gene. Since there are 20 different amino acids, any given group of three letters must represent a specific amino acid. GUC, for example, corresponds to « *valine* », and CAC to « *histidine* ». The decoder which enables the cell to translate the three-letter words into amino acids is called the genetic code. When ribosomes read a sentence in three-letter packets, they know exactly which of the twenty amino acids is assigned to each three-letter word and in which order. Ribosomes assemble amino acids one after another in order to finally obtain the completed protein. The result is a new protein: the one which had been « *ordered* ». Any sequencing error or wrong amino acid would render the protein useless. That is why such mistakes are practically never made. Once production is complete, the protein leaves the ribosome to go carry out its mission. It will be allowed to leave the cell, and will once more undergo security tests.

Mitochondria

Mitochondria are the structures which produce energy within the organism's cells, allowing them to function, enabling them to repair their lesions and care for themselves. Mitochondria fulfill several cellular functions, the best known being production of ATP (adenosine triphosphate), our cells' fuel. Mitochondria are therefore an essential element of cellular respiration, which enables us to produce the energy we need. In some ways, mitochondria can be compared to a car's engine. A cell cannot function without mitochondria, just as a car could not without an engine… They have their own DNA, and their own genes take part in mitochondrial operations. They always come from the mother, the male gamete in principle only carrying nuclear DNA.

2.3 - Cellular Language

Communication: the key word! Computers communicate through the Internet, dolphins through sound, human beings through their sensory organs, plants through specific molecules - they even have a social life! The study of these communication systems has given birth to a new biomedical specialization: « *Signaling* ».

Cellular signaling is a complex communication system which governs cells' fundamental processes and coordinates their activity. The capacity cells have to perceive their microenvironment and to respond to it correctly is the basis of homeostasis. This is why malfunctioning of the processing of cellular information might be responsible for illnesses such as cancer, auto-immune diseases or diabetes. Cells receive information from their neighbors through a class of proteins called receptors.

A cell is first and foremost a protein production plant. These components which are essential to life are manufactured according to blueprints deposited as DNA in the cell nucleus. In order to accomplish this mission at the right time, the cell constantly receives and emits chemical messages communicating its position in space, the state of its « *production equipment* » or the quality of its environment. It also informs its neighbors when initiating cell division. All of these signals are transported, by hormones traveling in the blood, secreted by several endocrine glands, these hormones selectively activate some of the hundreds of receptors anchored on the membrane surface. The cell is therefore a production workshop as well as a colossal communications center. These different means of communication are facilitated by diffusible substances, which is why cells are equipped with specific receptors.

Transmission Error

Typically, when a signal protein becomes embedded into its membrane receptor, it changes the geometrical configuration of the site and the message is transmitted inside the cell. Within the cytoplasm, other molecules take over and send the information through several successive steps all the way to the nucleus. A transmission error can have dramatic consequences. It can shutdown the production of essential proteins or lead to the assembly of poor quality parts.

2.4 - Group Living and its Constraints

Dr. Richard Béliveau, a molecular biologist at the University of Quebec comments humorously on the evolution of cellular functioning.

«Today's cells are the result of the evolution of a primitive cell which appeared on earth 3.5 billion years ago and looked much more like a bacterium than cells do now. During this extended period, this ancestral cell was subjected to huge environmental variations which forced it to constantly search for modifications which could offer it better chances of survival. This considerable adaptive strength is due to its ability to modify its genes to enable the production of new, more efficient proteins in order to deal with new challenges: this is what scientists call «a mutation». The ability cells have to mutate their genes is an essential characteristic of life without which we would never have seen the light of day. About 600 million years ago, cells made a decision which would revolutionize life on Earth: they began to cohabitate and form the first organisms made of more than one cell. This was a radical change at the time, as this cohabitation implied that the survival of the organism would take precedence over that of the individual cells. Originally individualists, cells became altruistic and forewent the ability to transform their genes and initiate mutations whenever they wished as they had in the past. The advantage of this evolution was that tasks could be distributed and cells could specialize. In order to effect this specialization, cells modified their rules in order to form new kinds of proteins which would improve their performance. This power of adaptation is the basis for evolution.»

In human beings, specialization has reached record complexity: a skin cell has seemingly nothing to do with a kidney cell, and yet all of the cells in the human body have the same genetic baggage. They are identical, have the same genes, but don't use the same genes to carry out their duties; in other words, every cell in the human body only uses those genes which are compatible with its function: this phenomenon is called « *cellular differentiation* ».

2.5 - Programmed Cell Death (Apoptosis)

Maintaining cellular function is a fragile phenomenon which is constantly confronted with the « *rebellious* » motivations of cells wishing to regain their freedom of action. This is exactly what takes place throughout our existence: as soon as a cell endures an external aggression, its first instinct is to interpret this aggression as a test which it must face as best it can, by mutating its genes in order to bypass this obstacle. Unfortunately for us, these aggressions are common throughout our lives, to the point where several damaged cells may rebel and even forget their essential function for the whole of the organism. Thankfully, in order to avoid cells gaining too much autonomy, this system is strictly supervised, which makes it possible to quickly eliminate rebellious cells by telling them... to kill themselves. This is what scientists coyly refer to as « *apoptosis* ».

Apoptosis (or programmed cell death) is the process by which cells self-destruct in reaction to a signal. It is one of the potential avenues of cell death, which is physiological, genetically programmed and necessary for survival. It is in constant balance with cellular proliferation, which is yet another manifestation of homeostasis.

Cancerous cells are usually cells in which this mechanism no longer functions. They survive and multiply despite genetic abnormalities which have arisen during the cell's life, when they should normally have destroyed themselves by apoptosis.

Apoptosis or
programmed cell death

« *The weight of cells which we kill off every year is equivalent to the weight of our body.* » Nicole Le Douarin

Indeed, every living cell contains a genetic code for its programmed death which, if it is initiated, causes, with the utmost discretion, the cell's departure. This furtive death is referred to by the term « apoptosis » (in Greek, this refers to falling leaves). Cells which die by apoptosis begin by cutting contact from neighboring cells, then undergo major internal modifications: the content of their nucleus fragments itself while their cytoplasm is divided into small pieces: apoptotic bodies, quickly absorbed by neighboring cells. Death by apoptosis is thus quick and generally does not cause any inflammation or scarring. This is why it has gone unnoticed for so long. The decision to activate or repress apoptosis is controlled by certain genes, as well as being under the influence of mitochondria; they participate by discharging part of their contents into the cytoplasm: an enzyme, Cytochrome C, and a factor, AIF (Apoptosis Inducing Factor). Apoptosis is an essential element for the proper functioning of organisms, and in particular of homeostasis. Entire regions of our organism undergo rapid regeneration: our skin, the inner lining of our intestines and our blood, for example. The remains of dead cells are reused to build new tissue. We thus constantly fuel our bodies with part of ourselves. The regulation of cellular life and death is therefore crucial for the functional balance of our organism. It is part of the « social » life of the cells which form it. These discoveries have allowed us to understand the mechanisms responsible for a number of diseases. We now know for example tat that acute

liver failure, caused by viruses or alcohol, is due to the large-scale death of liver cells.

Apoptosis and Cancer

The abnormal blocking of programmed cell death constitutes a decisive step in the transformation of a cell into a cancerous cell. By disrupting the proliferation signaling pathways in their favor, cancerous cells can benefit from a dual advantage: ample proliferation and improved resistance to cell death. Protein p53 is able to induce apoptosis in cells with too many abnormalities or too much stress. Consequently the inactivation of p53 gives cancerous cells a powerful advantage for survival. Other proteins which initiate apoptosis are inactivated or their expression diminished in cancerous cells in order to increase their ability to survive the stress and damage which they are constantly undergoing.

2.6 - Systemic Biology

The history of cells seems to mainly center around the maximization of their intelligence. When cells have reached their maximum size and to become more intelligent, they group into multicellular communities. They then begin to divide tasks among themselves and specialize. The advantages of community life have led to colonies of millions of billions of socially-interactive cells… which have become mammals and human beings. « *We are the product of this cooperation, without it there is no life.* » (Lipton)

The study of these relationships is now a rapidly growing field called « *systemic biology* ». A classic example of the benefits of microorganisms for humans is our digestive system's bacteria, which are essential to our survival. It should be noted that there are 10 to 100 times more bacteria in our gut than cells in our body. When their environment is favorable to them, the bacteria in our gut kill the other organisms which are not in harmony with the symbiosis between us and them. This cooperation allows us to benefit from a very efficient protection system and offers our guests a well-adapted living space. Furthermore, a large part of our digestion is accomplished by this micro-flora. These bacteria are not our enemies; on the contrary, without them we could not survive. There still remains one step leading to closer cooperation: it would seem that organisms belonging to different species may share their genes. This fact turns our definition of species on its head.

> « *Scientists are realizing that genes are being transmitted not only between the individual members of a species, but also between members of different species. Sharing genetic information through gene transfer accelerates evolution since organisms can acquire experience 'learned' from other organisms* ».

Given this gene-sharing, we can no longer see organisms as isolated entities. « *There is therefore no barrier between species* ». (Daniel Drell).

This phenomenon of dispersion of the genetic pool has rather important consequences: One study has already revealed that when humans ingest genetically modified foods, the artificial genes modify the nature of intestinal bacteria, which work symbiotically with our cells…

Mammals are fundamentally cooperative beings. Ethology, the study of animal behavior in different species, amply demonstrates that the propensity to live communally can be found at every scale in evolution. « *Altruism and the capacity to live communally are also very important in the mammal world* » (Lipton). We know that mammals help each other constantly, in a spontaneous and disinterested way. A chimpanzee will help another chimpanzee even if they know that there won't be a reward.

What should we keep in mind? We are made of 60 trillion cells which are quasi-identical but incredibly complex. The cell is the constituent unit of living organisms; it is also their functional unit. Schematically, we could see the manufacturing of all of the specific proteins necessary for the perpetuation of homeostasis as the cell's primary mission. To this end, it has at its disposal an ultra-sophisticated and hyper-secured control center holding all of the manufacturing code, an energy plant providing all of the necessary energy for all chemical operations, all of the necessary logistics to transport and store raw materials and finished goods, and finally a protective membrane which filters all entrances and exits very selectively. Cells live in a community and their social rules are very strict. It is thanks to this discipline that they have been able to create more than 200 different cell families with the same genetic baggage. Any breach of the collective rules subjects the offender to the death penalty, in the interest of the community.

S O U R C E S

Bruce H. Lipton.
Biologie des croyances. Québec : Ariane Editions Inc. ; 2006.

M. J. Denton.
Nature's Destiny: How the Laws of Biology Reveal Purpose in the Universe.
New York : Free Press ; 1998.

Nicole Le Douarin.
Les cellules souches. Paris : Odile Jacob ; 2007.

Richard Béliveau, Denis Gingras.
Les aliments contre le cancer. Québec : Trécarré ; 2005.

Walter Whali, Nathalie Constantin.
La nutrigénomique dans votre assiette. Bruxelles : Éditions De Boeck ; 2011.

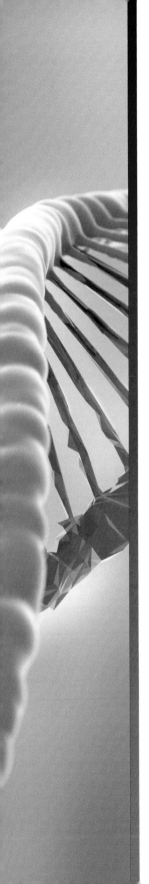

Conclusions

« Let us harness our cellular intelligence in order to climb another rung of the evolutionary ladder, where the most generous among us prosper »

- Bruce Lipton -

Our health, and consequently our longevity, are the result of the return to equilibrium of our body's cellular norms, this despite the constant changes caused by our environment. This continuous adaptation to change is achieved through the activity of our 60 trillion cells, each one with a specific mission.

Each and every one of us is in fact a cellular community made up of 60 trillion individuals! Each one of these intelligent structures, our cells, is composed of a membrane which surrounds 'miniature organs', called organelles, which are suspended in a gelatinous liquid (the cytoplasm). These organelles have functions which are very similar to those performed by our body's organs and tissues. Among these structures, we find the cell nucleus (the largest organelle), the mitochondria, the Golgi apparatus and the vesicles. Each cell takes on the equivalent of our body's functions: digestive, nervous, hormonal, respiratory, cardiovascular, excretory, and even immune function. Furthermore, each cell analyzes the thousands of stimuli found in its immediate environment, then triggers an appropriate behavioral reaction to ensure its survival. In addition to this, the cell is able to learn from the experience provided by its environment. It can thus build a cellular memory, which it will transmit when it divides itself.

The nucleus of each cell contains our entire hereditary capital, our genes. These genes hold the codes necessary for the assembly of more than 100 000 different types of proteins, which are essential for us to function properly. Each protein is a linear chain of amino acid molecules which is constantly bending and twisting under the influence of the electric charges found at each of its extremities. Its final form reflects a state of equilibrium between the charges. RNA, which is a temporary copy of DNA, is used as a template from which to copy the amino acid sequence which will constitute a specific protein's skeleton.

The supremacy of DNA has recently been called into question by a new field of study epigenetics; epigenetics literally means 'above genetics'. Epigenetics asserts that our genes do not make our lives an inescapable fate, a foregone conclusion. Indeed, epigenetics has shown that environmental factors can activate or deactivate our genes without modifying them. Even better, these epigenetic activations could be transmitted to future generations!

New research shows that our environment is the leading factor. Environmental signals are responsible for determining whether regulatory proteins will bond; those which form a sheath around DNA in order to open it up to be read and copied into RNA, and thereby trigger the assembly of the required protein. Recent studies show that these 'epigenetic switches' can produce more than 2 000 versions of a protein out of a single gene.

In this context, cellular biology now lends far more importance to the cellular membrane than before. Indeed, it is now seen as the cell's actual brain (Lipton). This relegates the nucleus to the level of a gigantic database, in charge, among other things, of the transmission of heredity. The cell membrane, thanks to its receptors, will analyze, and filter, hundreds of thousands of environmental signals, only letting in those signals which are useful to the cell's survival. The destruction of the cell membrane immediately triggers the cell's death, whereas if the nucleus is extracted, the cell will be able to survive for a certain amount of time, although it will no longer be able to divide

In a way, our clever cells could teach us how to live better, as they set an example of a community made up of 60 trillion individuals, able to live in perfect harmony.

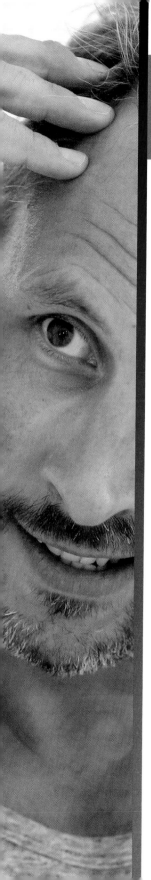

Part 2

A G I N G

- Part 2 -
Introduction

« Fundamentally no one believes in his own death, in the unconscious every one of us is convinced of his own immortality »

- Sigmund Freud -

Since 1960, theories regarding aging have evolved considerably. These theories, based on the knowledge of their time, have, in 55 years, made considerable progress. That which was regarded, not that long ago, as alchemy, became molecular biology; and that which was magical became genetics.

Today, we know that aging is not due to a singular cause. Aging is the direct consequence of a sometimes complex series of events, which will change from year to year, depending on our interactions with our environment. These events will bring about changes in gene expression, that is, in the activation or deactivation of certain genes, and this will cause the production (or absence thereof) of certain specific proteins.

Today we recognize that the cellular control of aging is linked to our DNA, to its ability to duplicate, as well as to telomere integrity. These two elements will be essential to the preservation of a stock of quality stem cells. DNA is the essential element of life, as it is the basis for every molecule in our body. Damage inflicted to our DNA by our environment, as well as by an unhealthy lifestyle, will lead to the appearance of a series of age-related illnesses, such as cardiovascular disease, diabetes or cancer. This damage, accumulating in our 60 trillion cells, will be responsible for aging, whereas our longevity will depend on the manner in which we are able to repair this damage, as well as how fast we achieve it. Our DNA is constantly duplicating throughout our lives, and, in optimal conditions, these copies are perfect - especially in younger individuals. However, starting as young as 35 or 40 years of age, our DNA, which is continually bombarded by an excess of free radicals, by radiation and subjected to a toxic environment, can no longer be repaired sufficiently or fast enough. Copies will be of poorer quality and certain bits of genetic code will be damaged. Proteins essential to certain functions will be missing, and this will lead to premature aging and the appearance of chronic, age-related illnesses.

Today we know that chronological age has very little to do with aging. Statistical values officially defining the age at which we become old have gone out of the window. Certain scientists, like Aubrey de Grey, are convinced that aging is a disease and a curable one at that. According to him, human beings age in seven different ways, all of which can be prevented. Indeed, he claims that aging is optional and that we would have to be « *crazy* » to choose to. Others think he should apply that word to himself!

It is quite probable, in fact, that aging is a complex illness which affects not only our body, our thoughts and our emotions, but also our families and our societies. Aging and death remain the two greatest mysteries which humanity has yet to solve.

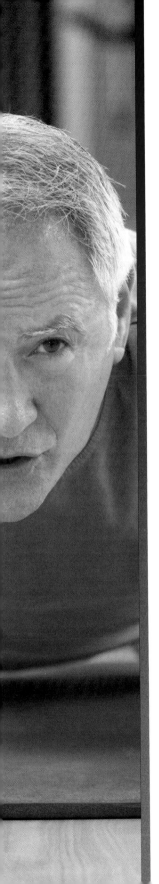

Chapter 1

Denying Old Age

« For everything there is a season, and a time for every matter under heaven. »

- Ecclesiastes, 3,1/8 -

Contrary to pregnancy denial, denying old age is not a pathology, only an attitude which affects a great many of us. If aging were enshrined in the laws of the Universe, we should logically accept it as such. And yet exactly the opposite is true! Indeed, most people consider death inevitable, but aging as unacceptable! The exploding sales of anti-aging cosmetics and of countless rejuvenation techniques are clear evidence of this.

This is why it is important, at least initially, to distinguish between longevity and senescence, and to concentrate on means of lowering the risk of contracting severe age-related illnesses in order to stay in top physical shape as long as possible.

« Aging is the sum of two criteria: the first is that the probability of dying increases exponentially with age; today, the probability of dying doubles in human beings every eight years; mortality is 32 times greater at sixty than at twenty years old, and 1024 times greater when we reach one hundred! The second criterion is represented by the appearance of external and psychological signs of aging, signs which categorize us as « elderly » (Radman).

We have even created an entire vocabulary with which to refer to old people. Here are a few examples: ancient, antediluvian, antiquated, archaic, dried-up, fallen, decrepit, faded, old-fashioned, outdated, dull, wilted, withered, fragile, graying, has-been, useless, vegetable, mature, Methuselah, ripe, past-it, withdrawn, resistant, wrinkled, wise, , worn out, venerable, veteran, dilapidated, old hag…

« Do all of these descriptions reflect how the elderly are judged by the rest of the population? In other words, does the value of human life diminish with age? How should we live in a world where aging is synonymous with failure, exclusion and decay? How should we tolerate aging when society and the media incite us to stay young and competitive? Why do some of us decide *to shorten our lives in order not to suffer the ravages of time? » (Marie De Hennezel).*

All of this depends on what we mean by « *aging* ». For some, it means social aging, the rules of which are dictated by society, such as retiring when we are sixty, and the consequences thereof, both direct and indirect. For others, it refers to the type of aging which we are all aware of and which we expect and dread every time we celebrate another decade, our 50s, then 60s, then 70s. And finally there is true aging, that which we experience and which we are surprised to actually discover, as it hardly corresponds to the idea which was fed to us during our lives. I must admit that as I write this book -I am 74 years old - my behavior and my ideas concerning this subject change every day. I feel like I am reliving my teenage years, but with a few advantages which add spice to this 'maturescence'.

Dr. Andrew Weil, a leading expert in the field of longevity, asked some of his patients what they thought of aging; here is what they said:

> «*When I was young I thought those who were fifty or sixty were... so old! Now that I'm there, I don't see it in the same way at all, but I still have some internal conflicts about age. I first accepted the idea that there are some things I cannot do anymore, like skiing, and I also accept that younger people can. There are times where I miss that energy I once had. I don't like the memory loss (am I getting Alzheimer's?). There is a kind of lack of control over the future that is unsettling to someone who is very used to being in charge. My sister had a stroke when she was sixty-eight - six years older than I. I realize that good health is 80 percent of the game. And some people have it and some don't. Some of it is luck; some of it comes through taking care of oneself. When I visit my sister in the retirement community, I shudder. I desperately do not want to be in one of those communities...*»

The simplest and most common way of denying aging is to deny the fact of it!

Some do it so well that they no longer even know their actual age. More and more fractures and sprains are due to people overestimating their physical capabilities. And let's not even mention the damage caused by anti-aging methods doled out by quacks.

Aging without being old, that is the challenge which this new generation has taken by cleaning up its life, a Generation Young which manages to take on years while remaining young. It knows that it will age differently than its parents, and has clear objectives: to keep aging in good health and wait for a new Nobel Prize winner to enable it to lose fifteen or twenty years and prepare for even greater longevity,(which we hope will happen in the next fifty years.)

«The path to aging well is full of obstacles, the most important being the penetrating fears we have when we think about it. The first is of course the fear of physically aging and no longer being attractive. It's true, our body has waned, wrinkles appear, we no longer receive compliments and above all we no longer feel the desire of others. Another fear is being a burden for our relatives, our children, our society, and it's true, it is a real problem. Most senior citizens who have been asked have trouble asking their children to house them, and yet on the other hand they don't want to live away from home. We are afraid of growing old in a retirement home; the heartbreak of leaving our home and the horror of confinement. In certain countries retirement homes are similar to boarding houses, with certain rules of conduct, in others they resemble prisons, in which we lose our freedom and risk being abused. In both cases we feel as though we have left the realm of the living.» (Marie De Hennezel)

Yet another fear is that of Alzheimer's, that of losing one's mind! This illness affects 47 million people around the world, with 7 million new cases per year, and it can unfortunately last years. This fear of dependence on others and the dread of psychological regression lead certain people to consider suicide, as a 'precautionary' solution. Aging also means getting closer to death, and in order not to think about it, we often prefer to be forgotten, and little by little we draw ourselves out of the world, we try to conceal our aging. Cutting ourselves off from work, choosing solitude, represents a public health problem: indeed, isolation and withdrawal, could predispose us to Alzheimer's disease.

For Marie De Hennezel, old age is, quite the contrary, another opportunity to face the reality of our existence. It presents us with the life challenges which we have not yet agreed to, and invites us to take them on:

> « *If we meet these challenges, old age no longer represents a stage of degradation which beats us down. It becomes an opportunity for growth, a way by which we can flourish even more. Just as it is for youth, growing older then becomes a way to widen the scope of our opportunities and capabilities. At that point we acquire the opportunity to live a fulfilling old age. And all of our energy can go towards this new life goal: to complete a life with which we can be fully satisfied, a life which was worth living.* »

Refusing to age, refusing to see ourselves age, is a reality which concerns many of us. We accept that death is inevitable, yet aging is unacceptable, because we live in a world where aging is synonymous with failure, exclusion or degeneration. This is why it is so tempting to deny the reality of it.

Aging without being old, that is the new challenge of Generation Young. But the road to aging well is full of obstacles: the fear of physically aging and no longer being attractive, the fear of being a burden for our family, the fear of losing our mind, the fear of solitude. Fears which so often inhibit us.

SOURCES

Andrew Weil.

Healthy Aging. New-York : Anchor Books ;2005.

Aubrey de Grey, Michael Rae.

Ending Aging. New-York : St. Martin's Griffin ; 1963.

Marie de Hennezel, Bertrand Vergely.

Une vie pour se mettre au monde. Paris : Carnets Nord ; 2010.

Miroslav Radman.

Au-delà de nos limites biologiques. Paris : Plon ; 2011.

Chapter 1 - Denying Old Age

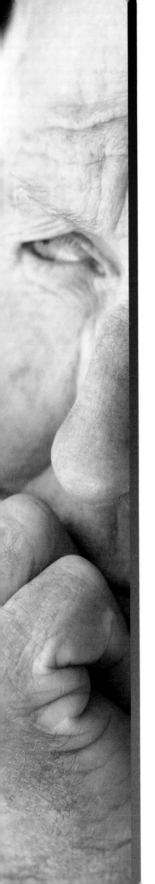

- Part 2 -

Chapter 2

Why Do We Age?

« We only see others age »

- André Malraux / Les chênes qu'on abat -

Today, the first thing of which we are certain is that chronological age no longer means much in terms of aging. Our 60 trillion cells will progressively age; this is what scientists call 'gradual senescence' which is essentially the growing inadequacy of the organism's defenses, and especially our DNA's, when faced with accumulating damage. When we age, cells also lose the capacity to multiply. This is essentially because of the shortening of our telomeres, which are no longer able to protect our chromosomes. This is what scientists call 'replicative senescence'. A third player completes this aging trilogy: stem cells, which are essential to cell renewal and proper maintenance. Stem cells are no longer able to get the job done if their DNA is seriously damaged and their telomeres are shortened. Our stem cell supply then shrinks, which compounds the problem.

2.1 - Gradual senescence, the accumulation of damage

Throughout their lives, living beings suffer many different kinds of damage which their organism attempts to rectify through its defense and repair mechanisms. At some point however, these mechanisms no longer manage to repair all of the damage fast enough. The damage then accumulates until it fatally obstructs the organism's functions. But where does this damage come from? It is important to know that every time a cell divides into two, its DNA does as well; this very complex process allows the DNA to read and copy itself on its own. This copying process is called 'replication' and the reading process 'translation'. A poor copy, or the accidental omission of certain sequences lead to a genetic mutation. This mutation can be responsible for the flawed assembly of proteins, and therefore lead to illnesses or premature aging.

It is estimated that between 70,000 and 100,000 separate occurrences damage DNA each day. Thankfully, our organism is able to repair this damage as soon as it appears, thanks to an extremely quick and efficient maintenance service. But starting around 30 years of age, things begin to change! Repairs aren't as quick anymore, delays build up, and when DNA duplicates, it now does so with mistakes which have not been fixed. Poor quality duplication also means poor quality proteins, with all of the negative consequences which that entails for our health.

These incidents have a dual origin: they are, on the one hand, due to external factors, through the interactions of living things with their environment and, on the other hand, due to internal factors, through the deterioration of the organism caused by its own operation.

2.1.1 - External Causes: The Environment

Michael Meaney and Gustavo Turecki, researchers at the Douglas Institute (Canada), have proven this in spectacular fashion in the past few years; according to Turecki, not only does the environment have an influence on mental and physical health, but it can also modify how genes, which we inherit at birth, function. Everything happens as though they were controlled by a series of switches. For example, what we eat makes us more or less vulnerable to certain types of cancer, nothing new there. But we now know that by activating epigenetic switches, food can alter the behavior of genes, and these modifications can then be transmitted from generation to generation. Our dietary indulgences can therefore negatively impact the health of our children! This discovery was published in March of 2009 in the prestigious journal Nature Neuroscience.

A Swedish study has even shown that a period of starvation can have repercussions, not only on the longevity of those living through it, but also on the life expectancy of their grandchildren! This new field called 'epigenetics' (the modulation of gene expression through behavior and particularly through nutrition) is regarded as a breakthrough in the understanding of all of the elements which may contribute to staying in good health and to slowing down the aging process.

Infections

Infections, even if they leave no lasting damage, always bring about the death of a certain quantity of cells. Each infection will demand the mobilization of a very large number of lymphocytes and our immune system sometimes finds itself entirely depleted, especially in the case of viruses like HIV.

Ultraviolet (UV) rays

UV rays can damage DNA, RNA (DNA's messenger) and proteins. Ultraviolet radiation emitted by the sun is classified into three types of rays: UVA rays, whose wavelength is between 400 and 315 nanometers, UVB rays, between 315 and 280 nanometers, and UVC rays, between 280 and 100 nanometers. A large part of UVB rays is filtered out by the atmosphere, whereas UVC rays are entirely absorbed by the ozone layer and never reach the earth's surface. The solar radiation to which we are exposed is therefore made up of 95% of UVA rays and 5% of UVB rays. How does UV radiation interact with DNA? We know that UVB rays chemically alter bases, in particular thymine. The genes which the DNA carries are thereby modified. This chemical reaction explains the strongly mutagenic properties of UVB rays. So for now, exercise caution when out in the sun, as even the 95% of UVA rays, which until recently were still considered harmless, have turned out to be harmful for genes. Let's not even mention tanning salons, where the ratio of UVA rays is even greater...

Poor Nutrition

The entire organism's activity depends on what it eats. Proper DNA replication, just like any other biological function, is therefore related to proper nutrition. Poor nutritional habits can lead to the activation of genes responsible for aging. And the opposite is also true; good nutrition fosters activation of genes responsible for longevity. Out of this a new field is born: nutrigenomics. A new branch of nutritional sciences aiming to study the interactions between the genome and nutrition, as well as the impact of these interactions on the way in which individuals, or populations, react to nutrition, on their predisposition to develop certain illnesses and more generally, on their health. In this way, nutrigenomics research attempts not only to explain in what way nutrients and all other nutritional components influence gene expression in individuals or populations, but also how the genome itself might influence the way in which an individual or a population reacts to food.

Pollution

Atmospheric pollution has become a major health problem. Polycyclic aromatic hydrocarbons (PAH) are a category of pollutants associated with vehicle exhaust, urban heating, and industries using coal and petroleum based products. More than 100 PAHs have been identified and are still produced in complex mixtures. The likelihood of DNA damage by PAHs leads them to be classified as mutagenic and carcinogenic.

> *Out of 10,000,000 existing chemical substances, about 100,000 are produced and used in large quantities. But toxic risks have only been studied for fewer than 3,000 of them and occupational exposure limits have only been set for 2,100.*

Every year, new chemical molecules are invented. They are generally complete unknowns for our organism and can all be potentially carcinogenic! It has now been proven that pollution is one of the leading causes of cancer. We know, for example, that asbestos is responsible for pleural cancer (mesothelioma), and that atmospheric pollution is one of the causes of lung cancer.

> *By tracking more than 16,000 men living in Oslo since 1972, Norwegian epidemiologists have been able to establish a link between the appearance of cases of lung cancer and air pollutants, nitrogen oxides in particular.*

Pollution related to vehicular traffic increases the risk of lung cancer. The worry is that today pollution is everywhere: in the air, in water, in the ground, in our food. No sector is left unaffected. We now find it in our everyday life – through the food industry in particular and its pesticides, insecticides, food dyes–they get into our plates, our glasses, our cleaning products, as well as the construction materials used in our houses and workplaces. The AFSSE (French Agency for Environmental Health and Safety) considers that pollution of urban areas by fine particulate matter is responsible for 3 to 5% of deaths in people older than 30 (several thousand people per year). The main illnesses caused by this particulate matter are cardio-pulmonary diseases, including lung cancer. These particles are released by road traffic, heating and certain industrial activities.

How do pollutants function?

There are several possibilities:

1 - Pollutants will stimulate proto-oncogenes and cause them to transform into active (procarcinogenic) oncogenes.

2 - A toxic substance's active metabolites can bond to a cell's DNA and cause it to modify itself, that is, mutate. During the DNA's next division, this leads to erroneous reading of its sequences, and therefore to mistakes in its reconstitution, and finally to the potential appearance of cancer. But this nightmare doesn't stop there, as the mutations which have been produced are inheritable, as has been shown in work published in the journal Science: « *Airborne particulate matter which pollutes the air causes inheritable genetic mutations. By exposing mice to the polluted environments of a highway and two steel mills, Canadian researchers have noted that males underwent genetic changes which they transmitted to their offspring.* »

This study is very troubling if it can be extrapolated to human beings, which is quite likely. This would mean that potentially carcinogenic or procarcinogenic DNA mutations, caused by pollution suffered by a father, could find themselves in his children and all of their progeny...

«A British team has brought to light the persistence of a genetic mutation in the germ line (sexual cells) of two successive generations, stemming from male rodents having been exposed to ionizing radiation. In Hamilton Harbor, Ontario, Canada, seagulls have a high rate of DNA mutation. These mutations have then been transmitted to the following generation. The

*exact origin has not been proven, but air pollution
and the polluted water in which contaminated fish
live seem to be the source. Studies have shown that
genetic transformations caused by pesticides in female
mice could be transmitted over several generations to
their offspring. They are therefore inheritable and these
genetic modifications could for example induce skin and
prostate cancer from generation to generation, because
of pesticides ingested by the grandmother mouse.»*

If, once more, all of this were confirmed for humans, this would mean that
mutations due to air pollution and ionizing radiation would be inheritable.
If this is the case, the number of cancer cases will keep growing, and, in
the future, they will affect ever younger individuals.

Electromagnetic pollution

Electromagnetic fields, generated by cellphone antennae, indirectly
cause breaks in DNA strands in human and animal cells. They can even
interrupt the synthesis of certain proteins. These are two key results of
the European Reflex study (Risk Evaluation of Potential Environmental
Hazards From Low Frequency Electromagnetic Field), which was
unveiled by the German foundation Verum, based in Munich. Funded by
the European Union, as well as the Swiss and Finnish governments, this
study brought together twelve laboratories during four years.

These results should however be handled with extreme care, in particular
as they come from in vitro experiments (on isolated cells) rather than in
vivo ones (on entire organs or organisms). The researchers insist on the
fact that these studies are not sufficient to determine whether a health
risk exists... (without excluding its possibility.) Prof. Franz Adlkofer, the
project's coordinator and the director of the Verum foundation, says that
the study proves the existence of a pathophysiological mechanism which
could explain the development of animal and human functional disorders
or illnesses. This claim is based, in particular, on the fact that the biological

impacts observed on the cells occurred at energy measurements– specific absorption rates, or SAR– below the threshold of 2 W/kg, which is currently recommended by the International Commission on Non-Ionizing Radiation Protection, and cited in French legislation.

Heavy Metal Pollution

It has been shown that toxic heavy metals increase free radical activity, which represents one of the major causes of aging. Heavy metals replace mineral cofactors, enzymes which are essential for our health. Heavy metal toxicity can also disrupt immune function. Arsenic, beryllium, cadmium, chromium, cobalt and nickel are carcinogenic heavy metals, found in nature, which inhibit our organism's ability to repair DNA. Mercury contaminates almost all fish products. For certain especially sensitive individuals, aluminum can also play a role in certain neurodegenerative illnesses, especially those linked to memory loss.

Tobacco

Smoking seriously harms your DNA; this indication could be prominently displayed on packs of cigarettes, next to smoking kills, smoking clogs your arteries or smoking can cause a slow and painful death. American researchers have just shown, in the journal Chemical Research in Toxicology, that a smoker's chromosomes are exposed to the adverse effects of tobacco right from the first few puffs. Essentially, you don't have to wait years, as one might think, before certain poisons in the smoke begin to damage your genetic material and cause cancer. Which is to say that all smokers, even casual smokers, or those who have just begun smoking, are affected. In order to reach these conclusions, which represent a serious warning for smokers; Professor Stephen Hecht and his team at the University of Minnesota tracked, in the organism of twelve volunteer smokers, a toxic substance, phenanthrene, one of the many polycyclic aromatic hydrocarbons (PAH) produced via tobacco combustion.

Previous studies had shown that phenanthrene only becomes carcinogenic after a biochemical transformation process which results in the production of a metabolite likely to cause DNA mutations and thereby initiate cancer. But no one had yet measured the speed at which these reactions take place in the organism. The results surprised the researchers themselves! Blood samples, taken every fifteen minutes, showed that smokers reach the maximum concentration of the substance only 15 to 30 minutes after having finished their cigarette. To make matters worse, this concentration decreases very slowly, levels remaining high six hours after the last puff.

The effect might be even more immediate, the authors, clearly not expecting such significant results, only having begun sampling fifteen minutes after ingestion. At which point they immediately found the highest value! The same experiment should be repeated to see what happens after one, then five minutes, says Prof. Bertrand Dautzenberg, a pulmonologist and president of the OFT (French bureau for smoking prevention) who also admits being astonished by the persistence of this toxic substance in the organism.

The dangers of tobacco are exacerbated by the fact that its combustion generates PAH nanoparticles and other toxic products less than a millionth of a meter in size which can penetrate the organism all the more easily, having been inhaled. Absorption is fastest through the lungs, taking place in a few seconds, compared to fifteen minutes or more through the skin or if taken orally.

Remember that lung cancer, 90% due to tobacco, is the deadliest cancer. Out of 12 million new cases diagnosed every year in the world, nearly 8 million will die from it. Specialists estimate that 100 million people have been killed by tobacco in the past century.

Stress

Chronic stress can have several negative consequences on health and can ruin one's life. A recent study indicates that persistent stress sustained over a long period damages our DNA and can thereby increase the chances of cancer and cause premature aging.

Stress :
Essential in the Short Term...

Stress is an absolutely essential phenomenon for our survival: detecting danger with our sensory organs (the smell of smoke, the sight of a menacing figure, the sound of a gunshot) puts the brain on high alert, which triggers a series of extremely complex processes together called the 'fight-or-flight response.

By activating the adrenal glands, your brain orders the release of action hormones into the blood, such as adrenaline, in order to accelerate your breathing, your heart beat, the flow of oxygen to tissue as well as your alertness and attention levels. What we commonly call the survival instinct is therefore essentially a stress reaction, a biologically programmed response which aims to mobilize our resources for combat, or a quick escape, when faced with a potentially fatal danger.

... But Detrimental
in the Long Term

Stress is generally short-lived, as the many physiological effects associated with it are extreme, and could have negative effects on the organism if they were to last. In fact, when it persists and becomes chronic, stress is known to foster the development of several disorders, including, among others, gastrointestinal disorders, such as stomach ulcers, certain cardiovascular diseases, and immune system impairment, which makes infections, depression and sleep disorders more likely.

Genetic Stress

American researchers have just shown that prolonged stress can also cause chromosomal anomalies. Indeed, they have established that the prolonged presence of adrenaline, as is the case for people suffering from chronic stress, causes a sharp increase in damage to the DNA structure. This harmful effect of adrenaline is due to the overstimulation brought on by cascading reactions responsible for the degradation of protein p53, one of the main protectors of the genetic material's integrity. This destructive effect of stress on DNA can even be seen at the level of sperm cells, suggesting that chronic stress, when suffered by men, could cause anomalies which could be transmitted to their children. Chronic stress is therefore not only harmful to our organs' proper functioning, but also causes DNA alterations which could lead to the development of a number of illnesses, including cancer.

Violence, mistreatment, sexual abuse, abandonment and other psychological traumas leave an indelible trace through adulthood. Since Freud, a series of clinical studies have confirmed that those having endured severe trauma during childhood are, on the whole, more likely to suffer from depression, substance abuse, asocial behavior, as well as obesity and cardiovascular disease. Even worse, this malaise can sometimes be hard-wired into us before birth! Indeed, other studies show that children whose mothers have undergone prolonged psychological stress or intense mental trauma during pregnancy, are at higher risk of becoming anxious, depressed, or even schizophrenic. A strong consensus has been established around this fact by psychologists; there is a clear link between psychological trauma and behavior. But what does this relationship represent concretely? How can negative experiences etch themselves into the organism to the point that they can lastingly affect behavior or health?

The secret of this biological marking could find itself right in the heart of our cells, where the effects of stress disrupt our organism by attacking our DNA. This strange power the mind has over the body has been demonstrated by Australian-American biologist Elizabeth Blackburn, winner of the Nobel Prize for Medicine in 2009, and Elissa Epel, a psychiatrist at the University of California. In 2004, by comparing the DNA of mothers with healthy children with that of mothers with children suffering from serious, chronic conditions, such as autism or motor or cerebral disabilities. The DNA of the latter, suffering from chronic psychological stress, showed signs of premature aging. As though it were being 'consumed' by anxiety. The telomeres of these anxious mothers were abnormally short, indicating accelerated aging, in the range of 9 to 17 years! We can therefore establish a clear link between emotions and what goes on at the cellular level, says Elissa Epel. And we have also shown that when the level of stress decreases, telomere length increases!

How could stress shorten telomeres? Probably because of interactions with cortisol, the stress hormone, which in high concentrations leads to accelerated cell division, and the more cells divide, the more telomeres shorten!

Sedentary lifestyle

According to the British journal The Lancet, lack of physical activity is responsible for one out of every ten deaths in the world, about as many as tobacco or obesity. In 2008 alone, physical inactivity would therefore be responsible for 5.3 million deaths out of the 57 million documented around the world. Between 60 and 85% of adults do not move enough. Average physical activity has fallen to one hour per day in 2000.

> *The role of physical activity continues to be undervalued despite evidence of its protective effects, says Harold W. Kohl (University of Texas) in The Lancet. He adds that much needs to be done to fully address this global issue.*

Moderate (at least 20 minutes three times per week) or intense physical activity (at least 3 hours per week) decreases by 30% the risk of early mortality. Furthermore, regularly engaging in sports improves emotional wellbeing, physical wellbeing, quality of life and self-perception. A beneficial role which is observed in teenagers and seniors alike. Several studies also show that the quality of life of those suffering from chronic illnesses also improves with exercise, as well as for those with certain types of handicaps, when coached by trainers specialized in these pathologies.

Doctor I-Min Lee (Harvard Medical School in Boston) highlights in The Lancet that 6 to 10% of cases of the four major non communicable diseases (cardiovascular disease, type 2 diabetes, breast and colon cancer) could be linked to exercising less than 150 minutes per week. That is the WHO's recommended average. The WHO recommends, for example, 30 minutes of brisk walking five days a week.

According to another study carried out in 122 countries and led by Doctor Pedro C. Hallal (University of Pelotas, Brazil), cited in the British journal, one third of adults and four teenagers out of five around the world don't get enough physical exercise, which increases by 20 to 30% the risk of cardiovascular disease, diabetes and certain types of cancer.

« *In most countries, inactivity rises with age, is higher in women than in men (34% compared to 28%), and is increased in high-income countries* », says Mr. Hallal. By promoting physical activity, life expectancy could grow by about 8 months, say specialists. In other words, decreasing global lack of activity by only 10% would amount to saving the lives of 533,000 people every year.

Why is lack of physical activity synonymous with premature aging? We know that a sedentary lifestyle leads, at the level of fat cells, to an epigenetic change which activates certain genes, or suppresses others, which protect our DNA.

2.1.2 - Internal Causes

Most damage sustained by our DNA is due to four main factors: oxidation, an ubiquitous feature of chemical reactions, leading to the presence of free radicals and oxidative stress; glycation due to excess sugar; chronic inflammation; and finally low or insufficient methylation, responsible for issues with gene expression.

Free Radicals

The human body needs oxygen to live. Most of our body's functions use oxygen to produce energy. This energy enables our organism to function and therefore live. However, part of this oxygen isn't used properly, and this small portion of oxygen produces what are called « *free radicals* ». These are harmful to a certain number of organic molecules, including our proteins and fats: proteins become stiff and lipids turn rancid. Free radicals are atoms with an uneven number of electrons, which therefore necessarily contain one 'bachelor' electron. This electron is said to be free as it has no opposite electric charge (from a proton) with which to join itself. Such an electron, by its very nature, is homeless, and tries to find a partner, even if it has to steal it from its neighbor! This is the dance of free radicals which go from molecule to molecule, strongly interfering with normal cell function. And the damage will progress to neighboring cells. In this way, free radicals are contagious, passing their bachelor electrons off to other victims. This damage may progress indefinitely and will only be stopped once the electron finds a partner. Ironically, the most common free radical in our body is oxygen, an element essential to our lives which, just as it performs its beneficial action, also hurts us.

Most of the damage sustained by the organism through its own operation is due to free radicals. One of their sources is the mitochondria. With time, DNA accumulates damage due to their activity. When mitochondrial DNA is damaged, the mitochondria begin to malfunction, the electron transport chains in particular, which then produce more free radicals.

Unsaturated fats are particularly vulnerable to free radicals. This is why the cell membrane, which is made up of a double layer of lipids, is often damaged. This causes poor cell receptivity. In the heart, this type of damage can lead to a reduction in the maximum heart rate which will continually decrease, throughout the aging process. Free radicals could also be responsible for cerebral aging. They could be responsible for the accumulation of a brownish pigment, lipofuscin, which stems from the oxidation of the cell membrane's phospholipids. By denaturing fats, these free radicals will bind them together, and these cross-links, along with lipofuscin, could clutter neurons and significantly interfere with the transmission of nerve impulses.

Free radicals denature structural proteins, such as collagen and elastin, by making them bond to each other. This mechanism leads to poorer tissue elasticity and the appearance of wrinkles, which then deepen.

Oxidative stress

When anti-oxidative defense systems are overwhelmed, the organism undergoes what is called 'oxidative stress'. It is estimated that DNA suffers around 3,627 lesions per hour. Without any repair mechanism, this would amount to almost 32 million lesions per year. A single cell undergoing all of that damage would be entirely incapable of replicating or assembling proteins, and would therefore be condemned to die. This is why these systems are closely watched. The cell has an entire group of enzymes designed to detoxify free radicals and has many substances which fight oxidative stress. The best known are SOD (superoxide dismutase) which reduces superoxide anions (O2) into hydrogen peroxide (H2O2); catalase, which completes detoxification by dividing hydrogen peroxide molecules into water and oxygen; and glutathione peroxidase which reduces peroxide radicals (ROOH) into alcohol (ROH).

Mitochondrial Aging

Dr. Bruce Ames calls mitochondria the weak link of aging. He says that mounting evidence shows that the deterioration of mitochondria is one of the major causes of aging. He thinks that the accumulation of destructive free radicals, by-products of a normal metabolism, which attack enzymes and other chemical compounds, is largely responsible for this deterioration.

When mitochondria age, the human organism loses the ability to stay young and healthy. This is because aging mitochondria have a negative effect on the cells which make up tissues and organs, which results in a significant slowdown of the entire system.

Glycation

If you heat sugar in a pot, it will first melt, and when its temperature reaches 170°C it will become brown. This can go faster if you add lemon zest or vinegar. This metamorphosis, called 'caramelization', is often used by chefs; it is actually a very complex chemical reaction, which they produce by mixing the sugar with corn syrup and butter, to make caramels. This mix of proteins and sugar is called the Maillard reaction, named after the

French scientist who first described it, in 1912. This caramelization is also observed in all living organisms, but it doesn't require high temperatures. It takes place when a sugar and a protein are present and is called 'glycation'. Glycation is one of the mechanisms of aging, still relatively unknown by the general public but with unquestionably important consequences, due to chronically high levels of sugar in the blood (glucose), and the consumption of overcooked foods. A reaction between a sugar (carbohydrate) and a protein, glycation generates 'glycated proteins' which can neither be destroyed nor released from the cell. This waste will therefore accumulate in our cells, polluting them and causing gene mutations. This gradual waste accumulation makes it more and more difficult for cells to function with age. In particular, it contributes to the progression of atherosclerosis, diabetes, kidney failure, Alzheimer's disease and cataracts. Glycation quietly entered the medical word thanks to tests for glycated hemoglobin levels (HbA1c), routinely used as a marker for hyperglycemia (excess sugar) to monitor diabetes treatments. Work done over the last twenty years show that glycated proteins, also called 'Advanced Glycosylation End products' or AGEs, play an important role in cellular and tissue damage brought on by diabetes, cardiovascular aging and kidney failure.

When cooking food in a pan or in the oven at high or very high temperatures (as low as 100°C but especially over 180°C), we can observe the autocatalytic destruction of glycated proteins which browns food and gives it a particular aromatic quality. The browned parts should not be consumed, as they pollute the organism which can no longer get rid of them. Eating a well grilled steak is nearly the equivalent, in terms of toxicity, of finishing at least one pack of cigarettes. It is therefore not surprising that the frequency of digestive cancers is correlated to that of grilled meat consumption. Grilled vegetables are less toxic but should still be avoided.

Consequences of Glycation

The consequences of protein glycation are many. Once glycated, proteins lose certain properties. This loss has important consequences for your metabolism and cellular functions. Circulating plasma proteins can also be glycated, among which albumin, insulin and immunoglobulins will mainly be affected, forming protein aggregates which can lead to lens clouding (cataracts).

Glycation of the proteins in blood vessel walls causes them to lose part of their mechanical properties as well as making them resistant to the enzymes which participate in vessel wall remodeling. It thereby contributes to the irreversible thickening of the arterial wall (arteriosclerosis). The alteration of fibrinogen and fibrin promotes fibrin deposition in vessels and the proliferation of smooth muscle fibers. The disruption of elastin's properties decreases the elasticity of large vessels, increases filtration through the carotid and leads to a lack of vasodilation.

Glycation disrupts DNA function, is responsible for chromosomal breakage, cellular aging and congenital malformations in diabetic pregnancies.

As for the skin, these glycated proteins accumulate in the cells and with age end up destroying the skin's support cushion made up of collagen and elastin. In other words, glucose will slowly surround collagen and elastin fibers, which will, over time, become rigid and even break. Little by little, glycation damages the subcutaneous substance which supports the dermis. And the latter will, accordingly, lose elasticity and tone. At the surface, wrinkles form and deepen, and skin hydration decreases.

Inflammation

The general public, as well as a significant portion of the medical community, is still generally unfamiliar with chronic inflammation. Illnesses such as cardiovascular disease, diabetes, Alzheimer's disease, obesity, certain types of depression and many others all have a clear inflammatory component. But researchers have recently discovered a new, rapidly growing epidemic: silent inflammation, which quietly eats away at your health and, many years later, becomes a chronic illness. It won't reveal itself through any kind of loud demonstration, as would a fever. Rather, it will cause general fatigue, aches and pains, headaches, in short, a whole series of annoyances which will make us underestimate the seriousness of the problem. This is why it is important and sometimes even vital, to recognize inflammation, in order to prevent or treat it.

The good news is that you can take back control, and permanently so, thanks to changes in lifestyle and nutrition. The key is our hormonal balance, and more specifically a particular group of local hormones called 'eicosanoids'. Keep them in balance and your future will be bright, let their balance fade and you will feel the consequences. Bad eicosanoids feed the inflammation which is responsible for practically all chronic illnesses. Silent inflammation is actually a sign of unbalanced homeostasis. It attacks our heart, our brain, our immune system before we can even feel its symptoms. Three hormones, if they are over-produced, can directly or indirectly trigger the silent inflammation process and lead to chronic illnesses; eicosanoid, insulin and cortisol. Each one of these three hormones contributes, alone or in combination with the two others, to this insidious chronic inflammation, when they are over-abundantly secreted.

Methylation

Most people have never heard of methylation, and yet we would all be dead without it. It plays an essential role in our organism's proper function. Yet it is a double-edged sword, and abnormal methylation can also lead to permanent health issues.

Methylation is a biochemical process which consists of the transfer of a methyl group, made of a carbon atom and three hydrogen atoms – CH3 (diagram)–, from one molecule to another molecule. Stated like this, this doesn't seem so stunning, and yet what results is of capital importance. Indeed, there is carbon in every organic substance on earth, and when carbon atoms change, a lot changes with them. In order to understand methylation, we have to go back to our genes. We have around 25,000 of them and they are identical in every one of our cells. But genes don't all act at the same time; actually, only about 10 to 15% of them are active at any one time. The expression or inhibition of genes occurs according to specific protein assembly needs at a given time, and the methylation process is in fact responsible for the activation and inhibition of the selected genes. The effects of this simple biochemical reaction on DNA synthesis, detoxification and our metabolism, in short on cellular homeostasis, are far-reaching.

Methylation is essential to proper DNA assembly. For example, when a cytosine (C) in a DNA segment is methylated, it becomes a thymine (T). This common mutation is called 'C-T polymorphism', from cytosine to thymine and can lead to very significant genetic changes. Placing a methyl group where there is none can lead to sometimes spectacular changes.

The organism also uses methylation to contribute to the elimination of heavy metals. When methylation is defective, these toxic metals accumulate and interfere with cell function. The liver uses methylation to contribute to the elimination of external toxins as well as that of its own chemical waste.

Methylation reactions are essential to normal brain function. They are essential, in fact, to the production of neurotransmitters, molecules used by brain cells to communicate with each other. These neurotransmitters are, among others, serotonin and melatonin, adrenaline and dopamine, as well as acetylcholine. Methylation errors have been linked to an increased risk of contracting Alzheimer's disease and depression. Finally, methylation is needed to produce one of the most important antioxidants, glutathione.

Methylation and homocysteine

The most direct way of determining whether your organism performs methylation properly is to measure the homocysteine levels in your blood. This metabolite–a molecule intended for disposal– is produced when you consume methionine, which is usually present in dietary proteins like those in red meat and poultry. Our organism uses the methylation process to detoxify homocysteine. In a 'normal' individual, this goes on without a hitch, but if there is a lack of methylation, the homocysteine then accumulates and becomes toxic.

High levels of homocysteine can be toxic for the outside of our arterial walls, and will fracture its internal walls. The organism seals these lesions with LDL cholesterol (the bad kind); homocysteine therefore worsens inflammation and increases the risk of thrombosis and heart attacks.

> *«A study of 15,000 male doctors has shown that even a slight increase in homocysteine levels caused the risk of a heart attack to triple and that of Alzheimer's disease to increase by 450%: equivalent to the risk posed by cigarettes. Taking certain nutritional supplements like vitamins B6, B9 (folic acid) and B12, and reducing red meat and poultry consumption can lower those levels.»*

Normal homocysteine levels should not be higher than 7, but a level of 9 leads to moderate risk, and there is high risk at 14/15.

2.2 - Replicative senescence

We have seen, in the first part, that aging was caused by the organism's insufficient defenses when faced with repeated and increasingly frequent attacks on our DNA, which will, by duplicating itself when it is inadequately repaired, produce deficient copies, which will then generate deficient proteins. A process of gradual senescence which is harmful to our health and to our longevity.

Unfortunately, even if this very significant problem had a solution, we would still find ourselves confronted with a second, just as significant one, called 'replicative senescence'. Our cells, at some point, refuse to continue replicating, commit suicide or become inactive. Why? This is the fascinating story of telomeres and of a very special enzyme which has gotten a lot of attention recently: telomerase.

Telomeres
and Telomerase

A story about shoestrings which revolutionized the world of science.

October 5th, 2009, San Francisco, early morning. Elizabeth Blackburn is still sleeping. Suddenly the phone rings and wakes her up. What she is about to learn will change her life; she and her two colleagues have just been awarded the Nobel Prize for Medicine, for their work on telomeres and telomerase. The life work of this Hobart native–(a small town on the island of Tasmania, Australia), now a molecular biology professor at UCSF, has just received its ultimate recognition.

All of this began in 1961 when a researcher at the University of Philadelphia, Leonard Hayflick, discovered that our cells eventually lose their ability to reproduce themselves. He noticed that after about 50 to 70 divisions, the cell loses the ability to regenerate itself and enters a state which scientists dub 'cellular senescence'. But Hayflick also observed that the cells' ability to duplicate was also influenced by the individual's age. The cells of a young, 30-year-old man multiplied more rapidly than those of a 60-year-old man, and his cells multiplied faster than those of a 90-year-old! What Hayflick discovered was a sort of inescapable clock mechanism present in all of our cells. This countdown was probably the product of accumulated cell damage, especially in our DNA; there was therefore something very specific in our cells which made us age and limited our longevity, but Hayflick did not yet know what.

Only 10 years later were researchers able, simultaneously in the United States and the Soviet Union, to offer an explanation of this surprising limitation. When a cell divides, the genetic material in the cell is also divided and must be copied. This is called DNA replication. These researchers suggested that the limitation would find its cause in this replication; in particular due to enzymes, responsible for the duplication of DNA strands, which would be unable to complete the duplication, for some as yet unknown reason. Consequently, each duplication would lead to DNA loss, as though copying an original, then a copy, then a copy of the copy, and so on, each time losing a little more detail.

This DNA loss with every duplication is a disaster for our life-sustaining proteins, and if this occurred regularly, we would all die after 70 divisions! But since this isn't the case, something else must be going on which stifles this process of programmed death.

Alekseï Olovnikov, a Russian biologist, was one of the first to describe telomeres in 1973. Telomeres, from the Greek word stelos (end) and meros (part), are a structure capping the extremities of the chromosomes' DNA strands, rather like the crimps on the end of a shoelace. These DNA sequences, resembling something like TTAGGG, are repeated hundreds of times, which means that even if, during every division, some DNA is lost at the end of the telomere, it has no immediate effect on the DNA's effectiveness, since the same sequence is found just before it, and before that one as well... until we run out of these sequences. This is when cellular senescence, and aging, begin.

Today we can measure telomere length. This is so simple nowadays that some labs in the United States and in Spain even offer this service to the general public. DNA and telomeres are organized into units, called nucleotides. These units are lined up like beads on a string, and their number can be assessed thanks to these specific tests. This is how we know that at the moment of conception, the embryo has telomeres 15,000 nucleotides long, and that at birth, telomeres have already shrunk down to 10,000 nucleotides. These telomeres continue to shorten with time, and when their length is of no more than 5,000 nucleotides, our cells become senescent, or simply go through programmed cell death (apoptosis).

What happens when a certain number of cells in our organisms are senescent? Recent epidemiological studies show that the presence of short telomeres is often linked with atherosclerosis, hypertension, cardiovascular disease, metabolic syndrome, Alzheimer's, infection, diabetes, fibrosis, and especially cancer risk factors. There is most likely a causal relationship between telomere shortening and global mortality.

« The length of telomeres has been analyzed in 150 people aged 60 or more. Those with the shortest telomeres were eight times as likely to die from infectious disease and three times as likely to have a heart attack. For the authors of the study, these results may reflect the fact that immune cells have to replicate quickly in order to combat an infection. Telomere shortening could slow down replication, thereby increasing the risk of infection. Short telomeres lead to chromosomal instability which often causes very aggressive carcinogenic mutations. »

Telomerase

In the 80's, Prof. Elizabeth Blackburn's research team discovered that telomere shortening isn't unavoidable. Many organisms, in fact, have the necessary tools to prevent it.

Elizabeth Blackburn made a surprising observation: our reproductive cells (sperm and egg cells) have long and stable telomeres, which never shrink. Our organism is composed of two types of cells: somatic cells, out of which all of the organs in our body are made, and reproductive cells, sperm cells in men and egg cells in women. These reproductive cells will give birth to future babies, and it is reassuring to know that our children don't come from old cells, with shriveled telomeres! Our germ line is a set of immortal cells, there since the dawn of time, since life has existed on earth.

All studies agree: sperm cell duplication does not shorten their telomeres, and this no matter our age; which means that an 80-year-old man has the same sperm as a young lad, with a telomere length of at least 10,000 base pairs (nucleotides). As for women's egg cells, their telomeres remain intact for a simple reason: egg cells never divide. A brand new egg appears every month of a woman's reproductively active years, and this is one of the reasons why a woman's reproductive window is constrained (by the existing supply of egg cells) whereas men have a theoretically unlimited capacity.

It therefore had to be discovered why, in a reproductive cell, telomeres remained intact, whereas in a somatic cell, telomeres shortened with every division. And Prof. Blackburn's team was the one to find the explanation, which earned them the Nobel Prize for Medicine in 2009. She discovered an enzyme which she called telomerase, which counteracts telomere shortening when activated. Indeed, it adds new nucleotides to the end of chromosomes. If telomerase is activated in a cell (geneticists refer to this as being expressed), it will immediately recreate the missing nucleotides and keep doing so as duplication continues.

The question we should now ask, obviously, is why? Why is this enzyme which is present in our body asleep in certain cells and active in others? Why do genes wake up, become active, and lead to the expression of telomerase? This depends on numerous factors, in particular our bodies' specific needs, the state of our DNA, and methylation, which enables gene activation. Some are never active but could be at some point, in case of a famine or some sort of significant shock.

In the case of telomerase, the gene which controls it is almost always inhibited (inactive) in somatic cells, and this prevents telomerase from being expressed. Why is this gene always inhibited? Probably in order to enable cancer-fighting genes to be expressed, if a risks exists (which it does every day).

> *In 2004, a study showed that chronic stress also has an effect on telomere length. A more recent study explains how this occurs: «Researchers from UCLA have studied lymphocytes (immune cells) taken from healthy donors (men and women) aged 25 to 55. These cells were treated with different concentrations of cortisol, the hormone which the organism releases when it is stressed, or with DMSO (as a control). After three days, the cultures treated with cortisol had fewer cells than the control cultures. Whereas the treatment with a cortisol concentration equal to that normally found in the human body had no effect on telomerase activity. Concentrations close to those found in an organism under stress reduced telomerase activity up to 50% compared to control cultures. »*

This discovery explains how stress reduces telomerase, accelerating cellular aging through increased cortisol production.

2.3 - Stem Cells and Aging

Adult stem cells are of major importance to tissue function. They insure homeostasis, that is, proper balance between the death of cells and the life of those meant to replace them. But they only produce the types of cells present in the tissue they inhabit. In this way, stem cells present in the blood provide blood cells, those in the skin provide epidermal cells etc. In certain organs, such as the lungs or the liver, stem cells only step in in the event of very severe damage. They can then enable the full regeneration of the damaged tissue, or even of part of the organ. This regenerative capability of organs, which is very limited in humans, is much more developed in certain lower-order species, thanks to their sizable stock of stem cells (on occasion reaching 30% of the organism's cellular mass).

We therefore have a pool of adult stem cells, spread out throughout the body but especially present in the blood, the marrow and abdominal fat; it is essential to our health and our longevity that this capital remain intact. Yet just like all other cells, stem cells endure constant attacks from free radicals, glycation, or inflammation. Their telomeres therefore also shorten, making the cell senile or forcing it to commit suicide. This is another major blow for the cell and its DNA which find themselves under attack from all sides.

Adult stem cells have three main characteristics: they multiply very quickly, they can transform into any cell type which is part of the embryological category to which they belong, and finally, they send signal molecules, called growth factors, which trigger regeneration processes within the cell. The danger inherent in the aging of stem cells is the same as for any somatic cell, but with one particularity: they will age faster if they are frequently used, as is the case for red blood cells. Indeed, rapid duplication leads to accelerated telomere shortening and senescence, or programmed cell death. We are therefore confronted with an entire mosaic of adult stem cells, whose cellular age will vary according to their location. However, we will see later on that it is now possible for us to reinvigorate our adult stem cell pool.

We can no longer consider natural death as a universal law of nature. Faced with this new 'reality', many scientists have become fascinated with understanding the biology of aging. All experts agree that the causes of aging are at the cellular level, and that it is through cellular biology that solutions are to be found. This field has now established that living beings exchange molecules with their environment and are constantly renewing themselves. They are therefore forced to constantly adapt themselves to their environment. It all comes back, as always, to the concept of homeostasis, of constant dynamic adaptability. Aging results from a homeostatic imbalance which begins with the DNA, causing a series of cascading imbalances. After a certain age (between 30 and 40 years old) DNA damage is no longer being repaired quickly enough, and the gap between damage and damage repair therefore only widens. The damage itself results from an imbalance between oxidation and anti-oxidation, followed by an imbalance in adult stem cells which ensure cellular homeostasis, that is, the balance between dying cells and the life of those meant to replace them. Human beings therefore undergo gradual senescence, aging being the result of insufficient defenses against their own deterioration. Consequently, it is only possible to overcome aging by regeneration or immediate repair.

Replicative senescence plays the leading role in aging. Telomere shortening leads to cellular senescence which will cause further damage by disseminating its toxic waste; the best case scenario is for the cell to commit suicide (apoptosis). Aging is the result of a homeostatic imbalance between cellular senescence or apoptosis on the one hand, and the replacement of old cells with new ones, produced by stem cells. Unfortunately, stem cells are also damaged in this way and their numbers shrink with time. This is the aging trilogy: degraded DNA, shortened telomeres and destroyed stem cells.

SOURCES

Miroslav Radman.

Au-delà de nos limites biologiques. Paris : Plon ; 2011.

Nicole Le Douarin.

Les cellules souches. Paris : Odile Jacob ; 2007.

Barry Sears.

The anti-inflammation Zone. New York : HarperCollins ; 2005.

Joseph C. Maroon.

The Longevity Factor. New York : Atria Books ; 2009.

Joseph C. Maroon.

Jeffrey Bost. Fish oil. Laguna Beach (Californie) : Basic Health Publications ; 2006.

Michael Fossel, Greta Blackburn, Dave Woynarowski.

The Immortality edge. Hoboken (New Jersey)
John Wiley & Sons, Inc. ; 2011.

Vincent C. Giampapa, Frederick F. Buechel.

Ohan Karatoprack. The gene makeover.
Laguna Beach (Californie) Basic Health ; 2007.

Vincent C. Giampapa.

The basic principles and practice of anti-aging medicine & age management.
Publication universitaire ; 2003.

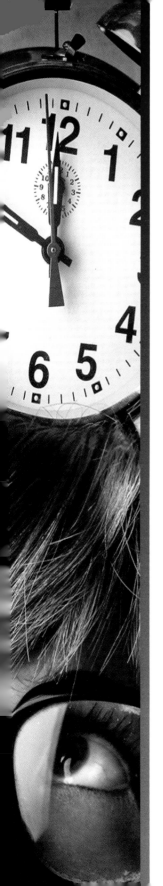

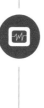

Chapter 3

How Do We Age?

« You know you're getting older when everything hurts,
and what doesn't hurt doesn't work! »

- Georges Burns, centenarian comedian -

Generally speaking, aging is directly related to the loss of homeostasis, of adaptability when faced with more and more frequent attacks. This begins with DNA and ends with very poor quality proteins, causing visible damage at the molecular, cellular, tissue and finally clinical level, when it becomes visible to the naked eye!

Two organs in particular age very visibly: facial skin and the brain, and aging is particularly harmful for one function: the immune system.

3.1 - Skin & Facial Aging

Skin owes its elasticity and its resistance to the different layers of tissue which constitute it: the epidermis, the dermis and the hypodermis. The epidermis, the skin's outer layer, makes it waterproof and makes it resistant. It is mostly made up of keratin, a fibrous protein produced by keratinocytes, and melanin, the main cutaneous pigment, produced by melanocytes. As time passes, keratinocytes are renewed more slowly and their terminal differentiation slows down.

Fundamental changes take place in the dermis, the skin's support structure, made up of 80% of elastin and collagen fibers, entirely enveloped in a gel made of glycoproteins. The main dermis cells, fibroblasts, are specialized in elastin and collagen fiber synthesis. Between 20 and 80 years of age, the fibroblast population - which ensures homeostasis of the synthesis, maturation and degradation of elastin and collagen fibers - is halved. The loss of fibroblasts causes an imbalance, which degrades the collagen and elastin fibers, and leads to diminished dermis elasticity and tonicity, and therefore the appearance of wrinkles.

Collagen fibers are distributed throughout the layers of the dermis. They are made of proteins, responsible for tissue cohesion and resistance. They are able to store water and contribute to skin hydration. A reduction in the quantity of collagen and/or a change in its quality cause the appearance of deep wrinkles.

Elastins are proteins arranged into fibers which are responsible for tissue elasticity and solidity. With age, elastin fibers become rarefied, and the skin thins and wrinkles.

Skin Renewal

Skin is an organ in constant renewal. Just as in bones, skin cells die and reappear every day. When functioning normally, they are renewed every 28 days, for a maximum of 50 cycles. But, with time, renewal slows its pace and the skin ages. The oldest cells may then accumulate and give an uneven complexion and thicker skin, revealing a dryness which often precedes skin aging. If this dryness is not corrected, wrinkles could make deeper marks in the skin, which also will likely thin and blemish easily. Facial volumes and aspect gradually change while wrinkles deepen.

Oxidation and Skin Aging

Our skin is constantly facing a multitude of external aggressions which can accelerate its aging process. It is particularly susceptible to free radical attacks, generated both by the normal functioning of our organism and by aggressive external elements, such as solar radiation, pollution or tobacco. These free radicals are dangerous molecules, often responsible for changes in tissues and cells causing skin aging.

However, the skin has an anti-oxidant defense system which brings together an entire arsenal of molecules, including enzymes such as superoxide dismutase, catalase, glutathione peroxidase or glutathione reductase. This arsenal also contains anti-oxidants provided by our nutrition, such as vitamins C and E or beta-carotene. But the organism's natural anti-oxidant defenses ultimately end up overwhelmed, and become less effective. This is how years of accumulated free radical damage can lead to very significant changes in skin appearance and health: the epidermis is less able to repair and renew tissue, collagen is less soluble, elastin fibers gradually deteriorate and become damaged, in particular in areas of skin damaged by the sun, where elastin has even more structural anomalies. Glycosaminoglycans are no longer able to properly interact with water, as fat content decreases. All of these changes, due to the passage of time, result in wrinkled, dry, tired skin; it becomes gray, less elastic and unable to properly heal itself.

Hyaluronic Acid

Skin is the main reservoir of hyaluronic acid, indispensable to life and to its beauty. But this acid is very fragile, and easily degraded. Synthesized by fibroblasts and keratinocytes, it is one of the essential components of the extracellular matrix. It has an important structural function, one of the key elements being the maintenance of dermal density and therefore skin firmness. It also acts literally like a sponge; capable of storing more than one thousand times its weight in water, it is essential in maintaining skin tissue hydration. These properties will also allow it to store other substances, like electrolytes, nutrients or growth factors, as well as ensure the evacuation of metabolic waste.

With age, the synthesis and quality of hyaluronic acid decreases, which explains in part skin dehydration and loss of firmness, along with the appearance of wrinkles.

Lipofuscin

I am sure that you have all already heard about what are called 'liver spots', and that you have already seen some. Most doctors will tell you that they have no pathological importance, and yet we can find the same components composing these spots in different parts of the body, including the brain. This brown pigment is actually lipofuscin, a mix of proteins, fats and metals, iron in particular. Lipofuscin is a cellular pigment made of molecular debris, and comes from aging lysosomes present in every cell in our body. When lysosomes age, they can no longer degrade on their own, as they have no more enzymatic activity. They become residual bodies which can remain in the cell for a very long time, as lipofuscin deposits. Today we consider lipofuscin to be a biological age marker. This pigment starts to accumulate right after birth and keeps doing so, more and more quickly, as time passes. It could be the cause of a serious eye disease called 'macular degeneration' which causes blindness.

The neurons, heart and skin of elderly people contain particularly high levels of lipofuscin, but it is likely that lipofuscin is not only a consequence of aging but also a cause.

The Role of the Environment

In the past few years, specialists have noticed that a harmful environment (sun, tobacco, stress...) can alter the genetic capital of skin cells, making them multiply less efficiently and become more fragile. It is therefore essential, in order to age well, to avoid these environmental factors as much as possible, particularly the sun, tobacco, pollution, all the time making sure to have a balanced diet and generally lead a healthy life.

The sun is the number one enemy of our skin and its deleterious effects are now well known. Ultraviolet rays, responsible for weakening skin cells, foster the development of skin cancer, limiting the production of good, elastic skin (the dermis is more rigid). Finally, excessive UV exposure increases the rate of skin cell degradation and inhibits their production. The skin thus becomes thinner and less resistant.

Tobacco is another powerful enemy of the skin, almost as harmful as solar radiation. The toxic products which cigarettes contain cause the fundamental structures of the dermis, hyaluronic acid in particular, to deteriorate and foster the improper production of elastin.

Air pollution plays a role in accelerating skin aging by weakening its immune system, lowering its hydration and decreasing its rate of desquamation. Although stress is unfortunately a difficult factor to avoid, it seems nonetheless true that it directly increases free radical production in the skin, these oxidized molecules destroying cells and potentially changing the structure of our DNA.

3.2 - Cerebral Aging

The brain begins to age very early, and as soon as we reach 25 years of age, the number of neurological connections begins to decrease. From the age of 50 onwards, the weight of the brain decreases on average by 2% every ten years. This natural development has its consequences, and this reduction in neurons will gradually slow down our mental and motor functions (in our movements and our reflexes).

This slowdown is also directly related, besides the decrease in neurons, to a drop in impulse speed, the actual transmission of information between neurons. This is why the more we age, the more time we need to process information. A global slowdown then takes place, which impacts on cognitive and intellectual function, and particularly memory. Indeed, the drop in processing speed can lead to the disappearance of information, before it can even be processed, which can in large part explain forgetfulness.

Furthermore, aging sensory organs (hearing, sight, smell...) provide poorer sensory perception, and get in the way of proper information capture, thereby diminishing our ability to memorize it properly. Very many senior citizens complain about their declining memory. These complaints often betray a fear of the most famous and most publicized disease linked to memory loss: Alzheimer's. Yet despite what is often believed, it is wrong to assume that decreasing intellectual and memory performance is necessarily linked to a pathology like Alzheimer's.

It is indeed perfectly normal for intellectual capabilities to decrease with age, simply because the brain ages, just like the rest of the body. Certain cognitive functions (intellectual functions: language, memory, attention, abstract thought, spatial representation, judgment, reasoning...), will be more susceptible than others to aging. This is the case in particular of attention and memory.

3.3 - The Immune System & Aging

With time, the immune system becomes less efficient. This process begins when the thymus starts to atrophy, which begins right after puberty. The immune system's decline therefore starts very early on, but its first symptoms are rarely discernible before we reach our fifties. The size of the thymus, as well as its activity, progressively withers with age. The organ's weight diminishes by two thirds and its lymphocyte content by 90%. The levels of thymic hormones in the blood also decrease after puberty and reach their lowest levels starting at around sixty years old. This increasing scarcity explains the deterioration of immune system performance observed in the elderly. Indeed, aging reduces our resistance to tumors and is often accompanied by more frequent infections and higher related mortality. In older people with poor immune response, all-cause mortality is twice as high as in young subjects. Cancer mortality is for its part three times as high, as are lung infections, whose propagation is helped by the decrease of the cough reflex. Latent infections like shingles, herpes or measles can resurface, but the most frequent risk is that of repeated urinary infections which gradually become resistant to antibiotics.

3.4 - Cardiac and arterial aging

They say we are only as old as our arteries, and, with few exceptions, this is true!

The most tragic aspect of cardiovascular diseases, and heart attacks in particular, is their brutality! One minute everything seems fine, the next we are overcome with pain, we panic, even worse, we die suddenly, without warning. Our arterial networks take years to age and can remain silent for a long time, without exhibiting any clinical symptoms. There are occasional warning signs of course, pain which flares up during physical exertion... But we often blame it on the physical effort itself.

Although the term 'cardiovascular' is often used, it is important to understand that the vascular system is the first to deteriorate, shutting off blood flow and depriving the body of oxygen, and leading to kidney, heart or brain damage.

The more we age, the more our arteries harden: this is what we call arteriosclerosis. But this hardening is often accompanied by cholesterol plaques which cling to the walls of the blood vessels. When this happens, as is most often the case, it is called atherosclerosis or atheromatous disease. Vascular walls are made up of several layers of cells. The first to be damaged is the one in direct contact with the blood stream, which is made of endothelial cells. These cells weaken with time and progressively lose the ability to synthesize collagen and elastin, two substances which are essential to arteries' flexibility. They become more and more rigid and less and less able to react to the heart's constant requests for them to expand or shrink depending on our body's oxygen needs. As damage accumulates, every layer of the arterial wall becomes inflamed, leading to scarring which will serve as an anchor point for cholesterol. This will continually deposit itself until it completely plugs the artery's lumen; circulation is then partially or completely stopped and oxygen and nutrition are no longer transported downstream. If this plumbing issue takes place in the renal arteries, it leads to kidney failure; in the coronary arteries (those which irrigate the heart), it leads to heart attacks, the severity of which will depend on the degree of obstruction; in the carotid arteries, it leads to strokes (Cerebrovascular Accidents or CVAs), resulting in the paralysis of the limbs on the side of the body opposite the damage, with or without aphasia (speech impairment). Our organism has however designed a cholesterol cleanup system, which we can measure via HDL (High Density Lipoprotein) blood levels, but it unfortunately also has a system which promotes cholesterol accumulation, measured in LDL (Low Density Lipoprotein) blood levels.

Hypertension is another consequence of arterial wall rigidity, and is assessed via two components. Systolic pressure, which reflects pressure variations during peak cardiac contraction; this value isn't constant as it is influenced by stress, anxiety, whether we are standing or sitting, physical activity and many other factors. Diastolic pressure reflects how our heart behaves when it refills with blood; it is more stable and a better indicator of our arteries' condition. Arterial pressure is measured with a sphygmomanometer or blood pressure monitor, the normal range being between 120 mm and 140 mm of mercury for systolic pressure and between 70 and 90 mm of mercury for diastolic pressure (these values vary from country to country).

3.5 - Hormones & Aging

There are two main activities we think of when talking about hormones. The first is intracellular and intercellular communication; this communication's quality depends on hormones which will interact not only at the level of the cell membrane, but also within the cell. The second is cellular homeostasis, that is, the preservation of a permanent balance of all functions.

Hormones are therefore essentially there to coordinate organ function. They are essential to our metabolic balance, and their concentration is also important. Transported through the blood, they travel deep into cells and activate production chains for cellular components. They build new ones and induce reactions which release the energy necessary for life.

This is all directed, of course, by the brain, specifically by the hypothalamus, which coordinates the activity of all peripheral hormones via two glands: the pituitary and pineal glands. These peripheral hormones will, in turn, influence the glands which emitted them by biofeedback control. Furthermore, a peripheral hormone can influence another by stimulating or inhibiting it.

The levels of certain hormones decrease with age. The thymus, which produces some of our hormones, also disappears around 40 years of age. Some consider this decrease to be a sign of aging, and that the measurement of hormone levels in the organism would be a reliable means of evaluating our biological age, independently of how old we are.

The following graph shows the average decrease, observed by some publications, of hormone levels with age. It varies depending on the individual, and is therefore truly only an average.

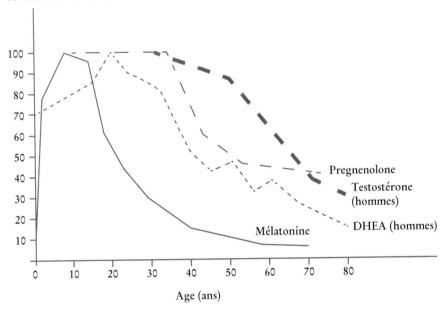

Taux relatif par rapport à l'âge
où le taux est maximal

Pregnenolone

Testostérone
(hommes)

DHEA (hommes)

Mélatonine

Age (ans)

Decrease in levels of certain hormones with age.
Source : Thierry Hertoghe

But is it this decline in hormone levels which causes aging or does aging cause the decrease in hormones? It has so far been assumed that the causal relationship goes both ways: the non-renewal of glandular cells caused by DNA damage and telomere shortening impacts the pool of stem cells meant to replace the aging glandular cells. Waste accumulates in the cells, which further stifles their activity. Hormonal deficiencies gradually appear, often very quietly. The concentration of most hormones in our blood plummets once we are 50, and the fact that every hormone is influenced by another leads to deficits through a lack of synergy.

3.6 - Other Signs of Aging

Aging-related anatomical and physiological changes start several years before the appearance of external signs. Several of these changes start appearing around our forties and continue to do so until our organism can no longer adapt itself. The process of senescence, on the physiological level, causes the decline of organic functions, followed by the aging of tissue and of the body's general appearance.

All of the organism's muscles, those in the torso and the extremities, in particular, atrophy with time, which leads to a general deterioration of muscular tone as well as a loss of power, strength, endurance and agility. Total muscle weight decreases by half from 30 to 70 years of age. Muscle aging is due to muscle fibers atrophying and an increase in intramuscular fat content. Muscles in the forearms lose the most strength.

Muscular strength, at 80 years old, has decreased by 30%. We have less strength and resistance, we lift lighter weights, we have less strength to open jars or for cleaning (mopping, vacuuming, moving furniture).

Our joints also undergo changes: ligaments calcify, ossify, and joints shrink through the erosion of cartilaginous surfaces. Whereas some joints become more rigid as they deteriorate, others become more flexible.

Even though they keep their appearance, bones also undergo changes. The process of calcium reabsorption becomes unbalanced and the bony tissue becomes more porous and fragile due to continuous demineralization. Osteoporosis is also one of the factors responsible for tooth loss, which is in fact connected to the inflammation and demineralization of the bone surrounding the tooth. Those teeth which remain become flatter, and the jaw atrophies, which makes the teeth appear longer and further apart. Bone resorption in the jaw and maxilla accentuates with tooth loss. The distance between the chin and nose shortens and teeth move backwards, in time changing the physiognomy of the elderly individual.

Height loss is another phenomenon which can be attributed to aging. It is actually due to the spine shortening (by 1.2 to 5 cm) through the slimming of the dorsal and lumbar vertebrae as a result of osteoporosis. This phenomenon, which is more pronounced in women than in men, begins during our fifties and is related to the interaction of different factors such as age, sex, race and environment. The shortening of the spine skews the body's proportions, the arms and legs remaining the same size, which causes a deviation of the upper thorax and accentuates the spine's natural curvature (kyphosis). In order to keep their balance, elderly people need to lean forward and slightly bend their knees in order to maintain their center of gravity. Cartilage wears out with time and these curvatures become permanent. The thoracic cavity becomes smaller and the ribs move down and out. The reduction of the rib cage is linked to the osteoporosis of the ribs and atrophying respiratory muscles. It decreases respiratory amplitude, which explains the posture which is often observed: « *torso pushed forward, head tilted back* ». This inward arching of the body changes our appearance, hinders mobility and accentuates the elderly person's shorter body.

For women, breasts sag and atrophy, and the nipples sometimes become inverted. The sebaceous glands which produce protective sebum become less active and lubricate the skin less, and it becomes dry and brittle as a result. The sweat glands become less active as well, and modify how body temperature is controlled by sweat.

The loss of subcutaneous fatty tissue is one of the clearer outcomes of aging. This phenomenon is common to all aging individuals and particularly affects the arms and legs. Tendons, veins and joints in the hands, as well as in our clavicles, protrude more, along with our ribs and knees. The cavities in our armpits and above our clavicles are accentuated. The maxillary bones are more visible, the cheekbones are more salient, and our eye sockets deepen. Our nose, ears and earlobes become longer, our eyelids and cheeks sag. In addition to atrophying and becoming less elastic, the skin undergoes other changes. Here are a few: the appearance of colored spots on the epidermis (lentigo senilis), of purpura, (bruising due to fragility of the dermis and blood vessels), the presence of senile telangiectasia (permanent dilation of small subcutaneous blood vessels), drying and flaking of the skin.

With age, changes in the balance of androgen and estrogen (hormones) occur, and lead to many changes: hair rarefies all over the body and falls little by little; in certain places, like the pubic area, armpits and extremities (feet and hands), hair loss is almost complete. Both men and women often see hair appear on the face however. For women, it mostly grows on the chin and upper lip, whereas for men, it will grow in the ears and nostrils; this unsightly hair is abundant and coarse, and often forces women to wax or shave it off; moreover, for certain elderly people, eyebrow hair becomes very thick and coarse.

The hair on our scalp also changes drastically during aging. Although hair loss is normal, it accentuates as we age. We have the most hair when we are 40. From this age onwards, the process reverses. Baldness, or the gradual thinning of our hair, is linked to racial and hormonal genetic predispositions. It affects men more often than women, and can begin as early as in our twenties. When we age, our hair changes appearance, becomes more scarce, thinner, weaker and has less volume. It gradually grays, half of people aged 50 or older having gray or graying hair. This discoloration is linked with lowered melanocyte activity. These cells produce melanin, a hair coloring agent. Nails also change. Their growth slows down, followed by the appearance of longitudinal striations and grooves on their surface, to which is added lowered peripheral circulation, all of which together make nails grow thicker, drier and more brittle; this phenomenon is even more pronounced for toenails.

The Body Slows Down

Reflexes, muscular coordination, balance and reaction time all decline. An elderly person walks more slowly, their gait becomes more halting, with smaller steps, and slippery sidewalks in the winter inspire greater apprehension. They need more time to cross intersections. They get into their bath very carefully. They get out of bed slowly, and getting dressed takes more time...

The eye lens is less elastic and focuses less accurately. This anomaly, called presbyopia, develops with age. The eyes gradually lose the ability to see objects with are very close or very far away (myopia) which makes progressive lenses necessary. Cataracts become more frequent with age. This issue is due to the yellowing, or discoloration, of the lens, which reduces the amount of light able to reach the sensitive area of the retina, distorts colors and makes vision and the accurate perception of objects more difficult.

Hearing loss appears with age and has many causes. Its incidence rate is higher in men than in women, at all ages. Most of this loss is selective rather than total and absolute. The hearing threshold for high frequency (high-pitched) sounds is more strongly affected than that of low frequency (low-pitched) sounds. The loss of high frequencies has serious consequences as it modifies the perception or the voices of others. Consonants being more high-pitched than vowels, normal speaking cadence and flow is deformed, and words blend with each other. The loss of high frequency perception is called presbycusis. Its frequency increases with age.

Food becomes blander and less appealing when we age. As tolerance to spices decreases at the same time, it isn't surprising that the loss of taste corresponds with the loss of appetite. Our diet can suffer from this. Our mucous membranes are generally less tolerant to irritation: friction from prostheses, overly seasoned food, liquids which are too hot or too cold, tobacco, and alcohol. All of this damages us, and healing is slower. Chewing becomes tiresome and uncomfortable. The alimentary bolus is therefore poorly masticated and its assimilation is incomplete. The salivary glands atrophy, which dries out the mouth, and gives it a metallic taste. Skin receptors generally remain intact. Transmission will more often fail at the level of the central nervous system, which explains why several studies have shown elevated pain thresholds for the skin.

The respiratory system becomes very vulnerable in the elderly. More abundant nasal secretions result in less permeability and limit breathing through the nose, which forces elderly people to breathe through their mouths. The nasal mucosa doesn't rid the air it breathes in of its impurities. Breathing through the mouth dehydrates the entire bronchial tree (mucosa).The bronchial system is enlarged through the trachea's dilation and atrophying mucosa, which increases the respiratory 'dead space' an unused, and unusable, volume of air, which is larger than in younger individuals.

Aging and Sleep

Gradual changes of the organism throughout the aging process also have an impact on sleep. Even for older people who are in good health, sleep is lighter. Falling asleep becomes more difficult and waking up happens more often during the night. Laboratory studies have confirmed these changes. Sleep efficiency (time actually spent sleeping compared to time spent in bed), which is around 95to 98% during youth, drops to 80 or even 70% later on. Furthermore, the duration of light sleep increases with age, whereas deep sleep decreases. And the waking threshold falls as well. Noises and other interruptions, even modest ones, are consequently more likely to wake us up. Certain studies seem to have shown that we need less sleep as we age, but most experts continue to think that we need just as much. The normal circadian sleep cycle (a 24-hour cycle) becoming gradually weaker, sleep increasingly tends to space itself out throughout the day, rather than concentrating itself during the night. Since we sleep less during the night when we age, we nap more and fall asleep reading or watching TV. All of these changes result in a phenomenon which elderly people often complain about: their sleep is shorter lived and less restful than before.

Be that as it may, there is no truly optimal amount of sleep. The ideal length enables us, when we sleep well, to not feel tired when we wake up, or drowsy during the day. The important thing is to find our own waking/sleep cycle to feel good during the day and at night.

All of our physiological functions will slow down, little by little. This is a complex and multifactorial process which affects all of our organs but whose progression varies a lot depending on the individual. Aging is directly linked to our loss of homeostasis, or our adaptability when faced with more and more frequent attacks. This starts with our DNA and ends with very poor quality proteins causing visible damage at the molecular, cellular, tissue, and finally clinical levels, where it can be seen with the naked eye! Two organs in particular age very obviously: facial skin and the brain, and aging is particularly harmful for one function: the immune system.

S O U R C E S

Alain Reinberg.

Nos horloges biologiques sont-elles à l'heure ? Paris : Le Pommier ; 2004.

Thierry Hertoghe, Jules-Jacques Nabet.

Comment rester jeune plus longtemps ? Paris : Albin Michel ; 2000.

Vincent C. Giampapa.

The basic principles and practice of anti-agingmedicine & age management. Publication universitaire ; 2003.

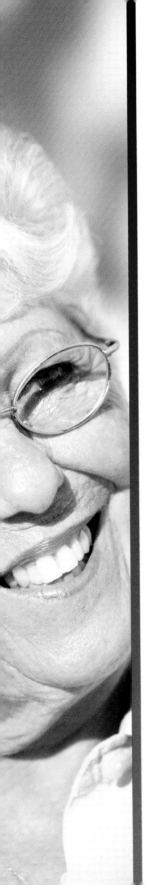

Chapter 4

Why Do Women Live Longer Than Men?

« Women develop symptoms, men develop behaviors »

- Alain Ehrenberg -

It's about time we put an end to the myth of men's supremacy over women. It's about time we seriously consider a well-established fact: no matter their age, men die in greater numbers than women. Statistically, women live on average 8 to 10 years longer than men; where can this weak spot come from? Are men more biologically vulnerable? Does their social conduct wear them out prematurely? The big surprise is that this assessment is worldwide. With few exceptions, this difference in longevity holds true in most populations, including in developing countries. Women are resistant to a point which men simply cannot equal!

«A team of Japanese biologists has just shown that a mouse born from two mothers lives one third longer than one born from a father and a mother. Tomohiro Kono and Manabu Kawahara of the Tokyo and Saga Universities actually managed to produce mice whose DNA comes from two females. Their scientific motivation was to understand why, in most animal species, females live longer than males. They even say that longevity could depend on a gene (called Rasgrf1) present in the 9th chromosome.»

A male fetus has fewer chances of surviving than a female one. At birth, a boy's lungs have fewer chances of surviving than those of a girl. In the United States, 20% of teenage mortality is due to violent deaths: suicide, homicidal behavior, murder. It would seem that boys have a 'physiological' tendency to die violent deaths. The brain regions responsible for judgment and decision making are less developed in young boys than in girls. Furthermore, social attitudes play a predominant role in this difference in survival rates; we encourage boys to be aggressive, to show off their strength, to never complain.

According to Anne-Sophie Cousteaux: « *the mostly 'preventable' causes of death to which 20 to 65 year olds are subjected: smoking, drinking, reckless driving, violent behavior, workplace accidents, are mostly confined to men. Furthermore, as they are used to regularly seeing gynecologists as a precautionary measure ever since their teenage years, women see healthcare as a preventative practice. For men, its purpose is mainly for treatment; they often wait a long time before seeing a doctor and avoid going to see a shrink! Women know themselves better, and better recognize and interpret their bodies' signals. In terms of health, they already know a lot due to their frequent role as the house nurse at home. They not only manage their own health but also that of those around them: children, grandchildren, husband, parents, in-laws and grandparents. They are responsible for any direct communication with doctors, hospitals or clinics. After spending so much time interacting with them, they learn a lot. After a certain age, health problems become the main topic of conversation among women. This allows them to exchange a lot of experience and knowledge gained through different events which they lived through themselves or at their loved ones' side. They consult doctors and treat themselves, even if this means resting more often and for longer than men, which enables them to live longer, with illnesses which are properly cared for.»*

Myocardial infarctions are a striking example. Early signs appear in men around 35 years of age, and this illness becomes the leading cause of death for men of 35 and older. But for women, the risk of heart attack only becomes significant starting at 60 years of age. Most women only begin to experience symptoms during menopause. Furthermore, men's immune systems are more fragile than women's, and statistically they suffer more from the ten most important illnesses which affect us.

As surprising as it might seem, the fact that men are more vulnerable than women has largely been ignored by the research community. Until 1980, clinical studies were practically only performed on men, perhaps due to the belief that what worked for men must necessarily work for women as well. Women were excluded for a variety of reasons, in particular during their reproductively active period. It was not until the 90's that researchers began to compare male and female data, and were continually taken by surprise! So much so that Columbia University decided, in 1997, to establish a brand new medical field, Gender Specific Medicine. Gender being understood as a generic term encompassing specific biological and chromosomal aspects, as well as the given social environment.

For millions of years, men were responsible for finding food and shelter, and for territorial protection. The surrounding environment required risk-taking and fighting off potential invaders. Then in the 19th century the industrial revolution took place and developed during the 20th century, and with it arrived technologies perfecting savings, effort and ergonomics. This progress allows a woman today to be a dockworker or a baggage-handler with a few flicks of a remote control. Nowadays, women can perform any and all activities usually entrusted to men, except, of course, when it comes to procreation. But this too could potentially change one day; some biologists wonder if the human race will always have the luxury of possessing two genders! The Y chromosome, which determines the male sex, seems to be degrading more and more every day, and this for the past 300 million years. In genetics labs, it is called the « *junk chromosome* ». It originally contained 1,500 genes, today these genes have disappeared or are hibernating. And this isn't surprising given how many cell divisions this chromosome supervises every day, being necessary for the production of 150 million sperm cells. The potential for mistakes during this process are simply astronomical. The Y chromosome will therefore dictate the evolution of the human race, as its mutations are frequent, contrary to the XX pair which defines the female sex and for which each chromosome can help the other.

4.1 - Impact of Social Changes

The world has completely changed in 150 years. Human beings no longer depend on their physical strength, and the Internet has no sexual preference. The field of robotics is full of promise, to the extent that a recent, intentionally provocative article, claims that dozens of women in New-York would rather have a good, custom-made robot than a needy man with which to share their life. Men aren't what they used to be, and neither are women!

4.2 - Male / Female Disparities

Today, research on male/female disparity shows that there are indeed huge differences between the two sexes, which express themselves from the moment of conception and last throughout their lifetime.

At conception, we know that the quantity and quality of sperm decreases with age, affecting sperm cells' mobility in particular. During pregnancy, males are at a higher risk of contracting an infection than females, as their immune system is less effective. During birth, mortality risk is 1.5 to 2 times higher for boys, and this disparity remains despite modern neonatal resuscitation methods. After their birth, and once these obstacles are passed for the little boy, boys and girls remain very different. I am not referring to sexual characteristics, but everything else, in particular the specificity of the male brain, due to the Sry gene in the Y chromosome. The differences in gray matter/white matter ratios are very significant: from 6 to 18 years old, boys lose 20% of their gray matter and gain 40% white matter, whereas girls only lose 5% of their gray matter and gain 28% white matter. Gray matter processes information whereas white matter transmits it, and these changes therefore inevitably cause behavioral disparities. During adolescence, different social aspirations between the sexes will have a strong influence on psychological development. Boys, in their prepubescent years, are hyper- aggressive, a trait absent from girls. Which leads some people to claim that the two genders should be schooled separately! They base this claim on boys' poor performance compared to girls during middle and high-school, even if their grades are good in math, physics and chemistry. Adolescence is a difficult period for boys; the suicide rate from 15 to 19 years of age is of 16 boys out of 100,000, whereas it is only 3.6 for girls. It is well known that high testosterone levels, which begin during puberty and plateau around 20 years old, promote violent and suicidal behavior. Furthermore, boys complete their suicide attempts four times more often than girls. During adulthood, depression becomes a greater threat, even if declared suicide attempts are two times lower than for women. The reason is that men have trouble talking about this issue and finding the words with which to describe the symptoms.

Sex and hunger are probably the two fundamental forces (or drivers) which impel men to act. They are meant to procreate, eat and survive. Biologically, a man's role is to inseminate a woman, and he is equipped accordingly. This is why he has a strong sexual appetite, especially between 18 and 30 years of age. His high levels of testosterone have something to do with it. Indeed, when it is expressed in women:

> «In a study led by investigators of the prestigious Massachusetts General Hospital in Boston, a testosterone patch in 75 women produced spectacular results: The percent age of women having sexual fantasies at least once a week doubled and the number of women who had intercourse at least once a week went from 23 percent to 41 percent. Desire, intensity of arousal, and the enjoyment and intensity of orgasm all increased significantly.»

When reaching the critical threshold of our forties, these differences become even more significant. Men suddenly realize their mortality, or their vulnerability, and their health may become their priority. The more they grow old, the more specific their fears become, especially as concerns cancer. Andropause is a state characterized by a gradual decrease in levels of testosterone and other hormones. Its intensity is in no way comparable to that of menopause, which is louder and more visible. The estrogen/testosterone ratio changes, which leads to breast growth in men, thinner bones (osteoporosis), decreased libido, and, as a bonus, higher rates of depression.

In the 1950s, Francis Madigan took an interest in the biological differences between the two sexes, and for him, the main reasons for the ever-growing gap between male and female longevity are not to be found in sociocultural factors. In order to test his hypothesis, he studied religious communities of both sexes which were isolated from the rest of society. Among the different factors which were explored, the role of sex hormones on cholesterol levels seems to be the most important biological factor.

In 1995, Ingrid Waldron reviewed the existing work on the effects of different biological factors, including sex hormones, body fat distribution, blood iron levels, etc. She reached the conclusion that female sex hormones decrease the risk of contracting cardiovascular disease, in part thanks to their positive effect on blood lipid content, whereas in men, high testosterone levels have a negative effect on cholesterol. According to her work, another factor seems to disadvantage men: their tendency to preferentially accumulate fat in the abdominal area could contribute to their harmful lipid levels, and consequently to their higher mortality from heart attacks.

Among the social, environmental and behavioral factors, smoking, diet and healthcare play a very important role. The main causes of this sexual differential, cardiovascular disease and lung cancer, are indeed linked to smoking. Among all of the studied populations, men smoke more than women, and among smokers, men are more often heavy users.

Why are women more resistant to life's wear and tear?

Just as popular belief suggests, there are fundamental differences between the two sexes, but contrary to this belief, men are not the stronger of the two. What then are the weaknesses which restrict men's resistance and the strengths which make the fairer sex actual superwomen?

Men have a genetic shortcoming which places them in weaker standing from the outset: their Y chromosome has aged, worn by the astronomical number of cell divisions needed to produce billions of sperm cells, of which only one will produce offspring. It would seem that this chromosomal stigma makes men more fragile, from conception to birth, during which they will accumulate shortcomings and risks of never seeing the light of day. If they are lucky enough to pass through this veritable obstacle course unscathed, they will emerge in an unfavorable environment, as they inherit their past duties as rugged men, more muscular than women, ancestrally responsible for the family's nourishment and protection, and for waging war. They are boys, therefore they will be told to «Be strong! Never complain.» These commandments will dictate men's behavior, and they will naturally become 'macho'; power, domination, occasionally violence are part of their male routine. But this behavior is a double edged sword. Being macho is sometimes a heavy burden, and since men don't have the right to complain, they keep it locked within them... Which leaves the door open to depression and its dreadful consequence: suicide. There is also testosterone, that magical hormone which makes men daydream of women and conditions their way of thinking. They will prioritize their professional career and stress will often rule their life. It should come as no surprise then that men do not stand up to wear as well as women. Women, in turn, are far more reasonable;

despite their duties as women and mothers, they manage their time far better. Chinese philosophy has clearly defined the opposite yet complementary roles of men and women. Men, closer to the Yang, have their heads turned toward the sky, symbolized by a circle, lost in their dreams and projects; whereas women, closer to the Yin, are focused on the earth, symbolized by a square, well aware of the problems of daily life which need to be dealt with. In more scientific terms, women are better able than men to maintain homeostasis.

SOURCES

Anne-Sophie Cousteaux, Jean-Louis Pan Ké Shon.
Le mal-être a-t-il un genre ? Suicide, risque suicidaire, dépression et dépendance alcoolique.
Revue française de sociologie, vol. 49, n°1, p.53-92 ; 2008.

Marianne J. Legato.
Why Men Die First. New York : Palgrave Macmillan ; 2009.

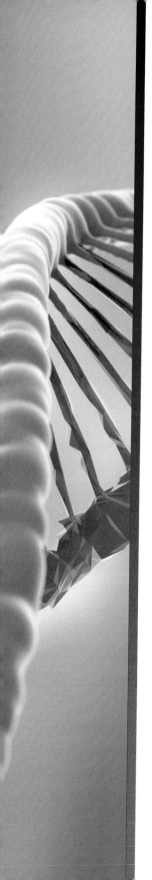

- Part 2 -
Conclusions

« The price we pay for sex is death »

- Bruce Carnes -

Modern science claims that natural death is unnecessary, just as individual immortality has no intrinsic value. Aging, for its part, is a complex illness which affects our body, our thoughts, our emotions, but also our families and our societies. Aging and death remain the two greatest mysteries which humanity has yet to solve. In this world of high-tech medical advances, these two scourges continue to curse us, just as they always have, promoting magical thinking, superstitions, alchemy and pseudoscience. Nevertheless, scientists are beginning to pierce some of the secrets of aging, and new fascinating discoveries are made every day.

Bruce Carnes, one of the greatest experts on aging, relates a discussion during which he was urged to describe his conception of life and death in a single sentence. His answer surprised everyone: « *The price we pay for sex is death.* » In his opinion, and that of many other experts, our reproductive system is extremely inefficient. Starting with the squandering of billions of sperm cells, sent off to die in order for a single one to win, down to the fact that all sexual reproduction is achieved at the expense of somatic cells, which are eternally doomed to die. In our system, the mortal somatic body is merely a vessel for our genes, which are for their part immortal, which leads Bruce Carnes and many others to say that our sexual nature is responsible for our mortality.

Demystifying Aging

There is a rift between most people's objective, to gain a few short years of life, and that of scientists, eradicating aging. Simply mentioning immortality, or hyper-longevity, causes knee-jerk reactions. Immediately we bring up overpopulation, the permanence of undesirable individuals, a two-tier system of hyper-longevity which only benefits the rich. These are of course legitimate objections, but we will have all the time in the world to find a solution to them. Up until now, aging and death have been considered inevitable and, psychologically, we had no other choice than to accept them. Living with, rather than being constantly haunted by those prospects. Furthermore, our rejection of aging is so deeply ingrained in us that it will be difficult to combat, even with objective proof, no matter how scientific. In addition to which, the idea of the existence of a biological clock is reinforced by the fact that all of the symptoms of aging, as well as those of age-related illnesses, occur at about the same time. But according to Aubrey de Grey, there could be another explanation for this, what he calls "a cascade of cause and effect chains». For him, if our organism experiences relatively silent anomalies, such as inflammation, oxidation or glycation, for long enough, each one of these will potentiate the others, in an accelerating process, until reaching a critical threshold, and, suddenly, all of the clinical signs will appear, almost at the same time.

What should we learn from this alchemy of aging? Everything revolves around DNA, whether nuclear or mitochondrial. There is every reason to believe that the main culprit is the oxidation of biological material. Especially when it attacks proteins, which ensure proper cell function. According to Radman, tiny differences, in a single amino acid within a protein, are enough to make it vulnerable to oxidation. This general oxidation of proteins increases with age, and the most fragile proteins within the cell will lose their functional capabilities and thereby plant the seeds of age-related illness. And with time, this damage will increase exponentially.

Finding a solution to all of the causes of aging, this is the very ambitious objective of a new generation of scientists. For Radman, we should invent a molecular system which could prevent cellular damage by protecting so-called repair proteins. For Aubrey de Grey, old age, sickness and death constitute collateral damage, the real tragedy being the deterioration of the human motor, but we will one day be able to permanently delay its expiration date. There is no genetic program which predetermines lifespan, we therefore have the opportunity to influence our longevity, until we one day take control of it. The human body is a patchwork of adaptation processes, all of which are characterized by their redundancies, over-mechanization, repair and regeneration capabilities, but our main strength is our astonishing ability to learn.

SOURCES

Jean-David Ponci.

La biologie du vieillissement. Paris : L'Harmattan ; 2008.

**Joël de Rosnay, Jean-Louis Servan-Schreiber,
François de Closets, Dominique Simonnet.**

Une vie en plus. Paris : Seuil ; 2005.

Miroslav Radman, Daniel Carton.

Au-delà de nos limites biologiques. Paris : Plon ; 2011.

Nicole Le Douarin.

Les cellules souches. Paris : Odile Jacob ; 2007.

Stuart J. Olshansky, Bruce A. Carnes.

The Quest For Immortality. New York : W.W.Norton & Company ; 2001.

Conclusions

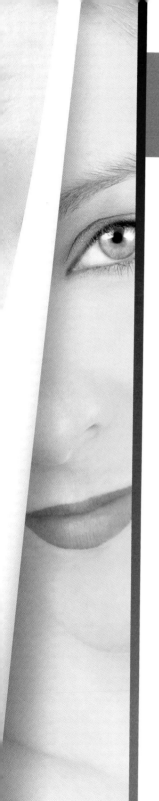

Part 3

REJUVENATING

At the end of the 19th century, Charles-Edouard Brown-Sequard, a famous physiologist, announces a miraculous discovery: the secret to eternal youth. He performs testicular ablations on domestic animals, extracts their « *vital essence* », and produces a concoction with which he inoculates elderly patients. His treatment seems to work, his patients have increased 'vitality' and surprising mental acuity. Brown-Sequard then injects himself with his concoctions at the age of 72, and claims to have better control over his bladder and bowels!

In 1920, Eugen Steinach, a physiology professor in Vienna, makes his fortune by performing vasectomies* on his elderly patients, or by transplanting the testicles of younger individuals! Many rejuvenation clinics quickly begin to offer rather surprising techniques: applying electricity to the testicles; exposing the genitals to doses of radium.

To this day, even though we live in a world of high-tech biomedical advances, aging and death still make the bread and butter of alchemists and quacks. And yet, in the last thirty years, science has made considerable progress in understanding aging and what can be done to reverse its mechanisms. This genuine scientific revolution calls into question quite a bit of data which was thought to be definitively substantiated.

As we have seen, the 'robustness' of our health is due to a constant balance between opposing but complimentary forces. This homeostasis is reflected in every aspect of our functions, even within our atoms, which constantly require opposing charges, in order not to become free radicals,

*A vasectomy is a sterilization method which involves the surgical cutting or blocking off of the vas deferens, which transport sperm.

which generate oxidative stress.

The hundreds of thousands of changes which take place each day demand that our body be perfectly organized in order to properly respond to these demands and immediately activate remedial processes which will lead to a nearly instantaneous return to equilibrium. These actions require the immediate assembly of specific proteins, controlled by genes which must be activated or deactivated as the case may be. This delicate balance between gene expression and repression manages our health's operating capital and, in the end, determines our longevity.

But let's go back to our DNA, which contains our genes. The key to health, quality of life and longevity can be found within it.

Having understood this, all modern cellular rejuvenation techniques focus on DNA reparation. They endeavor to maintain our specialized DNA maintenance department's power and speed precisely in order to avoid shoddy copying. The key to our longevity lies in our ability to continually improve the balance of our DNA's damage/repair ratio. It has been shown that faster and more efficient repairs mean greater chances for a longer life, and this balance is controlled by gene expression.

In practice, all life-extending methods are developed along three main vectors:

1 - Improving the balance between damage and damage repair, at the DNA level, and maintaining homeostasis. Anything which reduces genetic mutations improves DNA duplication quality, preserves our precious stock of stem cells, and consequently delays aging.

2 - Improving DNA function by controlling the oxidation, inflammation and glycation processes which severely damage it, and by improving the methylation processes, which specialize in gene activation and deactivation.

3 - Controlling and optimizing the environmental factors which have a direct impact on our DNA, e.g. nutrition, physical activity and the ability to handle stress.

We can separate methods to combat aging into two broad, complementary categories:

1 - Those which are designed to slow or delay aging. Their weakness resides in the fact that their effectiveness depends on the state of the organism is in when they are implemented.

2 - Those which are designed to rejuvenate in the true sense of the word. They can in certain instances 'reverse' the signs of aging.

Biologically, the difference between the two categories is a fundamental one: the former taps into our body's ability to heal and repair itself. The latter takes advantage of the amazing regenerative powers which our bodies have forgotten.

Regeneration! The magic word which would allow us to go back in time, erase our wrinkles, give us back the strength and vitality of our youth, all while preserving the maturity we have acquired, essential for our decision-making. Some scientists have even gone so far as to consider the possibility of immortality! That which would not that long ago have resulted in their being burned at the stake, today lends them very inquisitive ears, in particular among tech giants. Peter Thiel, the co-founder of PayPal, funds a number of foundations focusing on attaining immortality, such as the Methuselah Foundation chaired by Aubrey de Grey, Singularity University, or the SENS foundation (Strategies for Engineered Negligible Senescence). Larry Page, the co-founder of Google, established Calico, which is funding a new research center to combat aging, with a budget of 750 million dollars. Mark Zuckerberg, the co-founder of Facebook, launched the Breakthrough Prize in Life Sciences, which rewards research focusing on increasing our lifespan. Larry Ellison, the co-founder of Oracle, established the Ellison Medical Foundation to combat aging. A technological tsunami has been released, and immortality could be around the corner!

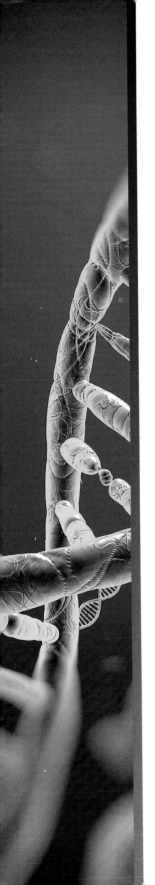

Chapter 1

Is Immortality Around the Corner?

« Every time a human being dies, a library burns »

- Anders Sandberg -

Each one of us carries within us a unique and complex universe of wisdom, knowledge, aptitudes, and experiences related to life and relationships. When someone dies, this colossal sum of information is lost forever. Why then should death be inevitable?

No, today we can no longer consider death as our inevitable fate. It is my sincere conviction that one of the main causes of this fate, as well as a means of thwarting it, can be found within our cells. Today, the combined action of new biotechnologies, of molecules derived from certain plants and lifestyle improvement can provide us with a second youth which we would not have even dreamed of a few years ago. The only concern would be: what do we need to do to extend our lives so as to benefit from as of yet unavailable, but ever more effective new strategies? Have we acquired the knowledge and technologies necessary to live forever? Not yet! But we can significantly lower the incidence of diseases and delay aging, and we can do so far beyond what people, including the medical community, imagine. We do not yet have the ability, however, to indefinitely extend human life.

In the opinion of Aubrey de Grey, a gerontologist and geneticist at Oxford University (United Kingdom), all we need is to regularly and effectively maintain our organism in order to repair DNA damage, just as we would a car! The amount of time which we spend on this earth is 30% determined by our genetic makeup and 70% determined by our environment. Our ability to manage this environment, in particular by improving our lifestyle, can change everything.

For Miroslav Radman, we need to protect the small molecules within the cell which repair damage in the cell's functional machinery. According to him, we need to concentrate on molecular damage; by limiting damage to protective molecules, they will be better able to carry out their mission. He considers protective molecules to be universal; those of resistant species can also protect other species. This is the case, for example, of polyphenols, which protect red grapes - and why not also humans? In this way, we could reclaim these protective molecules and benefit from them, which would allow our species to live longer.

For Caleb Finch, of the University of Southern California, Los Angeles, examples taken from nature suggest that *the human genome probably does not contain any absolute limit to its lifespan.* He notes that females of a North Pacific fish species, even when they reach 140 years of age, bear eggs, and abundantly so, while showing no signs of senescence. The fact that these animals seem not to age is, according to him, an indication that this process is not inevitable. *The plasticity of aging, he says, suggests that this phenomenon depends on environmental factors, rather than a genetic program.* If life expectancy is only moderately dependent on genetics, then we must conclude as Caleb Finch does that the environment determines most of the lifespan of living beings - our own, of course, but also that of other animals and plants.

The majority of researchers think that rather than those cells which are able to divide, it is the cells which rarely or never renew themselves, such as our muscles, heart and nervous tissue, which are most responsible for aging. *The idea of a strict limit to the human lifespan doesn't have a strong scientific basis,* says demographer John Wilmoth (University of California, Berkeley). He sees it as a myth. He doesn't believe that we could live forever, but stresses that no one has yet been able to find a strict limit to the human lifespan.

Against this background, a medical and philosophical revolution is already underway: death would no longer be inevitable, rather it would become a choice. *The idea that death is a problem in need of a solution rather than a reality dictated by nature or divine decree will become widespread,* says Laurent Alexandre, the founder of Doctissimo.

1.1 - Species That Live the Longest

Have you heard of George? He is a twenty pound, 140-year-old lobster. Destined to be eaten by some wealthy patron of a top New York restaurant, an employee told the press about this animal, which quickly became a news sensation. So much so that the restaurant announced, with great fanfare, that it would send George back into his native ocean, where, one assumes, he still lives a happy life.

Could lobsters be immortal? Not exactly, but they do not die of old age, because telomerase, the enzyme responsible for lengthening telomeres, is always activated in their organism. Therefore, their cells do not die, and they retain the ability to duplicate. Yet their shell remains susceptible to infection, which is why they still eventually pass away.

In Japan, Koi, a beautiful species of fish, usually white with red spots, and often found in ponds in Japanese gardens, are known for their long lifespan. They are so intrinsic to local culture that some have been given names, and their longevity has repeatedly been recorded, some living for more than 200years. One named Hanako, which has belonged to several people over the years, died in July 1977, at 226 years old!

Certain relatively primitive animals, such as sponges or coral, could live for 1,500 to 4,500 years, and probably even longer. Some of these invertebrates constitute larger organisms, made up of clones. The estimated age of some of them has already reached unprecedented numbers: the great red sponge of the Caribbean, *Xestospongia Muta*, could apparently live up to 2 300years old; the black coral generally found in tropical waters, *Antipatharia*, could easily live for more than 2,000 years.

Other animals, among them a majority of tortoises, renowned for their longevity, now only exist in books: *Adwaita*, a Seychelles tortoise, is said to have lived nearly 250 years. *Tu'i Malila*, a Madagascar radiated tortoise, reached 190 years old, whereas the Galápagos tortoise named *Harriet* lived to nearly 175 years old.

1.2 - Species That Elude Death

The Arthrobacter Bacteria

If conditions become unfavorable, these bacteria can lie dormant and release spores. These spores are specific, highly resistant organelles which can survive for a very long time (around 1,000 years) in extreme environments. They contain a copy of the mother cell's genome, and, when conditions improve, can give birth to new bacteria. This is called 'germination'. Yet this DNA repair mechanism is, unfortunately, not immortal. It sustains damage over time. According to Jean David Ponci, this places the Arthrobacter bacteria among those species which elude death, but are not immortal, in the biological sense.

The Hydra

When a part of its body is amputated, the hydra's body regenerates it in two or three days, which makes it potentially immortal. Indeed, the hydra seems to keep, within its body's central section, stem cells which are more potent than those which humans have as adults. If it sustains damage, these stem cells differentiate themselves in order to reproduce the missing cells and reconstruct the amputated section. The hydra's central section may therefore contain stem cells which undergo little or no aging, and as its extremities deteriorate, they may be replaced by stem cells which have differentiated themselves.

1.3 - A New Science: Regenerative Biotechnologies

But let's go back to the question of human longevity. Why can we find, within a single cellular mechanism, some elements which stand the test of time along with others which are very fragile? What is the biological difference which determines whether a human cellular organism is fragile or resistant? A new discipline, biogerontology, and its companion, regenerative medicine, may be able to answer these questions.

Could we ever fathom that a therapeutic action such as, for example, taking a pill, could significantly reduce the risk of cancer? That another pill could reduce the risk of stroke, or arthritis? Or that yet another pill could do all of this, and even reduce all risk associated with age-related illnesses, such as cardiovascular disease, diabetes, Alzheimer's, Parkinson's, hip fractures, osteoporosis? Would such a pill only exist in a fantastical utopia? Not at all, as it is already here. It is currently undergoing testing on animals, and a large number of scientists see its human application in the short term as realistic.

Gerontology was, until recently, a specialization which limited itself to managing the pathological consequences of old age and the study of palliative care. Biogerontology goes much further, as it focuses on the actual causes of aging. This has allowed biogerontologists to revolutionize our understanding of the biology of life and death. They have, among other things, clearly rejected the myths and commonly accepted ideas about age and its consequences, and have given us, for the first time, a solid scientific basis for increasing our longevity in the right conditions. Today, the idea of aging as an immutable process, set in stone by evolution, is undermined by biogerontologists whose research on the causes of cellular aging and knowledge of free radicals and telomere shortening has advanced by leaps and bounds. They are now able to impact cellular machinery and functions. For example, we know that our genetic equipment can be activated or deactivated via 'switches' which influence our longevity, and we also know how to adjust them. Biogerontology has the potential to do what no medical procedure has yet been able to.

This biomedical revolution has given birth to new health care techniques, called regenerative biotechnologies, whose goal is to apply the principles of regenerative medicine to repair damage sustained by aging organisms. In other words, these biotechnologies do not just slow down the accumulation of damage due to aging in our cells and tissues, but also replace damaged cells or repair cellular machinery. These new techniques will enable the actual rejuvenation of our structures and functions. Research centers focusing on this field are attempting to accelerate the transition of medical science from risk factor management towards a regenerative approach, based on the new tools which these biotechnologies can offer.

Restorative Biotechnology Targets

Decades of research on the elderly as well as animal testing have shown that there are only seven types of major cellular and molecular damage responsible for aging. According to Aubrey de Grey, this list is nearly definitive, as no substantial new elements have been uncovered for more than a generation, despite active scientific research in this field. The specific metabolic causes which generate damage are, at present, only partially understood. The good news, however, is that understanding these causes in detail isn't essential to the implementation of effective therapies. No matter the causes of the damage, regenerative biotechnologies will apply the same strategy; restore repair systems according to seven principles, which correspond to the seven types of damage. There is only one issue which can put a damper on our optimism; metabolic damage is repetitive, which consequently means that therapeutic strategies will have to be repeated... for as long as possible!

1 - Eliminating Extracellular Debris

Extracellular debris results from the accumulation in the extracellular space - that is, the space between cells - of bulky proteins which not only no longer serve any purpose, but also considerably impede the work of cells and tissues. The most famous of these protein debris are beta-amyloids. These compounds produce amyloid plaques, responsible for certain cognitive disorders as well as Alzheimer's disease.

2 - Eliminating Intracellular Debris

Cells possess an efficient system for the elimination and recycling of unusable materials and their subsequent ejection. The lysosome is the cell's incinerator, and contains all of the necessary enzymes to dismantle unwanted molecules; unfortunately, some molecules are so complex that the lysosomes are unable to cut them down into expellable pieces. They will therefore sit inside the cell until they begin to significantly obstruct first the lysosomes, then the entire cell from functioning.

3 - Eliminating Malfunctioning Cells

The activity of certain cells declines or even stops as they become ineffective or go into 'retirement'. This is the case of so-called senescent cells, such as skin cells, which no longer reproduce once their mission has been completed. The senescence program is activated once the risk of DNA mutation becomes too severe (risk of cancer), or when the inflammatory reaction is maintained beyond its assigned task, generating a risk of fibrosis, or finally when telomeres have become too short. These senescent cells excrete an abnormally large amount of proteins which will hyperactivate the immune system and damage neighboring tissue. At first

*Aubrey de Grey. www.jlife-sciences .com.

the damage isn't noticeable, but after decades of accumulation, it leads to severe metabolic dysfunction, which provides a foundation for cancer or immune system disorders.

4 - Disintegrating Reticulation (cross-linking)

Proteins are our body's worker molecules, they ensure the integrity of its structure and functions. The problem is that they are neither recycled nor replaced. Optimal tissue function therefore depends on the integrity of our proteins. Unfortunately, the sugar which circulates in our blood, glucose, frequently binds with certain proteins, creating a 'reticulated', or cross-linked structure. This reticulation handcuffs proteins which up until then moved freely, and chains two of them together virtually permanently, through chemical bonds. These two proteins, in these conditions, will no longer be able to carry out their mission. As time goes by, reticulated proteins accumulate and become a concrete, mechanical obstacle to the organism's function, such as in our arteries, lungs or even eyes and brain. One structure is particularly vulnerable to reticulation: elastin, responsible for the elasticity of blood vessels and the skin, whose performance will slowly diminish and lead to arterial wall rigidity and the appearance of wrinkles on the skin.

5 - Preventing Damage Due to Mitochondrial Chromosomal Mutations

The mitochondria are our cells' powerhouses. They will extract energy from nutrients in order to transform it into adenosine triphosphate (ATP), a type of energy which our metabolism can directly utilize. They are so important that they have their own DNA, which we only receive from our mother. Yet, just like any power transformer, mitochondria generate toxic waste, free radicals in particular, during the transformation process. This waste can affect the nearby mitochondrial DNA, which may lead to significant issues in the genetic code. Ideally, we would find a way to prevent the DNA's exposure, or fix it before it becomes harmful. But we are still a long way away from this! We therefore have to cut our losses and concentrate on eliminating damage as it appears.

6 - Rendering Cancerous Mutations Harmless

During aging, two types of damage accumulate in our genes: DNA sequence mutations, and epimutations, which affect the DNA's scaffolding. Both of these lead to abnormal genetic expression/activation, as they modify the amount of encoded proteins and their structure. What kind of harm can the modification of gene expression, caused by epimutations, lead to? For most people, cancer is the best known consequence, resulting from a series of epimutations which occur sequentially within the cell, and lead to uncontrolled growth. Other kinds of epimutations take place within our cells over time, and some scientists suspect that these non-cancerous mutations also contribute to age-related illnesses.

7 - Replacing Lost Cells

Every day, our cells experience damage which cannot be repaired or leads to cell death. Other cells commit suicide to avoid becoming cancerous or because their telomeres are too short. Some are replaced by stem cells, though these also undergo degenerative processes. The net result, after a few decades: tissues like our brain, heart, skeleton or thymus have lost so many cells that they become impaired. The answer lies in regenerative medicine and cell therapies, in tissue and potentially organ transplants.

These seven types of response to damage targeted by restorative biotechnologies are the basis for SENS (Strategies for Engineered Negligible Senescence) developed by Aubrey de Grey. He believes that we could live a thousand years if we were able to properly maintain our human machinery, just as we would a car. This is why it isn't unreasonable to believe that once proper therapies are designed, applicable to a middle-aged population of around fifty years of age and able to provide another thirty or fifty years of life expectancy, this same population will later be able to benefit from even more powerful remedies, which could extend their lives by fifty more years, and so on, indefinitely...

1.4 - Is immortality really around the corner?

Not yet! But we are getting closer. The technological revolution is modifying our relationship with death. It began with transplants, then cardiopulmonary resuscitation, enabling certain patients to survive for a number of years, then came stem cells, and telomerase activators, followed by the appearance of new fields of study: nanomedicine, epigenetics, nutrigenomics. An incredible technological revolution which is dramatically changing medicine and pushing back its limits. From the era of successful aging, we have moved on to cellular rejuvenation. The adoption of these new technologies will become a new way of life for the younger generations. The boundaries between man and machine are already blurred, and they may soon disappear! Our future will depend on the way in which we will manage to exploit this technological evolution.

□ R E M E M B E R □

Today we can no longer consider death as our immutable fate. The combined action of restorative biotechnologies, of molecules derived from certain plants, and lifestyle improvements, can provide us with a second youth which we would not even have dreamed of only a few years ago. Do we have the necessary knowledge and technologies to live eternally? Not yet! But we can significantly lower the incidence of diseases and delay aging, far beyond what people imagine. One problem remains: why can we find, within a single cellular mechanism, elements which stand the test of time and others which are very fragile? A new science, biogerontology, and its companion, regenerative medicine, may be able to answer these questions. These new disciplines will enable the actual rejuvenation of our structures and functions.

S O U R C E S

Axel Kahn, Fabrice Papillon.
Le secret de la salamandre. Paris : Nil Editions ; 2005.

Jean David Ponci.
La biologie du vieillissement. Paris : L'Harmattan ; 2008.

Laurent Alexandre.
La mort de la mort. Paris : JC Lattes ; 2011

Ray Kurzweil, Terry Grossman.
Serons-nous immortels ? Paris : Dunod ; 2006.

Miroslav Radman.
Au-delà de nos limites biologiques. Paris : Plon ; 2011.

Aubrey de Grey, Michael Rae.
Ending Aging. New-York : St. Martin's Griffin ; 1963.

Nicole Le Douarin.
Les cellules souches. Paris : Odile Jacob ; 2007.

Caleb E. Finch.
Longevity, Senescence, and the Genome. Chicago :The University of Chicago Press ; 1994.

Michael D.West.
The Immortal Cell. New York : Doubleday ; 2003.

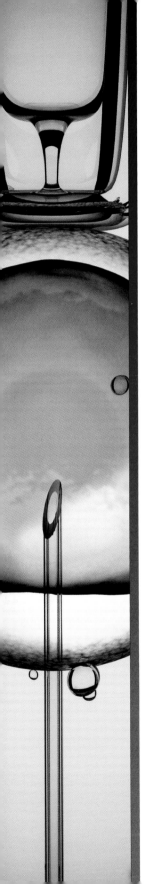

- Part 3 -

Chapter 2

Stem Cells, Regenerative Medicine
& Cell Therapy

« To regenerate is to brush up against immortality »

- Nicole Le Douarin -

Why does the heart of a zebra fish regenerate after a heart attack, and why is this not also the case in humans? Are our regenerative capabilities entirely absent or simply non-operational? If it is the latter, would it be possible to reactivate them? Salamanders and newts can regenerate their tails, eyes, legs or jaws after they have been sectioned off their body; the retina and lens can regenerate out of remaining optical tissue. According to Axel Kahn, hydras and certain worms can reconstitute an entire individual out of a single fragment. We know that this regenerative capability is mainly due to stem cell activity. Everything happens as if these cells were growing younger, as if they recovered a kind of virginity which would allow them to generate all of the different cell types anew, depending on the tissues in need of repair.

Nicole Le Douarin thinks that we human beings are entirely incapable of regenerating even the smallest bit of a limb. We do however heal; our wounds close, thanks to the partial regrowth of certain tissues... Which is to say that even if time has taken from mankind the ability to regenerate, it has left us the ability to repair ourselves. The knowledge acquired in this field allows us to foresee that so-called regenerative medicine will produce therapies via stem cells. A new challenge for medicine, which would no longer be simply remedial but now regenerative, capable of producing a source of new cells for our organs. We can already reactivate the mechanisms of regeneration in order to renew injured organs.

Stem cells are, as their name suggests, our body's first cells. The very first is called a 'zygote'; it emerges from the fusion of the mother's egg and of the father's sperm. This first, embryonic cell, will divide and multiply in order to create a group of cells, the blastocyst, which will give birth to the three embryonic layers, the ectoderm, mesoderm and endoderm, responsible for the production of all of our adult cells.

These stem cells are therefore split into two categories: embryonic stem cells, and adult stem cells. They are categorized according to their ability to reproduce through mitosis (cell division) and to differentiate themselves into an array of specialized cells. Mitosis is the process by which a cell, which has replicated its genetic material, divides into two in order to form two identical daughter cells, with the same genes. A stem cell can therefore produce clones of itself, simply through mitosis. But the special property which is particular to stem cells is that they can transform in order to produce cells which are different from the mother cell. This property is called 'potency' (in the sense of potentiality). Stem cells have different levels of potency depending on when they appeared during embryonic life.

Totipotent cells are embryonic stem cells which are derived from the zygote and the blastocyst. These cells can produce an entire organism, as they have the potential to give birth to all of the embryonic tissues.

Pluripotent cells are the descendants of the former, and have the potential to differentiate into almost every type of cell.

Multipotent cells can differentiate into a large number of cells, but only within a single family (e.g. bone marrow).

Oligopotent cells can differentiate into only a few types (e.g. within the epidermis, mesenchyme, fatty tissue or endothelium).

On the other hand **omnipotent** cells are not stem cells. They can regenerate, but only by dividing, and can therefore only produce a single type of cell: their own.

Theoretically, producing tissue with embryonic stem cells would be the most interesting option, as stem cells can multiply indefinitely and are pluripotent (or even totipotent). The only problem is that these cells come from human embryos, and bring about ethical considerations which have led to strict regulations governing research involving embryonic stem cells. But this ethical problem, due to the origin of embryonic stem cells, has recently been overcome by two researchers, and their results have earned them the Nobel Prize in 2012.

2.1 - iPS Cells

The Nobel Prize in Physiology or Medicine was awarded in Stockholm, in 2012, to two colleagues, from the UK and Japan, for their work on stem cells. They managed to obtain cells capable of producing every type of tissue in the human body, without their coming from an embryo. Biologist John Gurdon, 79 years old, and doctor and researcher Shinya Yamanaka, 50 years old, were awarded this prize for their research on nuclear reprogramming, a technique which allows us to transform specialized adult cells into non-specialized stem cells. This allows us to acquire stem cells which can serve as an effective substitute for embryonic stem cells, as the latter raise ethical questions.

This is the most promising way forward for the use of stem cells in regenerative medicine: induced pluripotent stem cells, or *iPS* cells. Reprogrammed specialized adult cells become pluripotent by reactivating the expression of certain stem cell genes.

What are the advantages of developing iPS cells?

First of all, they make it possible for samples taken from any individual to be cultured and reprogrammed, to then be reimplanted once transformed into pluripotent cells. In this way, it may soon be possible to reimplant neurons into people suffering from neurodegenerative diseases: Parkinson's disease, Huntington's chorea, Duchenne muscular dystrophy, amyotrophic lateral sclerosis etc. Another advantage is that implants would not be affected by the issue of histocompatibility, since the patient would be both the donor and the receiver. Finally, iPS cells contain the genes associated both with triggering an illness and its opposite, its cure. It would therefore be possible to study the progression of an illness in cell cultures and even to test medication designed to fight it.

2.2 - Fatty tissue, an unexpected source

Just this once, your fatty tissue may be good, or even excellent for your health. Indeed, it could allow us to harness the therapeutic potential of our adult stem cells. Against all odds, a team from the National Centre for Scientific Research (CNRS) in Toulouse, France, has just confirmed that fatty tissue, until recently considered to simply be a fat reserve, turns out to also contain an incredible wealth of multipotent stem cells, capable of giving birth to several types of cells. And early results show that their therapeutic potential is very promising.

French researchers have shown that it is possible to obtain functioning heart cells from fatty tissue cells, in vitro and in mice. These same researchers have also made use, in a model with mice, of cells derived from human fatty tissue to rebuild a damaged vascular network in a lower limb. This work allows us for the first time to consider the use of fatty tissue cells in cell therapy.

2.3 What are stem cells for?

Not only are stem cells able to transform into cells from other types of tissue, but they spontaneously do so every day. Every time our body undergoes an aggression, the damaged tissue secretes specific molecules which trigger stem cells into action. According to Christian Drapeau, this tissue also secretes molecules whose distress signals get the attention of stem cells. They will then circulate in the blood, go through the capillaries of the damaged tissue, and then, attracted by the signals emitted by the tissue, migrate towards them. Once there, they multiply by cloning themselves and at the same time transform into cells of the given tissue's type. The key to the success of this process is the amount of circulating stem cells.

Most of our tissues need to renew themselves regularly. Thanks to stem cells, they have a remarkable capacity to do so. Once more, this follows the homeostatic imperative, that is, the balance between proliferation and renewal on the one hand, and cell death on the other. These are the two fundamental processes of our organism's survival. Adult stem cells ensure cellular homeostasis, meaning the balance between dying and living cells. If stem cells do not find themselves able to carry out their mission effectively, the daily loss of cells may eventually lead to tissue degeneration and the appearance of illnesses.

2.4 Therapeutic Applications

The goal of regenerative medicine is to produce living, functional tissue which can replace damaged tissues or organs, or to cure congenital diseases. Regeneration can be performed *in situ*, through the stimulation of damaged organs, or in a lab.

Blood

Bone marrow was the first tissue to reveal the function of stem cells. Continually producing red and white blood cells and platelets, these cells were first transplanted in human beings in the late 50s. To this day, this transplant is still used to treat auto-immune diseases, immune deficiencies and leukemia, as well as 'solid' cancers. In order to minimize the risk of rejection, autologous transplants are performed whenever possible: once collected from the patient's blood, stem cells are stocked, sorted thanks to their surface markers to avoid potential tumor cells, and re-injected. They help to reactivate hematopoiesis, that is, the production of blood cells. But even though these are pure transplants, they remain imperfect. They cannot restore all of the blood cells on their own, and require the help of other cells, which also come from the bone marrow: mesenchymal stem cells. According to Patrick Laharrague, a researcher at the CNRS, these cells produce the necessary microenvironment to ensure the smooth functioning of the hematopoietic cells. The idea is therefore to combine blood stem cells and mesenchymal stem cells in the transplants. During the very first trials, which were performed on women having undergone heavy radiotherapy, the resumption of blood cell production was shown to be quicker. But this is not their only role. These cells also differentiate into fat, bone and cartilage, which explains their ability to repair bone and cartilaginous damage. Another prospect: the use of umbilical cord blood to avoid the use of very tricky lumbar punctures, as they contain more easily accessible immature stem cells, but their therapeutic use is once more limited by the small size of the transplants, too small to treat adults.

Blood donation

French researchers were able to inject a patient with red blood cells which were produced from his own stem cells. We have been trying to produce artificial blood for a long time, through different methods, such as re-programming skin cells or even with hydrogel molds. At the Pierre and Marie Curie University (UPMC) in Paris, Luc Douay and his team are researching the potential of stem cells for this purpose, and have just arrived at a remarkable result, presented in the journal Blood. This study was conducted in two stages. Using a human donor's stem cells, the scientists first managed to produce billions of cultivated red blood cells. For this, they used specific growth factors which regulate the proliferation and maturation of the stem cells into red blood cells. But the major step forward only took place afterwards, when this French team re-injected these cultivated red blood cells. *After five days*, explains Luc Douay, *the survival rate of these red blood cells in the blood was between 94 and 100%. And after 26 days, between 41 and 63%. These results are very promising, this rate being close to the average half-life of normal native blood cells of 28 days, which supports their viability as a possible transfusion source.*

This study is the first to show that these cultivated blood cells survive in the human body. For Luc Douay, this is a major breakthrough for transfusion medicine.

Skin

Tissue engineering, a rapidly evolving technology, aims to make skin substitutes which are as similar as possible to the 'real stuff'. They are already used in transplants for severe burn victims. To withstand the numerous external aggressions it faces - UV rays, chemical, bacterial and viral agents - our skin regenerates in its entirety every three weeks. The source of this perpetual movement: the epidermis' keratinocyte cells. Generated in its deepest layer, they multiply and slowly migrate towards the skin's surface to replace older cells. They have been routinely cultivated to be grafted onto severe burn victims for the past twenty years. You only need to harvest a few square centimeters of healthy skin from the patient and place them on a growth medium of fibroblasts, the dermis' cells. Only a few weeks are needed in order to gather a substantial surface of autologous (belonging to the same subject) epidermis. This is one of our most promising options: *cultured dermo-epidermal units*. Already used in pharmacotoxicological tests for cosmetics, this 'cultured skin', tested in animals, should soon go through its first clinical trials to stimulate healing in chronic wounds.

One of the skin's functions is to protect the body from the sun's ultraviolet, or UV, rays. This task is carried out by pigmented cells called melanocytes. By releasing melanin, the pigment which colors our skin, they protect the epidermis' other cells (keratinocytes) from the mutagenic effects of UV rays.

After having reconstructed an epidermis from pluripotent stem cells in 2009, a team of French researchers, led by Christine Baldeschi, has just given it its color: using the same strategy in vitro, they have managed to produce functional melanocytes, the cells which give skin its pigment and protect it from UV rays. This unlimited source of cells could someday be offered as a therapeutic alternative to patients suffering from genetic or non-genetic skin pigmentation disorders, such as vitiligo.

At present, cell therapy used to treat skin pigmentation disorders is carried out through autologous transplant. But this strategy is only effective if there are unaffected areas of skin near the hypo pigmented zones. This is the case for vitiligo, but unfortunately not for many other pathologies, such as albinism. In order to bridge this gap, researchers have considered an alternative strategy: using an external and unlimited source of perfectly controlled pigmented cells.

In 2009, Christine Baldeschi's team managed for the first time to produce keratinocyte cells - which make the constant renewal of our skin possible - out of embryonic pluripotent stem cells. These results, published in The Lancet (November 2009), have allowed the team to reach a new milestone by identifying the differentiation process which makes it possible to turn embryonic (hES) or induced pluripotent (iPS) stem cells into a pure and homogeneous melanocyte population capable of producing melanin and integrating itself into the epidermis.

The Brain and Nervous System

The old belief that our stock of neurons is set at birth no longer holds water. First identified in rats, neuronal stem cells have also been found in the human brain. Several teams are busy examining the behavior of these cells within the rodents' brains. But what about human beings?

A new type of stem cell, capable of differentiating itself into neurons, was discovered in adult brains, a discovery with the potential to heal brain injuries. By analyzing brain tissue collected through biopsies, biologists at Lund University in Sweden have for the first time discovered stem cells around small blood vessels in the brain. The function of these mesenchymal cells is still mysterious, but their plastic properties suggest they have great potential.

A biotechnology firm has just been given the green light for the first time from the British health authorities to attempt to treat the effects of cerebrovascular accidents, or CVAs, with fetal stem cells. Researchers are betting that the action of stem cells will be able to help affected areas to heal. Experiments conducted on rats by British company ReNeuron have shown that after injecting stem cells into damaged rat brains, the rats would regain control of their front limbs.

By injecting human embryonic stem cells into the brains of mice fetuses, researchers have produced mice with a few human neurons in their brain. This experiment, led by Fred Gage of the Salk Institute, shows that these cells do in fact become functional neurons. Notably, these stem cells grew to the size of a mouse's neurons, which are smaller than human neurons, and therefore assimilate themselves into their environment. Researchers will follow how these cells progress thanks to a fluorescent marker. Knowing that stem cells can become functional neurons is essential for the further development of human cures, based on embryonic stem cells.

Parkinson's disease

Parkinson's disease affects millions of people worldwide. But even if we are able to treat its symptoms, to this day we have no cure. This is why scientists are studying ways to prevent or treat this illness, through regenerative medicine and stem cell research.

People suffering from Parkinson's produce too little dopamine, a chemical substance which allows us to send messages to parts of the brain involved in motor control. This illness, which is also related to the aggregation of an abnormal form of the protein alpha-synuclein, forming what are called Lewy bodies, destroys the nerve cells which produce dopamine, called dopaminergic neurons, in an area of the brain called the substantia nigra. When their dopaminergic neurons die, patients develop tremors, muscle rigidity and slowness of movement. They can also lose their sense of smell, have trouble sleeping, and become depressed. Constipation and occasionally dementia can appear in the later stages of the disease.

Scientists still do not know what causes Parkinson's disease. In about one out of ten cases, the disease is due to a hereditary genetic problem which disrupts the production of alpha-synuclein. In the other nine out of ten cases, the exact causes have not been determined. This disease mainly affects individuals older than 40 years old, but can appear earlier. Men are at a higher risk than women. Certain studies have established a link with exposure to pesticides, whereas the consumption of tobacco and coffee seem to diminish the risk of developing the disease, although the exact reasons for this are unknown.

Current treatments for Parkinson's disease include a drug discovered in the 1960s, called Levodopa. It is converted into dopamine by the body, and acts as a substitute. Other drugs mimic the action of dopamine by stimulating nerve cells. Treatment also includes a healthy diet, physical exercise, occupational therapy, and physiotherapy. Deep brain stimulation, which is done by implanting electrodes, is used to treat patients for whom the illness has reached an advanced stage.

All of these treatments relieve the symptoms of the disease, but do not slow or reverse the destruction of the brain's nerve cells. Which means that even with treatment, symptoms often worsen with time. When they are first diagnosed, patients have generally been suffering from this illness for years and have already lost a majority of their essential nerve cells. An earlier diagnosis could be useful, but the goal of scientists is mainly to replace damaged cells. How can stem cells help in this regard?

Although the latent cause of this illness remains unknown, researchers know which brain cells and regions are responsible. They are already using stem cells to grow dopamine-producing nerve cells in the lab in order to study the disease. Since damage affects only one well defined cell type, we can consider replacing lost cells with new healthy ones.

Scandinavian scientists collected adrenal gland cells from four parkinsonian patients and implanted them into their brains. The adrenal glands are found above our kidneys and contain cells which secrete dopamine and analogous substances. Following the transplant, patients experienced some improvement in their health, which remained limited in scope and duration. This was the first transplant of dopamine-producing tissue into the human brain.

Scientists remain hopeful that the introduction of young cells into the brain will delay the appearance or progression of this illness. Induced pluripotent (iPS) cells could be produced in a lab from an adult patient's skin cells and used to generate dopaminergic neurons.

In 2010, in the United States, scientists treated rats with neurons derived from human skin cells produced via the iPS technique. The transplanted neurons diminished Parkinson's symptoms in rats. However, rodents (mice and rats) require fewer neurons than humans, and we do not yet know very well if this approach will function in patients. More studies will be necessary before we can be sure that these cells are safe, in particular in regard to the risk of forming brain tumors.

Anders Björklund as well as other researchers, in Sweden and in Italy, collected human skin cells and directly converted them into dopaminergic neurons. We do not yet know if these neurons will be able to survive and mitigate the disease's symptoms once they are transplanted into an animal. The long-term objective is to generate dopaminergic neurons from the patient's own skin or hair cells. Therapies for Parkinson's disease based on stem cells are not yet ready to be used in patients and more research is needed before clinical trials can be carried out.

Alzheimer's disease

Today, around 47 million people around the world suffer from Alzheimer's disease, and by 2050, over 100 million could develop it. Alzheimer's is the most common cause of dementia. The first signs of the disease often include memory impairment or trouble finding the right words. With time, symptoms such as confusion, sudden mood changes or memory loss settle in and progressively worsen. The cause of this disease is not yet clear, but researchers have noted that people suffering from it have abnormal accumulations of certain proteins in the brain. One of these proteins, beta-amyloid, aggregates into plaques. Another protein, tau, twists into neurofibrillary tangles. Scientists are still trying to find out if these changes in the brain are responsible for Alzheimer's disease. According to one of the proposed theories, the plaques might stop the brain's nerve cells from properly communicating with each other. The neurofibrillary tangles, for their part, might stop cells from acquiring the nutrients which they require. Regardless of the responsible mechanisms, it is clear that the disease's progression leads to the death of certain nerve cells. A growing number of them disappears as the disease progresses. This is why Alzheimer's disease is counted among the neurodegenerative diseases.

There is currently no treatment for Alzheimer's disease. The medication which we do have only temporarily mitigates certain symptoms. For example, by improving memory or the ability to carry out daily tasks. Most medication, part of a class called « *cholinesterase inhibitors* », helps prevent the degradation of a substance in the brain which transmits signals between neurons, acetylcholine. There is, however, no drug which can delay or stop the loss of neurons. Over the past two decades, the intensification of drug research and development efforts have allowed us to identify new substances which might have been able to reduce the accumulation of amyloid proteins in the brain. But extensive clinical trials for these substances have unfortunately failed. This raises new questions about our understanding of the disease, and how we simulate it in a lab environment. Until now, research has mainly focused on mice suffering from symptoms similar to those of Alzheimer's. But today stem cells can constitute new models for this illness. They could allow researchers to study it on human cells, and ultimately develop new treatments.

As part of one of the first studies of this kind, Korean researchers published results which show that adult stem cells can not only have a positive effect on those suffering from Alzheimer's disease, but also prevent the illness.

Scientists have recently taken advantage of iPS technology to grow neurons with some of the main characteristics of Alzheimer's disease. Researchers collected skin cells from patients suffering from Alzheimer's disease and reprogrammed them to turn into iPS cells. They then developed a method to grow neurons in a Petri dish from iPS cells. The lab-grown neurons release beta-amyloid proteins, which form plaques in patients' brains. This method allows scientists to study neurons similar to those affected by the illness in the brain, for example to better understand the causes and mechanisms of plaque and neurofibrillary tangle formation, as well as to research and test new drugs.

Stem Cells to Fix
the Spinal Cord

Thanks to stem cells collected in the brains of adult rats, a team of Canadian researchers managed to improve the motor functions of rats whose spinal cords had been damaged. Michael Fehlings (University of Toronto) and his colleagues' work also shows that this treatment must be administered rapidly after injury. Over one third of the stem cells was assimilated into the spinal cord's damaged tissue. Most of these cells became oligodendrocytes, which produce precious myelin, the sheath which surrounds nerve fibers and allows the transmission of nerve impulses towards the brain. According to Fehlings and his colleagues, 30% of the injected neuronal stem cells survive if the treatment is administered two or three weeks after the injury, compared to only 5% if it is applied six to eight weeks later. The scarring of the damaged area may explain, at least in part, this loss.

Muscles

How do we treat myopathies? The idea is to use donor stem cells which express the right gene. The problem is that this can lead to rejection if the patient is not receiving immunosuppressive treatment. But we can also use the patient's own cells, which have been genetically corrected in vitro before being reinjected.

The Heart

Research is quickly progressing in this field. Clinical trials are underway for treating post-infarction heart failure with cell therapy. Their goal: to regenerate the heart muscle's fibrous zones, which were modified by the infarction, by administering contractile stem cells. The debate on which cells to use is ongoing. Some prefer bone marrow stem cells; under certain conditions, they would be able to produce cardiomyocytes (heart cells);

others, among them Philippe Menasché, a cardiovascular surgeon at the Georges Pompidou European Hospital in Paris, favor the muscles' famous 'satellite' cells. A few weeks prior to the operation, these cells are collected from one of the patient's leg muscles and multiplied in a culture. They are then injected in different parts of the heart muscle. It would seem that these cells secrete cell growth factors which stimulate the original cardiomyocytes. Recently, another avenue of investigation has come into view: it appears that stem cells may be present within the heart muscle itself…

Researchers at the CNRS in Toulouse have shown for the first time that it is possible to obtain functional heart cells in vitro from fatty tissue cells in mice: after a few days in culture, in very simple conditions, some fatty tissue cells spontaneously differentiate into round cells which contract at a steady beat. These cells have all of the morphological and molecular characteristics of heart cells. The rhythm of the contractions can be modulated in vitro via the same nervous and pharmacological agents which modulate the heart rate within the organism. This first step is crucial, and opens up a new and promising path for regenerative therapy as applied to the heart muscle.

The Liver

When it is damaged, the liver's own cells, called hepatocytes, already provide it with surprising regenerative abilities. But the limited clinical trials involving the transplant of isolated hepatocytes have been disappointing: they do not proliferate well *in situ*.

As part of a project led by teams from Cambridge University and the Sanger Institute, in collaboration with a team from the Pasteur Institute and the Inserm (French Institute of Health and Medical research), researchers have shown for the first time that adult iPS cells, produced out of cells from patients suffering from a liver disease, can be genetically corrected and differentiated into hepatic cells in order to participate in liver regeneration in an animal model. This work, published on the journal Nature's website, represents a major proof of a concept, which allows us to foresee the future use of these stem cells in human patients.

Pancreas - Diabetes

The Inserm « *Cell Therapy of Diabetes* » team has for the past few years been carrying out transplants of pancreas cells responsible for insulin secretion (islets of Langerhans) in patients suffering from serious forms of type 1 (insulin-dependent) diabetes. Preliminary results already allow us to consider this French breakthrough as a significant step forward in combating diabetes.

Type 1 diabetes is characterized by the destruction, through an autoimmune reaction, of pancreatic beta cells, which produce insulin; this forces diabetic patients to have to receive multiple daily insulin injections. A potential path to curing this illness, according to scientists, is to grow beta cells *in vitro* out of stem cells. The idea is to multiply the patient's stem cells *in vitro* and specialize them into beta cells, then reimplant them while limiting autoimmune reactions. In order to accomplish this, the first step which needs to be mastered is the differentiation of stem cells into functional beta cells. This is what a Harvard team (United States) has just accomplished. Scientists established a very rigorous protocol which forces human stem cells to specialize into cells exhibiting markers specific to beta cells. Transplanted into type 1 diabetes mouse models, the cells which were produced regulate blood sugar just as well as normal beta cells, and are properly tolerated by the organism.

Testicles

According to a study published in the journal Nature, certain cells present in adult mouse testicles act like embryonic stem cells. According to the members of Gerd Hasenfuss' team, this could represent an alternative source of stem cells, which would bypass the reservations, and even outright hostility, expressed regarding research on embryos.

> *Gerd Hasenfuss (Georg-August University, Göttingen) and his colleagues have managed to extract these cells from adult males' testicles and differentiate them into several different tissues (skin, heart, brain...). These cells, called multipotent adult germinal stem cells, exhibit some of the characteristics of embryonic stem cells. If this work is one day successfully reproduced in humans, it would mean that adult males possess a valuable supply of stem cells!*

Japanese scientists have announced that they have, for the first time, succeeded in recreating functional sperm cells out of a mouse's embryonic stem cells. Progress which is likely to one day help in combating human sterility. *Sperm cells were used to fertilize eggs and the result was a healthy litter of mice which grew into perfectly fertile male and female adult mice, as the scientists from Kyoto University explained.* But this technology could not be used on human beings for another decade, say the authors. This experiment is nevertheless inspiring, as it removes one of the main biological barriers, that is, the recreation of sperm cells out of embryonic cells.

Intestines

For the first time, a team of Japanese scientists from the Tokyo Medical and Dental University, managed to reconstitute a damaged section of mouse intestine, with adult intestinal stem cells.

In order to achieve this regeneration, the team started by isolating a single intestinal stem cell in a healthy adult mouse. This cell was then cultured. After one week, it had multiplied into a million cells which reproduced the architecture and biological properties of the small intestine.

These cells were all transplanted into a mouse's damaged intestine. After one month, this transplant enabled the complete renewal of the intestinal mucosa. This new technique could one day allow us to treat certain inflammatory intestinal illnesses, such as Crohn's disease.

Arthritis

A true joint pathology, arthritis is characterized by mechanical pain during the day, which may hamper movement in some situations. It is due to deterioration of joint cartilage which ultimately leads to its complete destruction. Cartilage deterioration can be related to age, certain joint diseases, metabolic disorders, or excessive pressure on the joint, particularly when the patient is obese.

A European team, led by Professor Christian Jorgensen, (University of Montpellier, France), has developed an innovative project which aims to validate the use of fatty tissue stem cells to treat arthritis, an illness for which doctors only have symptomatic treatments. Stem cells are extracted from patients' fatty tissue, then treated, and reinjected into the affected joint, in order to activate cartilage regeneration. The first patient has been tested, and 18 others will follow as part of an initial cohort. 86 patients should be treated in the long run.

Under the influence of the environment of an articulation, fatty tissue stem cells injected into the joint can differentiate into chondrocytes, the cells responsible for cartilage formation. These newly formed chondrocytes can then repair the cartilage which was damaged by arthritis. Cartilage destruction is common in high-level athletes, who regularly receive stem cell injections. These injections are not considered doping by anti-doping agencies when cartilage damage is observed. If they were solely aimed at performance improvement, they would be illegal.

Teeth

Research on dental stem cells, which is very active in France, appears to be a promising field. Indeed, a team at the INSERM and the Paris Descartes University has just taken a further step in harnessing these cells to repair dental damage.

Odile Kellermann and her team worked with dental pulp taken from mice's molars. It is the 'living' part of the tooth, made of blood vessels and nerves. Up until now, scientists knew that dormant stem cells in the pulp would get to work in the event the tooth was damaged, but they still did not know how this process took place. In the future, the objective could be to develop therapeutic strategies which would mobilize the tooth's resident stem cells and amplify their natural restorative capabilities, says the INSERM. This could spell the end of capping materials (calcium hydroxide) and other biomaterials currently used by dentists to fill injured cavities.

Eyes

Embryonic stem cells, transplanted in 18 patients suffering from serious ocular pathologies, have improved the vision of more than half of them, according to the results of the longest study ever conducted in this technology, published in the journal *The Lancet*. The 18 patients all suffered from degenerative retinal diseases, and half of them from Stargardt disease, a major cause of juvenile blindness. The other patients suffered from the dry form of age-related macular degeneration (ARMD) which can also lead to blindness. There is currently no treatment for these two illnesses. Out of 18 patients followed over 22 months on average, ten demonstrated substantial improvement in their vision, as measured by their ability to read letters on a board.

Researchers from London University have just successfully transplanted cultivated stem cells into mice, which will become photoreceptors, receptors which give the eye the ability to perceive light .The scientists are hopeful that this will lead to a way to cure diseases such as retinitis pigmentosa, macular degeneration, Stargardt disease or diabetes-induced blindness. The British researchers have given themselves five years before they expect to initiate clinical trials on human beings.

Finally, A Rather Chilling Study

Live stem cells found in human corpses! Seventeen days after death, live stem cells can still be found in human corpses.

This scientific publication could truly trigger a wave of panic. A group of researchers led by Shahragim Tajbakhsh and Fabrice Chrétien (Pasteur Institute - Paris) has just published on the website of the journal Nature a rather surprising document. They have just discovered a never- before seen stock of live stem cells within the muscle tissue of a human corpse, **whose heart had stopped beating seventeen days earlier.**

How did this French team make such a pivotal discovery? Fabrice Chrétien tells us that the idea for these experiments came to him while he was examining muscle cells, which he had collected during an autopsy, under a microscope. While all neighboring cells were completely destroyed, these stem cells still looked good.

How could we explain these cells' survival, whether or not they are stem cells, within an oxygen-deprived environment? This is referred to as a state of quiescence: these cells get rid of their mitochondria, the organelles present in every cell which enable cellular respiration, giving cells their energy. Researchers are however unable to explain what compels the cells to rid themselves of their mitochondria. They are also unable to estimate how long this microscopic hibernation lasts.

Many questions remain concerning the therapeutic uses which could be made of these cells. Nevertheless, Professor Chrétien's team has already managed to transplant the offspring of the surviving cells and differentiate them into completely healthy muscle cells. And this from stem cells collected from mice which had been dead for fourteen days.

But before we can consider the medical potential of these advances, what impact will this research have on the perception of human corpses? The issue in this regard is the fear of declaring as dead people who are still alive. We should also consider the new possibilities offered by the ability to harvest organs from people who have died, but whose bodies are artificially kept alive. It nevertheless remains surprising that human cells can keep on living up to seventeen days (at least) after the signature of the death certificate and burial permit.

Stem Cells
and Aesthetic Medicine

Dr. Nathan Newman is a cosmetic surgeon and dermatologist; he practices his craft in Beverly Hills, one of Los Angeles' swanky neighborhoods. He is a pioneer of stem cell technologies. The idea of using stem cells instead of scalpels came to him more than ten years ago, as he was regularly performing liposuctions. Abdominal fat is rich in adult mesenchymal stem cells, which possess three very interesting characteristics. The first is their incredible ability to multiply, the second, their ability to differentiate into specialized cells as needed, and the third, their unique reparative and regenerative powers when injected into skin tissue.

The main problem was a technical one: the wand and high-pressure suction system used for liposuction offered no chances that the stem cells would survive. Innovations needed to be made: invent new wands and only use manual suction, via syringes. Thanks to these new instruments, it was possible to extract abdominal fat without altering the stem cells. The second step was to separate the stem cells from the fat; and this was made possible through custom-designed ultracentrifugation. All that was left to do was to reinject the stem cells, which had been concentrated, into the patient's face, the same patient from whom the fat had been extracted! In the case of autologous transplants such as these there is no risk of allergic reactions or of rejection. All of this takes less than three hours, and the patient can go back home having only received a small dose of local anesthetic to facilitate the penetration of the liposuction wand. To perfect his method, Dr. Newman has developed treatment protocols which have already taken the place of scalpels for most facial cosmetic surgery. His method, *Stem Cell Lift* ®, has traveled around the world!

The results are simply amazing. They are so remarkable that TV crews have come to film the entirety of the procedure simply to show that there is no trickery involved!

The main advantage of Stem Cell Lift ® compared to traditional plastic surgery, apart from the elimination of the scalpel, lies within the procedure's very nature: surgery cuts, augments, reduces, fills in or replaces; stem cells repair, regenerate, restore homeostasis, the face transforms naturally, curves reclaim their shape. The results are spectacular and genuine. Dr. Newman uses his method not only for cosmetic repairs, but also for reconstruction after nose jobs or jaw surgery due to cancer. These techniques which use fat as a stem cell source are increasingly used in the United States, in Switzerland and in Belgium, but less so in other European countries. Just like any new technology, it is hotly debated between those who advocate surgery and those who support the use of stem cells. Health authorities have not yet enacted any legislation in this field but it shouldn't take much longer.

The Use of Stem Cells
in Cosmetology

The past few years have seen the appearance of stem cell-based skincare products with such outlandish claims you might find them hard to believe. And you would be right, as they unfortunately do not work! Stem cells are live cells, and cannot survive outside of a very specific nutritional environment. This need cannot be met when we apply a cream or serum onto our skin. So, is it a scam? Probably, unless the product also contains other very effective ingredients.

There is a solution, however, which some laboratories use: growth factors. These are messenger proteins secreted by stem cells, which enable communication between cells. They bond to receptors located on the cell membrane and are then allowed to do their job that is activating cell proliferation and differentiation. At the level of the skin, these growth factors orchestrate intracellular healing, repair and regeneration. Researchers have already identified several hundred growth factors, each one with a specific mission, but their effectiveness depends on their synergy.

There is something magical about growth factors. We apply them to our epidermis, and yet the repairs are carried out in the dermis, where key compounds, collagen and elastin, are located. They are incapable of physically reaching the dermis, but can send a signal which, through cascading interactions, will reach it and make it possible to act on the extracellular matrix.

As we age, we observe a very significant reduction in growth factors, and therefore of collagen and elastin synthesis. This explains why we want to boost production of these growth factors in the skin, which requires the use of stem cells. Cultivated in a specific nutritional gel, they will rapidly multiply. During this phase, they will secrete very large quantities of growth factors into the gel. All that is needed then is to filter the gel, in order to eliminate the now useless stem cells, and what will remain is a gel packed with growth factors.

Growth factors produced by human abdominal fat stem cells are the most worthwhile. They offer more than 200 different growth factors, granting quick and effective synergistic activity. Unfortunately, their use is heavily regulated in certain countries. We can also produce growth factors with biotechnology, but their effectiveness is limited due to their instability and low penetrating power. Finally, certain laboratories in Switzerland offer plant-based growth factors made for example from alpine rose. These factors are excellent, but are limited in number, which means their synergistic power is almost null. The future lies in adult stem cell growth factors, but this means that health authorities will have to come to the right decision!

□ REMEMBER □

Human beings are incapable of regenerating themselves, but they do heal. Time has taken the ability to regenerate away from mankind, but it has left us the ability to repair ourselves. However, we are today able to reactivate the mechanisms of regeneration in order to renew damaged organs. Stem cells are, as their name implies, our body's first cells. They are divided into embryonic and adult stem cells . They are characterized by their ability to reproduce through mitosis and to differentiate into an array of specialized cells. Induced pluripotent stem cells make it possible to collect cells from any individual, culture and reimplant them once transformed. Adult stem cells ensure cellular homeostasis, that is, the balance between dying and living cells. If stem cells are unable to properly fulfill their mission, the daily loss of cells may eventually lead to tissue degeneration and the appearance of disease. The goal of regenerative medicine is to produce living, functional tissue, which can replace damaged tissues or organs.

SOURCES

Axel Kahn, Fabrice Papillon.
Le secret de la salamandre. Paris : Nil Editions ; 2005.

Christian Drapeau.
Le pouvoir insoupçonné des cellules souches. Québec : Les Éditions de l'Homme ; 2010.

Giorgio Maria Carbone.
L'enjeu des cellules souches. Paris : Salvator ; 2006.

Helena Baranova.
Nos gènes, notre santé, et nous. Paris : Armand Colin ; 2004.

Jean David Ponci.
La biologie du vieillissement. Paris : L'Harmattan ; 2008.

**Joël de Rosnay, Jean-Louis Servan-Schreiber,
François de Closets, Dominique Simonnet.**
Une vie en plus. Paris : Seuil ; 2005.

Nicole Le Douarin.
Les cellules souches. Paris : Odile Jacob ; 2007.

Andrew Weil.
Healthy Aging. New York : Anchor Books ; 2005.

Aubrey de Grey, Michael Rae.
Ending Aging. New-York : St. Martin's Griffin ; 1963.

Ray Kurzweil, Terry Grossman.
Serons-nous immortels ? Paris : Dunod ; 2006.

Michael D. West.
The Immortal Cell. New York : Doubleday ; 2003.

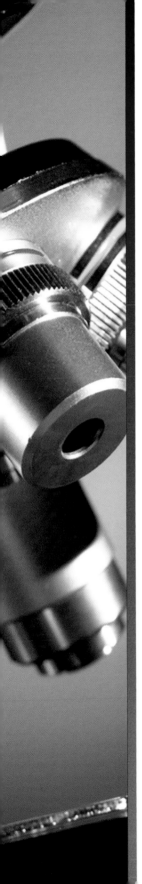

Chapter 3

Nanomedicine

« We are writing history with nanotechnologies,
but we do not know what that history is »

- Étienne Klein, physicist -

In 1966, a portentous film is released in the United States, its title: Fantastic Voyage. Here is its storyline. The United States and the Soviet Union have both developed a technology which makes it possible for matter to be miniaturized through a procedure which shrinks each atom separately, but this technology is of limited use, as objects return to their initial size after a maximum of 60 minutes.

However, Benes, a scientist working on the other side of the iron curtain, has found out how to make the transformation permanent. With the help of the CIA, he is able to cross over to the West, but an assassination attempt leaves him in a deep coma with a blood clot in his brain. The United States government is impatient to bring him back to life so that he can give them the secret to permanent miniaturization. In order to eliminate the blood clot, a group of scientists embark on board the *Proteus*, a miniaturized submarine which will be injected into Benes' body. Given how long miniaturization lasts, the team only has one hour to find and destroy the blood clot before their inevitable death, as once the miniaturized submarine begins to return to its normal size, it will be targeted by the subject's immune system and destroyed. The crew is plagued by many obstacles. A wrong turn forces them to go through the heart – which is temporarily shut off in order to avoid any deadly turbulence – then the lungs to replenish their oxygen supply. The crew members are soon forced to disassemble their radio equipment to repair the laser meant to destroy the blood clot; it soon becomes apparent that a saboteur has infiltrated the mission…

This film inspired Isaac Asimov, who wrote two books on the subject: *Fantastic Voyage*, the film's novelization, and a novel inspired by it, *Destination Brain*. Asimov's enthusiastic fascination with miniaturization was prophetic. Today, a team at UCLA (University of California, Los Angeles), in order to perform critical medical operations within the human body, has designed a submarine the size of a red blood cell, and called it Proteus. Within living systems, molecules carry out repetitive functions, just like a machine. Based on this observation, the team also created a 'nanocopter', a helicopter a nanometer wide with a « *motor* » the size of a virus, which utilizes the body's own energy, adenosine triphosphate (ATP). In a few years, nanotechnology will make it possible for us to repair our body and our brain, by partially rebuilding them. According to Ray Kurzweil, a worldwide specialist in modeling technologies, the 21st century will represent 20,000 years of progress, meaning it will be a thousand times more productive than the 20th. As a consequence, every aspect of our lives will undergo profound changes, in every area; from our health to our longevity, our economy, our society.

The 20th century was a century of grandiose achievements, the 21st will be that of the infinitesimally small. These technological revolutions have encouraged the emergence of nanoscience, of which nanomedicine is a part.

3.1 - Nanotechnologies

Materials whose properties were still unknown only a few years ago, ever smaller and ever more powerful computers, applications in every part of daily life; this is the invisible revolution brought on by these new materials measured in billionths of a meter (a million times smaller than a millimeter). The miniaturization of electronic devices has made our environment ever more receptive, interactive. Able to manipulate matter at the microscopic level, nanotechnologies will improve our daily life and make it more productive, as well as more comfortable. They are the key to our future, as they will touch on every aspect of our lives.

Scanning Tunneling Microscope

Thirty years ago, a new microscope was revolutionizing the scientific world. It allowed us to peer into a world never seen before, that of nano-objects, the invisible world of atoms and molecules. The scanning tunneling microscope (STM), was invented in 1981 by researchers at IBM, Gerd Binnig and Heinrich Rohrer, who were rewarded with the Nobel Prize for Physics for their work in 1986. It is a scanning probe microscope which takes advantage of a quantum mechanical phenomenon, tunneling. This microscope explores surfaces in the same way one would read a page written in braille. It uses a probe whose tip is made of a single atom. When it gets a few nanometers away from the sample, an electron exchange takes place with the nearest atom; this is what is referred to as quantum tunneling! By keeping the value of this current constant, the probe follows, atom by atom, the shape of the explored surface. Computer programs convert this data into images. With this microscope, we were able to see atoms and molecules for the first time, and this completely revolutionized the knowledge we had of them. But this microscope had something else up its sleeve: if its tip gets even closer to the surface, current exchanges intensify. Researchers have discovered that by using this energy they could move atoms, one by one, and literally modify matter.

Nanomaterials

Some of these applications are already being harnessed in our daily lives. Glass, for example, now has an extra feature which we cannot see: tiny groups of titanium dioxide molecule are deposited on its surface, and this addition makes it self-cleaning and self-disinfecting when exposed to light. Today, this is the most effective way of making all kinds of surfaces self-cleaning. The more than 15,000 windows of the Tokyo airport are all self-cleaning, made of Nano glass. Many materials today can benefit from features offered by nanoparticles. Titanium dioxide can also be found in public restrooms, surgical masks, highway noise barriers, and on the facades of many buildings. Certain applications will lead to radical modifications in urban architecture. This is the case for carbon nanotubes; when they combust, carbon atoms are assembled into a hexagonal structure which we can coil around itself, forming tiny cylinders. They can be reduced to a diameter of a single nanometer, a thousand times thinner than a strand of hair. Yet this is the strongest material we have ever produced, a hundred times more resistant than steel, and six times lighter.

We are therefore capable today of creating new materials the performance of which is unmatched anywhere in nature.

Nanoelectronics

These carbon nanotubes have also ended up being remarkable miniature semiconductors. A South Korean lab has designed a type of ink containing suspended carbon nanotubes. This ink, when used in a printer, will be able to reproduce full electronic circuits on materials such as plastic or paper. These electronic circuits can be found in our passports and highway payment systems, and they are also used in stock management. They have the benefit of communicating and being location-aware. They can receive all sorts of messages, whether chemical, biological, or physical, such as temperatures. These nanosensors can be embedded into our cell-phones or even our clothes. Nanofibers can replace all batteries, while providing a thousand-fold increase in the life of a charge (from what we have so far discovered). Thanks to nanosensors, it is possible to detect almost anything: fires breaking out, toxic leaks, but also to follow up on the propagation of a given danger within a system.

Nanocomputing

Computers have now existed for more than 70 years. They function by answering simple equations, through a series of cascading transistors. The miniaturization of transistors is precisely what revolutionized the IT industry. For more than a quarter of a century, the number of transistors we can embed onto silicon chips has doubled every two years. Unfortunately, the minimum size at which these components can be built is 20 nanometers. Below this threshold, physical phenomena make it impossible for transistors to function properly. But a new nanomaterial is on the cusp of breaking through this limitation: graphene, an unfurled carbon nanotube, only a single atom thick! This nanotube can conduct electric current a thousand times more efficiently than copper. An ideal substitute for current silicon chips.

3.2 Nanomedicine

Nanomedicine focuses more on prevention than traditional medicine, and is more customizable, by decoding our body's most secretive signals. This type of care is also less invasive and more effective against incapacitating chronic illnesses.

Nanomedicine makes it possible for diagnoses to be carried out far earlier. Current tests are based on complex protocols, which can only be performed in state of the art labs, which are few and far between, and too expensive to be used frequently.

3.2.1 - Molecular Signatures

According to Dr. Chad Mirkin, at Northwestern University (Chicago), early symptoms appear at the nanometer scale. In order to coordinate themselves, our 60 trillion cells are constantly swapping tiny messenger molecules, DNA fragments only a few nanometers long. The cascading reactions produced by these molecular messages are our cells' deepest form of operation. When a cell is sick, it emits a series of messages, which biologists call biomarkers. They are the molecular signatures of disease, and the detection of these elements is the cornerstone of our most sophisticated diagnostic systems.

According to Chad Mirkin, almost every illness has a specific genetic biomarker, and often a protein biomarker as well. Over the past twenty years, the identification of these markers has undergone a great deal of progress. Today, it is possible to elaborate tests which detect them and make it possible to rapidly determine the nature and stage of development of the illness, and consequently which treatment to implement.

This revolution is underway. The first diagnostic systems, coming out of Chad Mirkin's research have been in use for three years already, in about fifty American hospitals.

Chad Mirkin says that in 2009, when a new influenza virus, H1N1, appeared, his team was able, thanks to nanotechnology, to detect and identify the pathogenic virus , and accurately determine its nature; all of this took them about three and a half hours. Traditional methods, which require the virus to first be cultured, only after which a detection and identification process can be carried out, could take up to 14 days before obtaining any results. William Moffatt adds that «The big difference with nanotechnology is that it makes it possible to embed everything we need to completely automate tests in a simple, disposable chip. This technology is incredibly precise and sensitive, and at the same time very easy to use and cheap.»

3.2.2 - Gold Nanoparticles

Nanomolecular diagnostic systems take advantage of a fundamental property of the messenger molecules they are searching for. Nanomolecules systematically bond with complementary molecules, called ligands, in the same way a key is designed to open its complementary lock. By attaching these ligands to a specially-made device, we can therefore capture the corresponding biomarker if it is present in the sample. But these objects are so small that it is very difficult to see the test results, which explains the complexity of current devices. Chad Mirkin solved this problem, at the molecular level, by taking advantage of the properties of gold nanoparticles.

Gold nanoparticles are little magnets made of gold atoms. When they are less than 100 nanometers in diameter, we see them as red. This red coloring is so bright that any solution containing them, even if very dilute, will appear very brightly colored. Think of them as nanometer-scale beacons, which attach themselves to the desired molecules, and reveal, thanks to their powerful signal, the presence of a disease's biomarker. They can identify a disease's biomarker among a million other signals, with incredible precision – a near 100% success rate for most tests (Chad Mirkin).

Many of these types of systems will most likely show up in hospitals very quickly. But nanotechnology is progressing so quickly that it could, in the short term, produce even simpler and more surprising screening tools. In Italy, Dr. Silvano Dragonieri is hoping to detect the early signs of cancer thanks to a simple electronic system: a tool originally designed to carry out sanitary controls for the food industry, or to detect traces of explosives in a military context.

Over the past few years, we have discovered that our breath contains a mix of more than 3,000 volatile organic compounds. For example, patients suffering from lung cancer have a different combination of volatile organic compounds than that of a healthy person. We have already established that this 'bouquet' could distinguish asthmatic individuals from those who do not have asthma, just as for those diagnosed with lung cancer, as well as healthy subjects from those with chronic bronchitis (Silvano Dragonieri).

Chemotherapy is a classic treatment for cancer, which attacks diseased cells as well, unfortunately, as healthy tissue. A new type of treatment makes use of a procedure developed by Omid Farokhzad. Nanoparticles capable of exclusively targeting cancer cells can send toxic molecules as part of chemotherapy, without affecting the organism's other cells. According to Omid Farokhzad, during a classical chemotherapy treatment, only two percent of the product actually reaches the tumor. The rest goes into other tissues, where it is responsible for its well-known side effects. With this kind of targeted delivery, we can control with incredible precision the final destination of the molecules. Thanks to nanoparticles, we can multiply the number of active molecules directly attacking the tumor by twenty. With classical chemotherapy, the dose needed to produce similar results would be deadly. Thanks to targeted nanoparticles, we can completely eradicate tumors with very few side-effects.

These tests have also shown that this procedure makes it possible to deliver much stronger, and therefore much more effective doses to the cancer cells, without incurring any additional risks for the patients. According to Omid Farokhsad, the true potential of nanotechnology goes far beyond cancer therapies. We can develop far more effective treatments for cardiovascular disease as well as much more powerful vaccines. Indeed, another company a few miles outside of Boston is developing the concept of nanovaccines, based on the same techniques: nanoparticles attached to immune cells, emulating the size, shape and molecular signature of natural pathogens.

According to Werner Cautreels, what we are seeing today is just the tip of the iceberg. What is coming will be huge, too big to imagine for people today. What is certain is that the medicine we will be practicing in 30 or 40 years will be nothing like what we are doing today.

Nanomedicine is the product of nanotechnology and related research in the medical field. It will revolutionize early screening techniques by detecting molecular signatures. Furthermore, nanomedicine is developing nanomedications which will completely change how active molecules are distributed within the organism. The areas for their application are numerous, in particular for oncology, a field where their possible applications are the most abundant due to the potential to directly target tumors via nanoparticles. Nanovaccines are beginning to appear. Gene therapy also has many potential applications: nanovectors for gene transfers, microsurgery... Finally, as far as restorative biotechnologies are concerned, research on nanoimplants and prostheses could lead to revolutionary applications.

Chapter 3 - Nanomedicine

SOURCES

Bernadette Bensaude-Vincent.
Les vertiges de la technoscience, façonner le monde atome par atome.
Paris : La Découverte ; 2009.

Joël de Rosnay, Jean-Louis Servan-Schreiber,
François de Closets, Dominique Simonnet.
Une vie en plus. Paris : Seuil ; 2005.

Ray Kurzweil, Terry Grossman.
Serons-nous immortels ? Paris : Dunod ; 2006.

Aubrey de Grey, Michael Rae.
Ending Aging. New-York : St. Martin's Griffin ; 1963.

Ann B. Pearson.
The Proteus Effect. Washington D.C. : Joseph Henry Press ; 2004.

Eric R. Braverman.
Younger You. New York : Mc Graw Hill ; 2007.

Eric R. Braverman.
The Eedge Effect. New York : Sterling Publishing Co. Inc. ; 2005.

Paul Yanick Jr. Vincent C. Giampapa.
Quantum Longevity. San Diego, CA :
ProMotion Publishing ; 1997.

Ray Kurzweil, Terry Grossman.
Fantastic Voyage. New York : Plume Book ; 2005.

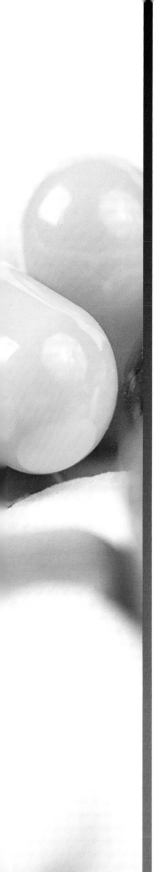

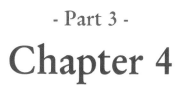

Chapter 4

Active Nutritional Supplementation

« Let your food be your medicine alone ! »

- HIPPOCRATES -

In an ideal world we would always eat healthily. Our food wouldn't be cultivated in soil filled with toxic heavy metals and pesticides. But even if we were given the opportunity to always eat healthy food, we would still be the same weak-willed creatures, addicted to sugar, French fries, grilled steak, chocolate mousse and whipped cream!

The sad truth is that the motivational speeches of nutritionists are not enough. We can no longer only depend on food itself to fulfill our basic nutritional needs. If we want to really step up to the plate and fight oxidation, silent inflammation and glycation, if we want good methylation to manage our genetic expression, if we want to protect our telomeres and stem cells, then we need to boost our nutrition with dietary supplements whose effectiveness has been demonstrated.

Today, doctors, nutritionists and other experts have a better understanding of nutrition and biochemistry. In the field of nutrition, the progress and discoveries made in the past few years have underlined the essential role of vitamins, minerals, medicinal plants and other substances for our health. Furthermore, numerous studies have shown that nutritional supplementation can help prevent cardiovascular diseases, cancer and osteoporosis, as well as other chronic illnesses.

Just a few decades ago, clinical studies attempting to prove the effectiveness of dietary supplements were relatively rare, whereas today we are seeing a huge surge in these studies, thousands of researchers studying the role of certain plants on our health and longevity. Omega 3, resveratrol, telomerase activators and antioxidants, anti-aging supplements have benefited from tens of thousands of in vitro and in vivo clinical trials. There is ample evidence that this principle of active supplementation, integrated into a better lifestyle, leads to a longer lifespan.

Despite this, the European Food Safety Authority (EFSA) and the European Commission remain surprisingly reluctant. They systematically refute all serious claims regarding dietary supplements, deliberately ignoring publications from the most important scientific journals (Nature, The Lancet, JAMA, Cells etc.) whose authors are often internationally acclaimed.

Good active dietary supplementation should be carried out in two steps.

The first, which is restorative, is meant to improve the system designed to repair the damage which our DNA undergoes every day. This can be achieved by fighting inflammation, oxidation and glycation, and by improving methylation. This supplementation should be permanent, as this damage takes place every day, 24 hours a day, 7 days a week!

The second step, which is regenerative, will attempt to revive the process of regeneration which was lost, in order to lengthen our telomeres and protect our stock of stem cells.

4.1 - Restorative Dietary Supplementation

There are many dietary supplements with protective or restorative properties, and which have demonstrated their effectiveness through double-blind clinical studies. We have selected a few which seem to be among the most effective.

Vitamins and Minerals

These dietary supplements cannot be ignored in terms of their anti-aging properties! There are hundreds of clinical studies demonstrating the positive effect of regular vitamin and mineral consumption. These studies show that the elderly have an excessively low vitamin intake, in particular for vitamins A, C, D, E, K and folates (vitamin B9). This would be improved by vitamin supplementation. The brain in particular is very metabolically active, and spends a lot of energy, which makes it very sensitive to any metabolic insufficiency provoked by a shortage in essential nutrients.

In 1996, the results of a double-blind study carried out over nine years, and published in the journal JAMA, demonstrated that selenium supplementation reduces the risk of cancer mortality by half. This same journal demonstrated the previous week that folic acid supplementation substantially reduces cardiovascular risk.

The same year, the American Journal of Clinical Nutrition also published an article showing that dietary supplementation increases human life expectancy. This study, carried out from 1984 to 1993 on 11 178 seniors, shows that taking vitamin E reduces all-cause mortality by 34%. It reduces the risk of dying from coronary heart disease by 63%, and cancer mortality by 59%. The combination of vitamins C and E reduces mortality by 42% according to this study!

The SUViMAX study, carried out in France, has shown that vitamin supplementation can lengthen our lifespan. This study was carried out in France on 13,000 volunteers who were monitored during eight years. Participants were given dietary supplements as capsules containing the following antioxidant vitamins and minerals, in the doses shown: beta-carotene (provitamin A): 6 mg; Vitamin C: 120 mg; Vitamin E: 30 mg; Selenium: 100 µg; Zinc: 20 mg. Other volunteers were given identical capsules containing a placebo. The doctors did not know which volunteers were being given vitamins and which weren't, and were thus able to impartially assess developments in their health. This protocol is what gives its name to double-blind studies. And its results are remarkable. They unambiguously show that the active pills manage to reduce cancer rates by 31% and all-cause mortality by 37%.

Vitamin D3

More than 90% of our vitamin D needs should normally be provided by sun exposure, yet in western countries, whether in France, Belgium, Switzerland, the United States, or Canada, vitamin D levels are far below where they should be. And especially so during the winter months. Scientists have shown the essential role which vitamin D plays in cell division and differentiation and its influence on the immune system. Low vitamin D levels are linked to almost every age-related disorder, including cancer and chronic vascular and inflammatory diseases. Research indicates that a 5,000 IU daily dose could have many beneficial effects. Other studies have shown that vitamin D, when combined with other natural substances, can have an effect on adult stem cells and thereby increase neurogenesis and improve cognitive ability.

Fighting Inflammation

Omega 3

This is the most important dietary supplement, as well as the best documented. We can say with certainty that we all need omega 3. Adults, children, seniors, pregnant and nursing women, newborns and teenagers... This list could go on forever! Nearly 18,000 scientific studies have reviewed the many health benefits of this essential fatty acid, which is crucial to our nutritional balance, and can only come from our diet.

The activity of omega 3 fatty acids is polymorphic, that is, they can spring into action in many different areas in many different forms.

In our blood : fish oils containing omega 3 reduce inflammation when they are present in the blood, and this activity is global, as the blood flow takes omega 3 far from its entry point. Inflammation reduction is a fundamental objective in combating age-related chronic illness.

In our cell membranes : cell membranes are mainly composed of phospholipids. Eicosanoids, a type of hormone only active locally, are synthesized from the essential fatty acids present in phospholipids: omega 3 and omega 6. Just as with cholesterol, there are good and bad omega fatty acids, and good and bad eicosanoids. Omega 3 are the good fatty acids. They will trigger the release of good eicosanoids, which are anti-inflammatory. Omega 6 are the bad fatty acids, which will cause the release of pro-inflammatory eicosanoids. Omega 3 and omega 6 are constantly battling it out in the cell membrane. Since we consume on average five to ten times more omega 6 than omega 3, we often end up with higher pro-inflammatory activity, with all of the negative consequences this entails for our health.

Within the cell : fish oils are active at many levels in gene expression, in particular for DNA. They inhibit genes involved in cancer, as well as activate protective genes. Several studies have demonstrated omega 3 fatty acids' antioxidant properties, even if we do not classify them in this category.

It has been shown that the activity of omega 3 is far-reaching: anti-inflammatory, anti-cancer, anti-hypertensive, effective in preventing and treating macular degeneration, arthritis, dementia, and Alzheimer's disease. DHA, the most important component of omega 3 fatty acids, directly affects eyesight and cognitive ability. The Rotterdam consensus, in 2003, determined that omega 3 intake, in the form of fish oil or dietary supplements, taken once a week, reduced the risk of dementia, and therefore of Alzheimer's, by 60%. Omega 3 improves learning in children and diminishes the risk of postpartum depression by half.

Telomeres and Omega 3

This might surprise you, but it has been shown, in vitro, that fish oil inhibits the activation of telomerase in cancer cells. This is good news, as cancer cells become immortal, in part because their telomerase is activated 24 hours a day, seven days a week!

These studies might come to contradict another one, published in the Journal of the American Medical Association (JAMA). The authors followed 608 participants with coronary artery disease over 5 years and monitored the amount of fish oil they consumed each day. They regularly measured telomere length and noticed that those consuming the most DHA and EPA (the two major components of omega 3 fatty acids) had longer telomeres, whereas those taking no omega 3 had shorter telomeres on average. Omega 3 can seemingly have two opposite actions. But they are not alone; they are called 'adaptogens', as their goal seems to be to bring a factor or a measure within its normal range. Ginseng, another adaptogen, can increase arterial pressure when it is too low, or conversely lower it when it is too high.

But why take dietary supplements derived from fish oil and not the fish itself, and why not other omega 3 sources?

Taking fish oils high in DHA and EPA is certainly possible, but there are however two obstacles: the first is that in order to reach proper doses of EPA and DHA we would need to consume large quantities of fish, the second is that our oceans are heavily polluted by mercury and polyvinyl chloride (PVC). The only way to acquire non-contaminated oil is to extract it and immediately perform a molecular distillation which will eliminate all heavy metals, without altering the oil.

For vegetarians, we could use vegetable oils such as linseed oil, chia oil, or even purslane oil. But these oils do not contain EPA or DHA but rather alpha-linolenic acid which is the precursor of omega 3. It can produce EPA and DHA, although four times less than fish oil.

Krill is a type of small cold-water shrimp which feeds on plankton and which whales are very fond of. Krill oil is very high in omega 3, EPA et DHA included; it has been the subject of many studies which, although very positive, do not surpass results achieved with fish oil. The main obstacle is strictly environmental. Krill is a part of a fragile ecosystem which runs the risk of being disrupted if we extract krill from it on a massive scale.

Careful though, we should not confuse oil from fatty fish with fish liver oil. The latter contains vitamins A and D, and prolonged use could expose you to the serious consequences of an overdose.

The omega 3 content of food is indicated on their label. One gram of omega 3 represents: 50 g of farmed salmon, 60 g of canned salmon, 65 g of canned sardines, 75 g of fresh mackerel, and 130 g of canned tuna. Are there any issues, or even side effects, to taking large doses of omega 3 fatty acids?

The most common issue with fish oil is unpleasant belching which smells of 'rotten' fish. In the vast majority of cases, this is due to oxidized oil. Knowing this, most major brands prevent oxidation as soon as the extraction takes place (most of the time on a fishing boat or on the farming grounds), after which they immediately freeze the oil. Quality oil therefore does not lead to this kind of issue.

Some users may notice more frequent nosebleeds. This is due to the thinning effect of omega 3 on the blood. If you already take anticoagulants or aspirin, talk to your doctor about taking omega 3.

Finally, some people who are allergic to fish or shellfish may be allergic to fish oil; they should use vegetable oil.

Fighting Oxidation

Polyphenols

In November of 1991, CBS News's 60 minutes runs a story suggesting that red wine consumption in France explains the lower rate of heart disease in that country. The report dubs this phenomenon: « *The French Paradox* ». Red wine is now known to contain polyphenols such as resveratrol, quercetin and catechins, among others. They all have high antioxidant activity, and take part in preventing many illnesses including heart attack, cancer and stroke. Polyphenols are the most abundant antioxidants in our diet and they improve health through a variety of gene activation mechanisms. Some polyphenols give red wine its color, chocolate its dark browns, green tea its emerald hues. Grapes, apples, onions, soy beans, peanuts, berries and many other fruits and vegetables are high in polyphenols. Resveratrol, a highly active polyphenol, which can be found in high doses in the skin of red grapes, now plays a major role in aging management practices.

The secret of these ingredients dates back four million years, when our ancestors were exposed to high levels of stress following important environmental and climatic changes. In return, and in order to improve their chances of survival, certain specific genes were then activated, including those which control the metabolism of carbohydrates, proteins and fats. In times of plenty, our body first burns dietary carbohydrates and stores energy as fats; whereas when food is scarce, these genes first mobilize stored fat. Plants which were contemporaries of our ancestors also endured environmental stresses, such as droughts, infections, parasites and thermal aggressions provoked by the sun. In order to survive, these stressed plants activated their own survival genes, and produced natural molecules which boosted their cellular defenses as well as their repair mechanisms. The molecule found in the skin of grapes meant for red wine production (resveratrol) is produced to fight off invaders. Lab mice which have been given this plant molecule also benefit from this same reaction to stress. This means that ingested plants communicate with the cells of the organism which ingests them, take advantage of the language of molecular genetics and activate survival genes.

Resveratrol

In 2002, David Sinclair and Joseph Baur of Harvard University publish their revolutionary discovery in the prestigious journal Nature: a substance called «resveratrol», extracted from red wine, could activate certain genes in animal cells and lead to spectacular clinical improvements , including improvements in memory, shrinking fat cells (even with a calorie-rich diet), energy and endurance in stimulated muscle cells, increases in muscular strength and reduced fatigue, coordination and mobility improvements. But what is even more remarkable is that these molecules are very effective in decreasing the rates of certain cancers, vascular diseases and brain degeneration, and extend the lifespan of treated mice by 25%. These little molecules present in red wine activate the sirtuin genes (our survival genes!) in the absence of calorie restriction, which is normally required for their activation, in order to produce the same cardioprotective effect as wine, without the alcohol!

In order to test resveratrol's ability to activate sirtuins in living creatures, the research team at Harvard, led by David Sinclair, selected a yeast, a monocellular organism which is closely related to animals and humans. They noticed that, even when used in small doses, resveratrol increases the lifespan of yeast cells by 60 to 80%. Yeast treated with resveratrol lived for 38 generations on average compared to only 19 for untreated yeast. Additional experiments on human cells have shown that resveratrol activates a similar pathway necessitating the SIRT1 gene, enabling 30% of human cells to survive gamma radiation, compared to 10% for untreated cells.

The activation of the SIRT1 gene by resveratrol stimulates a wide range of processes, in particular immune defense mechanisms, neuronal protection and metabolic optimization in the liver, muscles and adipocytes. Resveratrol has other effects including stimulating the production of cellular energy, adenosine triphosphate (ATP), in mitochondria as well as the modulation of insulin growth factor (IGF-1) which increases insulin sensitivity and thereby lowers obesity. Furthermore, there is considerable evidence for resveratrol's antioxidant properties; it inhibits the oxidation of low-density lipoproteins, or LDLs, and neutralizes harmful hydroxyl radicals. Perhaps one of the best free-radical neutralizers, resveratrol has beneficial consequences for longevity.

Resveratrol is present in nature in two forms: the bioactive form, trans-resveratrol, and cis-resveratrol, whose activity is seven times less. The 'trans' form is therefore strongly preferred.

We currently know of three sources for resveratrol.

    1 - Synthetic (poorly assimilated).

    2 - Extracted from Japanese knotweed, Polygonum cuspidatum: this is the most common source!

    3 - Extracted from grape skin, which contains all of the cofactors present in grapes. This guarantees perfect assimilation.

What is an appropriate dose of resveratrol?

Some products have a dose of a few milligrams and others of a few hundred milligrams. Which is right? Is this dosage arms-race beneficial for our organism?

A glass of wine contains around 0.10 to 0.65 mg of resveratrol. For long-term protection, a dose of 30 to 75 mg of trans-resveratrol per day is enough. For quick protection, a dose of 100 to 500 mg will be effective, but only for a relatively short time (one to two months).

Rejuvenating Our Mitochondria

The mitochondria are the powerhouses of the cell. When we age, they decrease in number, and those which remain are less and less effective and produce more and more waste. The result is a huge loss of energy, constant physical and cognitive issues, and the acceleration of cellular degradation. This major energy deficit is involved in most age-related degenerative illnesses. However, a nutrient has just been discovered which makes it possible, not only to improve the function of existing mitochondria, but also to increase their numbers.

PQQ (pyrroloquinoline quinone)

PQQ makes it possible, not only to improve the function of existing mitochondria, but also to increase their numbers, which is an exceptional advancement! Indeed, there is currently no way to increase mitochondria numbers. By generating new mitochondria, this dietary supplement ensures the longevity of all cells. Due to its high stability, PQQ turns out to be a powerful antioxidant, far superior to conventional antioxidants for protecting mitochondrial DNA; it is 30 to 5,000 times stronger than most ordinary antioxidants such as vitamin C. By transferring large numbers of electrons, it neutralizes the main free radicals hindering mitochondrial function, without suffering from molecular degradation. It also protects brain cells against oxidative damage following cases of ischemia, inflammation or oxidative lesions. In this context, PQQ significantly reduces the expanse of damaged cerebral tissue. It improves memory test performance and also interacts positively with cerebral neurotransmitter systems.

PQQ in Synergy with CoQ10

Recent studies have shown that when these two nutrients are paired rather than taken separately, they offer better cardiovascular and cognitive performance in particular. This is no surprise since the heart and the brain are by far the two organs which use the most energy. A Japanese study carried out in 2007 showed that PQQ, taken in 20 mg daily doses, enhances memory, attention and cognitive function. The performance of the group receiving a PQQ supplement was twice as strong as that of the placebo group. The simultaneous ingestion of 300 mg of CoQ10 enhanced performance even more in memory tests. Mental ability and quality of life can therefore be improved in older individuals, in addition to which this treatment also helps prevent cognitive decline in elderly people.

Fighting Glycation

Glycation is the third fundamental mechanism of DNA destruction and aging, after oxidation and inflammation. It is also the least well known. We also age because our proteins caramelize, which leads to chronically high blood sugar levels. A lot of research over the last twenty years shows that glycated proteins, also called Advanced Glycosylation End products or AGEs, play a very important role in cellular and tissue damage brought on by diabetes, cardiovascular aging and kidney failure. Dietary supplements with L-Carnosine in particular can help prevent this phenomenon.

L-Carnosine

Carnosine (or L-Carnosine) is a molecule naturally found in muscles and the brain. Cells with long lifespans (such as neurons) contain high levels of carnosine. Furthermore, muscular carnosine concentration is positively correlated with longevity, which makes it a potential biomarker for aging. It is present in high concentration in those muscles which actively contract and in very low concentrations in the case of certain muscular diseases such as Duchenne muscular dystrophy. Its muscular concentration decreases with age. Its strongest effect is anti-glycation, as it reacts with sugars such as glucose and galactose, forming glycated carnosine. It interrupts glycation in its early stages and forms completely harmless products which are easy to eliminate. Carnosine therefore makes it possible to decrease protein glycation and the formation of advanced glycosylation end products. Carnosine is an antioxidant which protects and stabilizes the cell membrane, just like vitamin E. Indeed, supplementing with carnosine increases your vitamin E levels.

According to a recent study, daily doses of carnosine taken by 20 healthy volunteers over one to four months did not lead to any side effects; on the contrary, half of the subjects noted improvements in facial appearance, muscular resistance or general well-being, and even, for some, in sleep and libido. These benefits appeared within a short period of time, whereas the expected aging-prevention effects will only arise through long-term supplementation. Taking 500 mg three times daily during meals is therefore strongly recommended in order to counteract excess sugar intake.

Improving Methylation

Methionine, SAMe

Methionine is an essential amino acid provided by our diet. Some methionine-rich foods include meat, eggs, nuts, corn, rice and grains in general.

When ATP and magnesium are present, it is converted into its active form, S-Adenosyl methionine (SAMe) which is the universal donor of the methyl group (CH3) responsible for around one hundred biochemical reactions in our organism. The methylation of DNA helps maintain its integrity, and contributes to gene expression and fixing replication errors. Methylation is an extremely important operation, on many levels: for neurotransmitter synthesis, the metabolism of phospholipids which govern cell membrane quality and message retrieval, and for putting unexpressed sections of the genome on standby.

All molecule types undergo methylation. Protein methylation is therefore essential for communication between cells, as it activates membrane receptors, while the methylation of phospholipids (fatty acids in cell membranes) helps maintain membrane flexibility and permeability, which are qualities essential for interaction between cells. Methylation is also necessary for the production of our most important antioxidant, glutathione. Responsible for adrenalin production out of norepinephrine and melatonin, itself out of serotonin, methylation largely regulates brain activity, influences sleep and positively affects mental processes. Other than the brain, the liver also uses methylation to help in detoxifying the organism.

All of the organism's methylation reactions therefore require the presence of a molecule, S-Adenosyl methionine (SAMe), produced in the body out of methionine and adenosine triphosphate (ATP), the energy creating intermediary produced by the cell.

SAMe being the supreme methylation substance, anything which might deplete the supply of SAMe will decrease methylation. Anything which might obstruct ATP synthesis (e.g. alcohol) will deplete the supply of SAMe, just as the lack of vitamin B6, B12 and folic acid (B9) will.

A good dose is of 400 mg, taken twice daily.

4.2 - Regenerative Dietary Supplementation

Its goal is much more ambitious than that of restorative supplementation, indeed it strives to reactivate this cellular regeneration we have talked so much about, mainly by addressing the issues of telomeres and stem cells.

Telomerase Activators

What Is Telomerase?

Telomerase is an enzyme which lengthens telomeres. Made of a protein and an RNA strand (DNA's messenger), telomerase is constantly busy repairing the extremities of chromosomes and thereby maintains the integrity of the telomeres. We can find active telomerase in sex cells and in some stem cells, but it is disabled in almost every one of our 60 trillion somatic cells.

In 1997, scientists introduced telomerase into skin cells which were cultivated in a Petri dish. They noticed that, not only was the telomerase active, but the cell had become immortal; it could multiply indefinitely without losing any of its vitality. Even better, the telomeres, which at first were quite short, had quickly lengthened.

A few years later, these same scientists deliberately injected telomerase-activation genes into human skin cells with very short telomeres. Then they transplanted these cells into the backs of mice. Those which were not given these genes showed clear signs of aging, with wrinkling, dry, withered skin, whereas those which had benefited from the telomerase-activation gene maintained youthful skin. For the first time, researchers had just demonstrated the process by which we age!

In November 2008, other researchers cloned mice out of cells containing the telomerase-activation gene; the lifespan of these mice was extended by half compared to those which had not been given the gene. We had just proved that it was possible to reverse the aging process at the level of the entire organism, by allowing telomerase to exert its effect.

Ronald DePinho, then a researcher at Harvard University (USA), published in the highly reputable international scientific journal Nature, an article presenting his findings on telomerase. It turns out that the stimulation of telomerase can regenerate organs and tissues. Mice suffering from Alzheimer's disease have for example had their mental abilities return to normal and their cerebral volume go back to that of a healthy mouse. Other studies have shown that if telomerase is activated, we can observe the regeneration, and therefore the rejuvenation, of skin, hair, nails and organs exhausted from continuous wear and tear.

Telomerase and Cancer

Cancer starts when everything is going wrong in a cell and it is straining to control its growth and duplication. The cancer cell begins to multiply chaotically, ignoring chemical signals ordering it to stop. Most of the time, thankfully, telomeres continue to shorten and the cell reaches the end of its life. But in certain cases the cancer cell will find a way to lengthen its telomeres. When this happens, the cancer becomes uncontrollable and very aggressive. In 90% of cases, this is achieved by activating the telomerase gene. This is why anticancer research is focused on telomerase inhibitors and many molecules are currently being studied.

If this is the case, then why do longevity specialists want so badly to find ways to lengthen telomeres? This is because, although it is true that cancers need telomerase to grow, it is just as true that telomerase does not lead to cancer in healthy cells. This has been abundantly demonstrated in at least seven large studies which all agree on the fact that telomerase does not induce cancer. Scientists explain it like this: generally speaking, we know that when telomeres shorten this is bad news for our health. This means that cells become senescent and this brings about chromosomal instability. This instability will cause mutations which are often linked to cancer: the deactivation of genes responsible for tumor suppression and the activation of genes which promote tumors. If, in this context, the telomerase gene is activated, then the cancer will become devastating!

Paradoxically, the fact that cells need telomerase to become cancerous nevertheless does not make it carcinogenic. We have discovered rather the opposite, that telomerase could contribute to preventing the appearance of cancer, not just because it eliminates chromosomal instability, but also because it increases immune cell longevity and thereby strengthens their ability to destroy cancers.

According to studies published in late 1999 in the monthly journal Nature Genetics, Dr. Woodring Wright, of the University of Texas, has clearly demonstrated that adding telomerase to cultured human cells does not make them evolve into cancer cells. Over the course of their work, Dr. Wright's team managed to multiply human cells in a lab setting to over two hundred times their normal life expectancy, without causing the appearance of cancer cells. They cannot be differentiated from 'young cells' and they show no signs of chromosomal anomalies or dysfunctions in the cell cycle checkpoints.

In a parallel study, Dr. Choy-Pik Chiu's team, noted that adding telomerase to mouse cells did not cause the appearance of any malignant tumors. For Dr. Wright, the anomalies seen in cancer cells are due to other mutations. Telomerase simply makes it possible for cells to continue to multiply. Telomerase therefore does not appear to be oncogenic. If this were the case, young people would have far more cases of cancer than older individuals. What we see is rather the opposite: a much higher rate of cancer in elderly people who also show signs of cellular senescence and whose immune system is starting to have trouble fighting off cancerous attacks, which occur daily.

Re-establishing Telomerase Activity

Even if adult somatic cells have stopped producing telomerase, they still possess its component parts. All that is needed is to force one of these components, the catalytic subunit hTERT, to re-establish telomerase activity. By introducing this TERT gene into human primary cells, we can therefore lengthen telomeres and dramatically alter cell growth.

A study carried out for over a year on vascular retina cells has shown that cells which produce telomerase keep dividing, whereas those not producing any become senescent. Another study on genetically modified mice in which telomerase was entirely absent showed that these creatures age at an accelerated rate, become infertile and suffer from diabetes, osteoporosis or neurodegenerative pathologies, and die very young. Furthermore, reactivating telomerase for a month in another group of these same mice led to surprising results: the recovery of fertility, of spleen, liver and kidney vitality, and finally the reversal of the effects of aging on the brain. The brains themselves grew and their neurons became active again.

All of these studies make it possible for many scientists to affirm that any substance which increases telomerase activity therefore allows us to lessen age-related pathologies.

What Substances Activate the Telomerase Gene?

A number of molecules have been studied and experimented with in humans for the past few years. Research done on these substances clearly shows that they are able to stimulate the telomerase gene, increase the number of telomeres, significantly lengthen them, and consequently to reverse certain mechanisms of aging by driving back cell death, once believed to be inescapable after a certain number of divisions. These molecules are likely to be only the very first of a list which will certainly grow over the coming years.

The most interesting substances come from a plant which has been used in traditional Chinese medicine for millennia: dried Astragalus root (*Astragalus membranaceus*). According to recent studies, this extract is able to activate telomerase in cultured keratinocyte cells, fibroblasts and immune cells. Although the average length of telomeres does not grow, the proportion of short telomeres significantly decreases. Since the primary goal is to prevent telomeres from shortening below the critical threshold beyond which cellular senescence begins, this is a very promising start!
An Excellent Telomerase Activator: TA-65®

Studies carried out on individuals taking TA-65®, the commercial name for this Astragalus root extract, have shown increased T-cell counts, improved immune function, greater bone density, but above all the lengthening of the shortest telomeres via telomerase activation. TA-65® has shown itself to be a transient activator, which does not cause any permanent genetic mutations. TA-65® preferentially affects the shortest telomeres, those which would halt cell division and lead to senescence.

Preserving Our Stock of Stem Cells

The Concept of an Organ's Functional Reserve

This is an organ's capacity to mobilize its margin of defense or functional capacity when exposed to an aggression or to stress. This margin enables it to return as quickly as possible to its normal function. For example, when we are twenty years old, we are lucky enough to possess 300 to 400% more functional reserve than is strictly necessary. From forty to fifty, we only have 150%, and when we reach our sixties we fall below 100%, which creates the risk of a loss of functionality for the organ in question in the presence of a stress, even a small one.

Our stem cells are responsible for producing this functional reserve. Naturally activating stem cells would therefore be a very promising step in combating aging and increasing lifespan and quality of life. Although it is now possible in certain countries to receive adult bone marrow stem cell injections, it is still far from being a common practice.

Hence the appeal of studies carried out in the past few years by some researchers who have managed, through the use of nutrients and plant extracts, to stimulate and increase the amount of adult bone marrow stem cells. Scientists are indeed prioritizing the use of bone marrow to achieve this regenerative effect since its cells evolve every day by producing new stocks of red and white blood cells and platelets. The mature cells are then released into the bloodstream where they perform their vital and regenerative functions.

Fucoidan

Well known in Japan for its immuno-stimulating and anticancer properties, Fucoidan is extracted from a type of algae, *Laminaria japonica*, which is part of the kelp family. This sulfated polysaccharide is in fact capable of strengthening the immune system, helping it fight off different kinds of viruses more effectively, and encouraging apoptosis in cancer cells, thereby improving the organism's defenses. In fact, it seems that people who consume large quantities of this substance have a longer lifespan, which is reflected in the longevity of the residents of Okinawa, for whom this type of brown algae is part of their daily diet. Scientific research on Fucoidan started in the 70s, and it has been the subject of nearly 700 publications since. Their findings, along with the pragmatic data provided by the longstanding use of Fucoidan-rich brown algae in Japan, as well as in Hawaii and Tonga, seem to indicate that Fucoidan is capable of mitigating a large number of health issues and increasing life expectancy. Just like other active ingredients extracted from algae, Fucoidan, in certain concentrations, has been shown to have stimulating properties for bone marrow stem cells. A clinical study in which healthy volunteers ingested three grams of Fucoidan daily for fifteen days showed significant increases in peripheral blood hematopoietic stem cell ratios. No side effects were observed.

4.3 - Hormones

When we talk about hormones, we mainly think of two fundamental issues. The first, inter and intracellular communication. This communication depends on the proportions of certain hormones which will interact with the cell membrane as well as with the intracellular milieu. The second issue is homeostasis. Hormones manage the integration of information among the different systems and organs, and work towards their optimal operation. They will, among other functions, maintain a constant balance between the brain, the immune system and the digestive system. Our functions communicate via a 'web'-like network, whose communication medium is made up of hormones. The brain coordinates this system. It sends out messages and in return receives information (this is called feedback). This back and forth exchange makes it possible to control communications between the brain and organs or between different organs; the result is continued health and optimal quality of life. This is the reason why it is essential to maintain optimal function of our hormonal neurotransmitters.

Pregnenolone :
The Memory Hormone

Pregnenolone is the precursor of most hormones, naturally synthesized in our body out of cholesterol. The synthesis takes place in the cells' mitochondria, under the effect of specific enzymes. Pregnenolone is a precursor of DHEA, progesterone, aldosterone and cortisone. For its part, DHEA is a precursor of testosterone and estrogens.

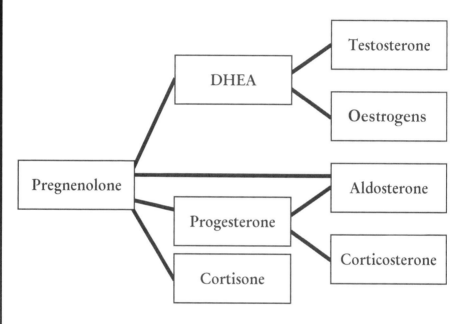

The organism produces hormones out of other hormones. Source: Thierry Hertoghe.

Pregnenolone levels decrease with age. Statistics show that around 75 years old, our levels are about 40% of those we have when we are 30. However recent studies by the European Institute of Aging show that concentrations of 20% or less are frequent in healthy individuals Pregnenolone is extremely important to brain function. Its concentration in the brain could be ten times higher than that of other hormones. Pregnenolone testing is not done in all labs, but more common tests showing low levels of hormones derived from it may warn of a potential deficiency. A blood count below 2 ng/ml is too low. Your doctor could prescribe, depending on the severity of the deficiency, between 5 and 50 mg of pregnenolone daily, taken orally, but watch out for excessive dosage!

Testosterone : Important, and Not Just for Men

Men synthesize around 10 to 20 times more testosterone than women (or at least until andropause, that is, as long as they are sexually active). During puberty, testosterone levels considerably increase and are responsible for sexual, bone and muscular development in men, as well as for behavioral changes. Testosterone levels then decrease with age, both in men and women. Contrary to popular belief, no study has ever shown testosterone to increase the risk of prostate cancer, nor that it would promote its development. On the contrary, studies on this subject note the positive effect of testosterone supplementation on prostate health. This seems logical, since testosterone levels of older individuals suffering from prostate cancer are generally very low, whereas this type of cancer almost never appears in young men with high testosterone levels. Total blood testosterone levels of 6 000 pg/ml for men and of 200 pg/ml for women are considered insufficient and therefore require a prescription. Testosterone is available as a topical gel, capsules or injections.

DHEA : A True Anti-Age Hormone

DHEA is the most abundant steroid hormone in the human body. Its levels are highest when we are twenty years old, and then sharply decline. DHEA is the subject of an impassioned debate concerning its anti-aging properties and its use as a routine supplement, as is often the case in the United States. One of the fundamental reasons for this controversy is due to the fact that the effects of DHEA are observed in the long term. It has almost no short-term effects (within a week, for example). However numerous studies have shown a correlation between DHEA and longevity in older men. Osteoporosis, AIDS, breast and other cancers, autoimmune diseases, cardiovascular diseases, Alzheimer's disease, thyroid diseases and diabetes are far more common in individuals with low DHEA levels. Studies on individuals over the age of 90 show that those who reach that age have higher than average levels of DHEA. Blood DHEA levels in young adults is on average between 150 and 400 µg/dl. In women, levels below 150 µg/dl and, in men, below 200, suggest a deficiency and could lead your doctor to prescribe oral DEHA supplements, of 5 to 25 mg/day for women and 25 to 50 mg/day for men.

Melatonin : The Sleep Hormone, but Also an Essential Antioxidant

Our organism produces thirty to sixty times more melatonin at night than during the day. It's our sleep hormone, which makes us fall asleep naturally. Melatonin is also a powerful antioxidant, boosts the immune system and inhibits cancer. Animal studies have shown that mice whose pineal gland (which produces melatonin) has been removed have more tumors. Melatonin supplementation prevents their appearance. Melatonin levels rapidly lower with age, being at their peak during adolescence.

Several studies have shown that melatonin stimulates the immune system, especially in older animals, or those who are stressed or sick. Melatonin stimulates the production of T-cells and natural killer cells. Thymus redevelopment has even been observed in older mice (remember that the thymus disappears in humans around our forties).

The sleep cycle, which is essential to a balanced life, is linked to the secretion of this hormone, whose role in health has been made abundantly clear. Decreased secretion, which is followed by sleep reduction, can lead to the early onset of age-related diseases. Melatonin is naturally produced by the epiphysis (or pineal gland, at the center of the brain) which plays a crucial role in the sleep-wake cycle. Normally it is released at nightfall to facilitate falling asleep. Secretion peaks between 2 and 4 AM and decreases during the second half of the night, in preparation for waking up. In the elderly, melatonin production is often insufficient, which can lead to sleep disorders. It might then be useful, in order to regain a healthy, restorative sleep cycle, to take melatonin, which 'resynchronizes' our internal clock.

Supplementation can start with very weak doses which can be adjusted according to results. Most often, 0.5 to 1 mg are enough, taken fifteen minutes before going to bed.

Melatonin doesn't make sleep last longer, but rather improves the quality of sleep. It is recommended in particular as an aid in withdrawal from hypnotics. In this case, melatonin is prescribed as Circadin® (or equivalent), a 2 mg sustained-release dose which is delivered throughout the night.

For jet lag, one tablet every night for three to five days on the way out and for six to eight days after the return trip are recommended. Some doctors also offer it as a night cream. These creams help repair aggressions endured by the skin during the day, as melatonin is a powerful antioxidant. Melatonin is a hormone, and should therefore be used with care. On the internet we can find supplements with 5 mg doses. Avoid them! This kind of overdosage leads to a crash in morning cortisol levels. Immunity is built up at night thanks to melatonin, but we need cortisol in the morning in order to mobilize our immune capabilities. Incorrect melatonin dosing could therefore disrupt the immune system. Furthermore, high doses modify thyroid hormones and cause nocturnal awakenings, the exact opposite of the desired effect.

We can naturally increase melatonin secretion with light. We need sufficient retinal cell stimulation during the day for melatonin to be secreted at night. A 20% increase in melatonin production has been demonstrated in elderly individuals suffering from cataracts (lens clouding) after surgery. Serotonin or tryptophan-rich foods, like milk, nuts or bananas, are beneficial to melatonin levels. Eating a banana between 4 and 6 PM makes it easier to fall asleep.

If we want to combat cellular aging effectively, we need to take good dietary supplements. Research and clinical studies have shown that it is possible to affect every level of cellular aging through appropriate supplementation. The latest advances made in understanding the role of telomerase, which have been awarded a Nobel Prize, lead us to believe that we are now entering a new era; the era of cellular regeneration, thanks to the combined action of telomerase activators and stem cells. Finally, we now have technology powerful enough to demonstrate the positive influence of dietary supplements on gene expression and therefore on our longevity.

SOURCES

David Servan-Schreiber.
Guérir. Paris : Laffont ; 2003.

David Servan-Schreiber.
Anticancer. Paris : Laffont ; 2007.

Dominique Rueff, Maurice Nahon.
Stratégie longue vie. Archamps : Éditions Jouvence ; 2013.

Richard Béliveau, Denis Gingras.
Les aliments contre le cancer. Québec : Trécarré ; 2005.

Thierry Hertoghe, Jules-Jacques Nabet.
Comment rester jeune plus longtemps ? Paris : Albin Michel ; 2000.

David Stipp.
The youth Pill. New York : Current, Penguin Group ; 2013.

Joseph C. Maroon, Jeffrey Bost.
Fish oil. Laguna Beach (Californie) : Basic Health Publications ; 2006.

Michael Fossel, Greta Blackburn, Dave Woynarowski.
The Immortality edge.
Hoboken (New Jersey) :
John Wiley & Sons, Inc. ; 2011. ProMotion Publishing ; 1997.

Ray Kurzweil, Terry Grossman.
Fantastic Voyage. New York : Plume Book ; 2005.

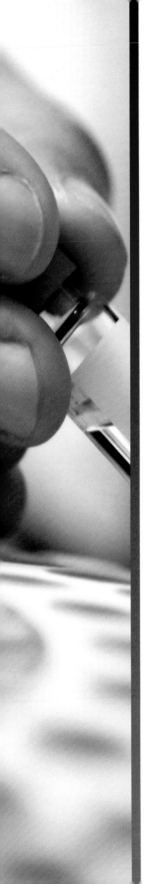

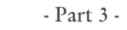

- Part 3 -

Chapter 5

The Promise of Epigenetics

« Genetics proposes, epigenetics disposes »

- Prof Walter Wahli -

Sequencing the entire human genome propelled our knowledge of genetics to a new level and led to the creation of new terms ending with the suffix « *ome* », meaning complete. The term genome therefore designates the entirety of the genetic material contained within our chromosomes. Genomics refers to the set of technologies which analyze our genes; transcriptomics describe the analysis of active genes; proteomics, the global analysis of all proteins.

Almost 99.8% of human DNA is identical in all of the human species, and our DNA differs from that of apes by only 2%; and yet... the differences are obvious! Similarly, this 0.2% variance between humans is what makes us all different, all unique, excepting monozygotic (identical) twins, who have exactly the same DNA. Not that long ago, we believed that everything came from our genes! We inherited our genes from our parents, which were mixed like we would shuffle a deck of cards, and the result of this mix gave birth to our own genes, which made us, in a way, by blending, gave us a unique personality. And that was it, our genes would stay static throughout our life. In actuality, this is not exactly right! It is true that the codes within our genes which are used to assemble our proteins are nearly written in stone within our 23 chromosome pairs, these libraries kept within the nucleus of each of our cells; but this big book of life, when read, is subject to our interpretation; just like a Beethoven symphony might be masterfully or blunderingly interpreted depending on the conductor and the musicians.

We have around 20,000 to 30,000 genes, very few of which are « *coding* » genes, that is, having assembly instructions. Some are active 24 hours a day, and manage those proteins which are essential to life: the heart, brain, kidneys. Most are inactive, or suppressed, and are only activated, or expressed, when necessary. But who decides when and where genes are activated, and how does this happen? Contrary to the widespread notion that we are programmed by our genetic code, scientists have shown that it is actually an index of datasets which can be activated or not, according to circumstances. Did you know that we therefore communicate with our genes every day, and that our genes are heavily influenced by what we tell them, and will act accordingly? Today, many researchers note that our actions, our experiences, our emotions, constantly shape gene expression. In fact, our 'biological fate' is only 30% determined by our genes, and 70% by our environment; this reality has led to a new field of study called «*epigenetics*», which literally means «*above*» genetics. A gene can therefore be activated or deactivated, and the implementation of the instructions it carries will only take place if it is ordered and supplied with the necessary energy.

5.1 - Epigenetics

«The difference between genetics and epigenetics can probably be compared to the difference between writing and reading a book. Once a book is written, the text (the genes or DNA: stored information) will be the same in all the copies distributed to the interested audience. However, each individual reader of a given book may interpret the story slightly differently, with varying emotions and projections as they continue to unfold the chapters. In a very similar manner, epigenetics would allow different interpretations of a fixed template (the book or genetic code) and result in different read-outs, dependent upon the variable conditions under which this template is interrogated.» Thomas Jenuwein (Max Planck Institute of Immunobiology and Epigenetics, Freiburg, Germany)

There are therefore factors besides the genetic code itself which guide and determine cell growth. What exactly influences the presence or activity of the cell's worker proteins in this way? We have learned that these influences operate at the level of individual genes by activating or deactivating them. Different organs and tissues do not have the same active genes. In brain cells, the genes which put heart cells together are inactive, and the opposite is true in heart cells. In this way, only 10 to 20% of genes are active in each type of biological tissue. Only those genes which perform tasks which are common to all cells, such as absorbing food, transforming it, growing and dividing, are active in all cells. The question which remains is through which factor, which process do genes become active or inactive depending on their environment?

Our body's functions are therefore governed both by our genetic code and our epigenetic configuration, also called its genomic imprinting. It consists of a set of switches which activate or deactivate genes. Epigenetics therefore allows us to escape to some extent from our genetic fate (Wahli). The interaction of their genotype and environment will determine an individual's « *phenotype* », that is, all of the anatomical, physiological and molecular characteristics which make each of us unique, even though we share an identical 99.8% of our genes.

Switch Molecules

The switches which control gene activity are small molecules which attach to certain parts of our DNA. Scientists have discovered that DNA could be epigenetically modified by small molecular groups bonding either directly to the DNA itself or to the histone proteins associated with it. During the DNA methylation process, enzymes (yet another kind of protein!) present within the cell drop a small molecule onto a gene in order to deactivate it, like placing a cap on a pen. This molecule makes the gene unreadable. The gene's activity is therefore controlled by the presence or absence of these proteins, which are themselves regulated by environmental signals. Epigenetics has deeply changed our understanding of cellular life. It is already possible, says Bruce Lipton, to create more than 2,000 protein variants out of a single genetic matrix. Even more importantly, a large number of studies have shown that environmental factors, diet, stress, and emotions in particular, can not only alter the duplication of genetic material, but modify the genes themselves.

The fact that our environment changes our genetic configuration shows that it is not static. All we need is to change our circumstances, our diet, exercise regimen, stress levels, for it to decline. But the opposite is also true. We can modify and improve, through a healthy lifestyle, an imperfect epigenetic configuration which finds itself unable to provide good health.

Stress and Epigenetics

Violence, mistreatment, sexual abuse, abandonment, leave an indelible trace in adulthood. A multitude of clinical studies have confirmed that those who have endured severe trauma in childhood are, on the whole, more likely to suffer from depression, substance abuse, asocial behavior, as well as obesity, diabetes and cardiovascular disease. Worse still, other studies have shown that children whose mothers have undergone intense psychological stress or trauma during pregnancy are at a higher risk of becoming anxious or depressed. This is an established psychological fact: there is a very clear link between psychological trauma and behavior. But what is this relationship embodied by? How can negative experiences etch themselves into the organism to the point that they can lastingly affect behavior or health?

Scientists from the University of California compared the DNA of mothers with healthy children with that of mothers with children suffering from serious chronic conditions, such as autism, or from chronic psychological stress, showed signs of premature aging. In particular, their telomeres were abnormally short, indicating accelerated aging in the range of 9 to 17 years!

But that isn't all. On top of attacking telomeres, the stress also makes its mark directly onto our genes, by modifying certain kinds of behavior in a targeted and lasting way. These epigenetic modifications are like small 'labels', methyl groups, which tell the cellular machinery which genes it should make use of or ignore. Biologists now see that psychological stress and trauma lead to epigenetic labeling mistakes in the hippocampus, the part of the brain which controls emotion.

A team led by Michael Meaney, at McGill University (Canada), has proven this by comparing the brains of baby rats which were nurtured by their mothers to those of neglected rats. Neglect leads to epigenetic changes

which block the gene used to produce corticoid receptors in the hippocampus. These receptors control the stress response by decreasing levels of corticoids, the hormone released in case of stress, in the blood. The neglected rats have fewer cortisol receptors and are therefore less equipped to deal with stress. They are always anxious, suffer from memory disorders and exhibit signs of depression. Even in adulthood, unexpected events are taken entirely out of proportion.

We have seen a proliferation of studies in the last few years which confirm the role the environment and life experience play in the onset of mental disorders.

In 2008, Canadian researchers at the Center for Addiction and Mental Health compared the brains of individuals suffering from schizophrenia or bipolar disorder to those of a control population. 40 genes were found in the former which had abnormal methylation. For most of them, these genes were involved in brain development or transmitting messages between neurons.

Scientists are still far from being able to clearly distinguish nature from nurture in psychiatric illnesses. But some of the data is quite troubling, and we sometimes need to go back quite far in an individual's personal history, before their birth, to find the origin of their illness. *I think that most chronic illnesses such as asthma, cancer, diabetes, obesity, and neurological illnesses (autism, bipolar disorder, schizophrenia) are partially the result of poor epigenetic management during the first developmental stages*, says Randy Jirtle, the director of the epigenetics lab at Duke University, in the United States.

While an individual's genome remains quite stable during their lifetime, all of their epigenetic markers which regulate gene expression, their 'epigenome', is constantly being modified as a reaction to external variations. And this is precisely its role: *the epigenome is an interface between our genes, which are static, and our environment, which is always changing,* says Randy Jirtle. In this way, the genetic 'orchestration' remains the same, but its interpretation may vary over time, depending on its epigenetic marking.

But if the epigenetic marking is dynamic, could it be reversible? An experiment by researchers at Rockefeller University in New York suggests this may be the case. They managed, in November of 2009, to cancel out the epigenetic effects caused by stress in the brains of young mice, by giving them Prozac, an antidepressant. Thankfully, positive emotions can also leave a mark. In 2008, work carried out at *Massachusetts General Hospital* showed that eight weeks of relaxation were enough to modify the expression of several hundred genes, in direct opposition to the effects brought about by stress. Furthermore, a new study done at Saarland University in Homburg has just shown that physical activity slows down telomere shortening in white blood cells.

But the epigenetic marking of our genes may also be transmitted to our offspring, and cause them to experience the weight of our past. This was demonstrated by a famous study, carried out it 1992, on the famine which had struck the Netherlands in 1945. In reaction to the lack of food, children conceived during this period were smaller than average, and had a higher risk, as adults, of suffering from diabetes or cardiovascular disease. Nothing unexpected so far. But what is surprising is that their own children also suffer from low birthweight and poor health. The problem: the epigenetic mark left by famine which was transmitted over two generations. Epigenetic markings are certainly reversible and malleable, but they can also be transmitted, almost identically, to our offspring.

5.2 - Nutrigenomics

Nutritional genomics, or nutrigenomics, focuses on the direct impact of food on genes and their expression, that is, the way in which they are activated. For example, if you eat a pizza, we will study how this pizza selects a portion of your genes, activates them, and influences your metabolism. In this way, every type of food has its own sort of 'genetic signature'. The constituent parts of your diet act as signals which regulate gene activity. How? Micronutrients in your diet are either incorporated into cells and transported to the nucleus where they will bond to transcription factors, or directly influence gene expression.

'*Nutrigenetics*' does the opposite. It focuses on our genes' influence on our diet and our way of eating. Why, for example, do some people get fatter while eating very little, whereas others may stuff themselves and not gain a single pound. Thanks to modern technology, we can define subpopulations of individuals with a genetic make-up rendering them susceptible to certain illnesses, in order to attempt to better adapt their diet. These genotypes have been identified for a large number of ailments, such as, for example, lactose intolerance, which affects 1 to 5% of Northern Europeans and nine out of ten Africans and Asians.

The Promise of Nutrigenomics

Today we better understand the influence of our genes on the appearance of our illnesses and aging. But at the same time, researchers are increasingly faced with the incredible complexity of this genetic influence. Furthermore, the risk of developing an illness is highly dependent on environmental factors. In this way, genetic and environmental factors both contribute to the appearance of a metabolic imbalance; but their respective contributions remain very difficult to determine.

This is the context in which nutrigenomics and nutrigenetics are working, and they will be playing an increasingly essential role. Nutrigenetics brings to light new 'candidate genes', which can predispose us to certain diseases. Nutrigenomics, meanwhile, allows us to understand the importance of our diet in the appearance and progression of a disease.

The health risks of coffee consumption have repeatedly been researched, and the results are contradictory to say the least, some studies saying that coffee is bad for your heart and others stating the opposite. The nutrigenetic approach has given us a definitive answer. Coffee consumption leads to an increased risk of myocardial infarction in individuals with a specific polymorphism leading to the loss of cytochrome P450 1A2, a caffeine detoxification protein.

Diet has a considerable influence in the prevention, or conversely, in the promotion, of many age-related illnesses: cancer, degenerative diseases and silent inflammation. Nutrigenomics is useful during the early stages of a disease, where it helps in slowing the progression of initial symptoms, and promoting a return to homeostasis. To achieve this, it needs reliable biological markers, which are able to detect any deviations, no matter how small. Nanotechnology is starting to produce this generation of biological markers.

Nutrigenomics is behind the emergence of a predictive, individualized form of healthcare. This type of care, which aims to evaluate health risks individually before they appear, and detect, via biomarkers, molecules indicating the early stages of disorders, is then able to formulate dietary recommendations.

Beyond this, interactions between drugs and food are very numerous and must be taken into consideration when determining the conditions necessary for introducing drugs to the market. Certain nutrients may bond to certain drugs and render them useless. The calcium and iron in food, for example, decreases the absorption of some antibiotics, and vitamin K can interfere with certain types of anticoagulants. Taking anti-inflammatory drugs (or aspirin) may give us heartburn if taken in conjunction with certain types of citrus. Thanks to nutrigenomics we can already determine dietary constraints, the nature and proportions of which will make it possible to develop very effective weapons to improve treatments such as chemotherapy or antiretroviral drugs to combat AIDS.

5.3 - Genetic Tests

A great many companies have recently mushroomed on the web, offering individualized advice based on saliva samples. After analyzing their genotype, these companies will offer a consulting service to incite interested clients to change their lifestyle or take drastic measures, as Angelina Jolie has. These tests have not, for now, had a lot of impact on consumers, but the rapid progress being made in this field will certainly pique the public's interest, and it is therefore crucial to identify the objectives, benefits, and dangers of such tests, and what they entail.

Although their scientific foundation is solid, it would seem that these tests are not yet ready to enter the market. A recent evaluation of the recommendations given by seven internet-based companies has shown that they severely lacked conclusive scientific evidence. This led to them being termed « *genetic horoscopes* ». The evaluation covered three key elements: the tests themselves, their interpretation, that is, the validity of the correlations made to the risk of developing a disease, and finally their recommendations.

5.4 - Genetic Polymorphisms

We are all different. This is obvious morphologically, but it is also true metabolically. Although our DNA is 99.8% identical to our neighbor's, the remaining 0.2% makes us 'unique'. Geneticists refer to these variables of our genetic make-up as genetic polymorphisms. We have three billion nucleotides (the basic unit of DNA) in our genome, and, on average, one nucleotide out of every one thousand changes from one individual to the next. If one of these differences is found in more than 1% of the population, it is called an SNP, a Single Nucleotide Polymorphism.

We have already identified several million SNPs, responsible for our eye color, our corpulence, as well as our potential to develop certain diseases. Identifying the profile of SNPs allow us to define groups of individuals who are at-risk for certain diseases and adapt their diet and potential treatment. Thanks to new technologies, in particular DNA microarrays, we are able to examine, in one go, several hundreds of thousands of SNPs in an individual, and thereby define a 'genotype', that is, their comprehensive genetic composition, that which will be transmitted to their offspring, and which might include predispositions to certain diseases.

Nevertheless, this does not mean we can conclusively call a polymorphism good or bad in and of itself: it entirely depends on the environment within which it arises. For example, many polymorphisms will be good or bad for us depending on our diet. This is how different human genotypes lead to individualized reactions to environmental factors: diet, medication, pollutants... and influence our longevity.

Epigenetics is a new field of study that is shaking up everything we know about genetics. All experts used to agree that our genes determined 100% of our fate. We now know that they are only 30% responsible for it. The other 70% depend on our emotional, social, and physical environment, on the quality of the air we breathe, the water we drink, the food we eat, our physical activity, pollutants, toxins etc. There are therefore other factors besides the genetic code itself which guide and determine cell growth. The realization that our environment alters our genetic configuration shows that this configuration is not static. All we need is to change our circumstances for it to decline. But the opposite must then also be true. An epigenetic expression which finds itself unable to keep us healthy can be modified and improved through a healthy lifestyle. Nutrigenomics, or nutritional genomics, focuses on the direct impact of food on genes and their expression, while nutrigenetics does the opposite: it focuses on our genes 'influence on our diet and our way of eating. Diet has a considerable influence in the prevention of many age-related illnesses. Thanks to nutrigenomics, we can already determine dietary constraints and requirements which will represent a very effective weapon to improve treatments such as chemotherapy or antiretroviral drugs to combat AIDS.

SOURCES

Frédéric Dardel, Renaud Leblond.

Main basse sur le génome. Paris : Anne Carrière Éditions ; 2008.

Helena Baranova.

Nos gènes, notre santé, et nous. Paris : Armand Colin ; 2004.

Walter Wahli, Nathalie Constantin.

La nutrigénomique dans votre assiette. Bruxelles : Éditions De Boeck ; 2011.

Brandon Colby.

Outsmart Your Genes. New York : Perigee Book ; 2010.

Vincent C. Giampapa, Frederick F. Buechel, Ohan Karatoprack.

The Gene Makeover. Laguna Beach (Californie) : Basic Health ; 2007.

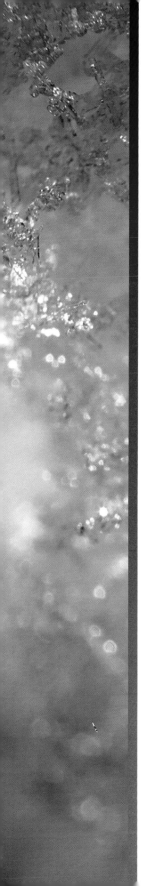

Chapter 6

And What about Cryonics?

« Death is not when life turns off. People can and have survived being - turned off - »

- Alcor Life Extension Foundation -

Cryonics is a process of cryopreservation (low-temperature preservation, □ 196° C) of all or part of living beings, in the hopes of one day resuscitating them. Current medical knowledge and know-how is not capable of reversing this process. In the United States, it can only be performed on humans for whom a death certificate has been signed, and only if their clinical death is not too advanced. It is forbidden in France. Cryonics is part of the broad field of low-temperature biological matter preservation, and hopes to interrupt all biological processes and preserve tissues and organs from aging. It isn't freezing but rather vitrification, a sophisticated process which uses cryoprotectants in order to prevent the formation of ice crystals in the tiny structures within tissues (cryosuspension).

Cryonics advocates try to justify this method through three criteria, the scientific validity of which is not yet well established.

1 - Life can be interrupted, then resumed, provided that its basic structures remain intact during cryopreservation.

Cryonics specialists point out studies which suggest that cryoprotectants, when circulated in the brain in high concentrations before being cooled, could prevent it from being damaged and conserve the cells' fine structure, the supposed seat of memory and identity. For opponents, we cannot justify the practice of cryonics, given the current limitations of this technique; indeed, we are only able to reversibly cryopreserve the cells, tissues and blood vessels of small animal organs, embryos and sperm. Certain frog species can indeed survive a few months in a frozen state, a few degrees Celsius below zero, but this is no longer the case if they are cryopreserved. Supporters respond that reversibility does not have to be demonstrable yet; if it is already possible to preserve the information contained in the brain, we have, theoretically, prevented its death, until its restoration is later made possible.

2 - Vitrification, contrarily to freezing, may be able to perfectly preserve the integrity of our functions.
The problem lies in the fact that cryonic operations cannot be carried out until legal death has been declared, that is, after cerebral death has been observed; cardiac arrest is not enough. But blood flow is interrupted when the heart stops, leading to ischemic injury: without a supply of oxygen and

nutrients, cells, tissues and organs begin to deteriorate. If the heart takes too long to restart, the oxygen which is reintroduced can cause even more damage due to oxidative constraints, which is known as reperfusion injury. Cryonicists are working to minimize reperfusion and ischemic injury by cooling the body down and putting it on life support as soon as death has been declared. Antioxidants and anticoagulants, such as heparin, may also be injected.

3 - Methods by which to repair possible damage may soon be available.

Cryonicists are basing their hopes on the progress of nanomedicine but it is universally agreed that cryopreservation reversibility will not be achievable in the short term. Optimists look to bioengineering, or molecular nanotechnology. Returning to life requires the reparation of damage caused by the lack of oxygen, cryoprotectant toxicity, thermal constraints, and ice crystals forming in tissues which were unsuccessfully vitrified; in many cases, this will require substantial tissue regeneration. Current scenarios for achieving this generally envision using microscopic organisms or machines to restore cellular structures at the molecular level, and if possible prior to warming the body. 'Mind transfer' is another approach, in the event that a technology able to scan the memory of a preserved brain one day appears. It may take us centuries to find a way to reverse the current process, combining neurovitrification and cooling. It may even remain impossible.

Neuropreservation

Neuropreservation is the cryopreservation of the brain, most often along with the rest of the head. To achieve this, we first have to surgically separate it from the rest of the body. Sometimes abbreviated to 'neuro', it is one of the two choices offered to candidates, the other being the preservation of the entire body. The basic argument in favor of neuropreservation is that our memory, personality and identity are all stored in the brain's chemical structure. It is also justified by the idea that if future technologies were able to repair the damage caused by cryonics and reverse the process, they would probably also be able to regenerate the rest of the body.

Beyond the scientific aspect, and the likelihood of achieving the outcome hoped for by the proponents of this technology, cryonics is confronted with social, cultural, moral and symbolic obstacles. Death has a very particular status in all cultures, as do corpses. The respect owed to the dead is in fact the reason why cryonics is prohibited in France.

The cost of cryopreservation varies tremendously, going from 28,000 American dollars to preserve an entire body at the Cryonics Institute, to 80,000 for Neuropreservation and 200,000 for the cryopreservation of the entire body at Alcor or the American Cryonics Society.

☐ REMEMBER ☐

Cryonics still finds itself within the realm of science-fiction even if certain scientific facts may lead to its validation. It remains a field of clinical experimentation, with only a few hundred participants who pay a small fortune to participate in this program, arguing that they are better off being in the experimental group than the control group!

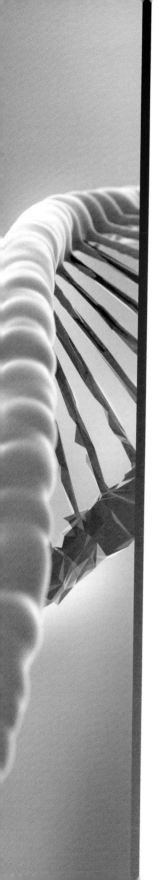

- Part 3 -
Conclusions

« *Death is a problem to be resolved, not a*
reality imposed by Nature. »

- Dr Laurent Alexandre / La mort de la mort -

Existing knowledge and technology already make it possible for us to live longer, all while remaining healthy. Since the beginning of the 20th century, we have continually extended our life expectancy, by three months each year, or by 25% today! Or even by six hours each day! Since our ability to lengthen the human lifespan has been established, the key question is whether we can do it better and faster. The answer: « *Yes, we can do it better! Yes, we can also do it faster!* » But this depends entirely on us.

Science generally moves forward by small, successive steps, and rarely makes spectacular discoveries. But we have reached a point where our knowledge and our technologies can add twenty years to our lifespan, long enough for a new Nobel Prize winner to make a discovery just as groundbreaking as that of telomerase activators, and add another twenty years, and so on... For now, the most effective strategies combat age-related chronic illnesses: diabetes, cancer, cardiovascular diseases, Alzheimer's disease, macular degeneration, and many others! We will gain those extra twenty years thanks to the progress made in this field. Additionally, recent studies make it possible for us to produce molecules which protect the cellular machinery from nuclear and mitochondrial DNA damage, oxidative damage, the harmful effects of inflammation, and the negative effects of glycation.

With stem cells, we are moving into an as-of-yet unexplored field: cellular regeneration, the possibility of providing new, young cells where they are needed. This new biotechnology will revolutionize medicine. Athletes today can see their professional careers extended by several years thanks to stem cell injections in their elbows or knees. In the same way, a patient can avoid having knee prostheses. Type 1 diabetes will soon be cured, also thanks to stem cell injections. We are already targeting Parkinson's and Alzheimer's disease. New technologies which use iPS cells make it possible, out of a simple skin cell, to recreate every type of living tissue to then transplant them, or even to use them in therapeutic trials, costing ten times less money and time than traditional methods.

Thanks to telomerase activators, a human cell can become immortal. The only unresolved obstacle is that we do not yet know how to achieve this for tissues or organs, let alone the entire body. Tens of thousands of individuals regularly take TA-65®, the only activator whose effectiveness has been clinically proven. But others will soon follow. Measuring the length of telomeres is no longer exclusive to academic centers, it is now an option for the general public.

The advances made in genetics, epigenetics and nutritional genomics are already tangible. We know what impacts certain molecules have on gene expression and understand the relationships between certain foods and gene expression. Very soon, we will be able to provide anyone with individualized menus according to their epigenetic profile. Epigenetic biomarkers and genetic polymorphism tests will very soon be able to give us real information on our health risks.

Nanomedicine already makes it possible for us to build or repair, molecule by molecule, and soon atom by atom, anything which potentially could be damaging. Even better, this nanotechnology will make it possible for us to make a molecular, or even atomic diagnosis, to then target treatment at the same level.

The exponential increase in computing speeds along with the emergence of artificial intelligence will allow us to better understand the brain and vanquish the scourges which plague it.

Even more revolutionary, all of these new technologies cross-pollinate. By reaching the nanometer scale, we will be able to create communications between neurons, atoms, genes and computers, and each element of the system will become a communicating part of the whole!

But the greatest part of it all is that we can ride this technological wave. We can play our part alongside restorative biotechnologies and regenerative medicine. Let us finally decide to take charge of our genetic expression. Let's work on our lifestyle, the way we eat, move, think, feel, and the way we talk to others. By doing this, we will repress our bad genes and activate those which are good for us.

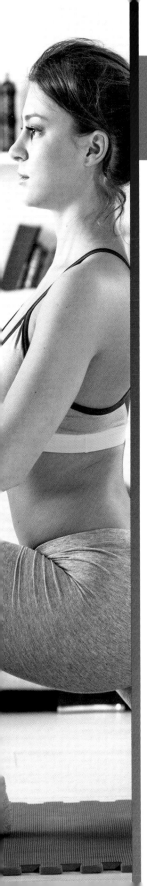

Part 4

LIFESTYLE AND LONGEVITY

Introduction

Chapter 1 : Nutrition and Longevity

Chapter 2 : Physical Activity and Longevity

Chapter 3 : Stress and Longevity

Conclusion

Introduction

« By the time we learn to live it's already too late.» »

- Louis Aragon -

Dr. Dean Ornish, from the University of San Francisco, followed up men with slow-growing prostate cancer for twelve months. During a three day long intensive workshop, these men learned the importance of taking their health into their own hands. They learned to eat differently: very little saturated fat and an almost entirely vegetarian diet, with lots of fruits, vegetables, pulses and whole-grain starches. At the same time, they reduced their processed sugar and white flour consumption. They performed moderate exercise (walking or equivalent) for at least thirty minutes a day, six days a week, and learned how to manage stress through breathing exercises or relaxation methods such as yoga or meditation, at least six days a week as well. They also took daily dietary supplements containing soya protein, fish oil, vitamin E, vitamin C and selenium. After six months, the cancer had stopped its progression in more than 70% of patients. Even more astonishing is that after only three months, telomerase activity grew by 30%, thanks to this diet.

Today it has become obvious that our health is determined by the quality of the air we breathe, by our diet, by tobacco, by drugs and toxic substances, by physical exercise, by mental strain, by the stress we undergo, as well as by the love and friendship which we receive. In the past few years, science has confirmed the validity of these obvious truths. Scientific proof showing that quality of life, psychologically as well as in terms of our environment, modify the state of our genes by activating or deactivating them. Most geneticists now believe that our genes' behavior can be modified by our life experiences, and that these changes can even be transmitted to future generations. Genetically identical twins with significant differences in lifestyle were studied, for example. As they grew and developed, they were exposed to different experiences, in different physical and psychological environments, and their appearance changed. One stayed healthy while the other contracted cancer. How was this possible? This can be explained by an epigenetic mechanism linked to living conditions. Cancer-protection genes were deactivated in one and not the other. Although they are genetically identical, this is not the case epigenetically. Dr. Arturas Petonis, from the University of Toronto, believes epigenetics may hold the answer to certain unsolved mysteries: why would one monozygotic twin develop a chronic illness and not the other? Why are certain diseases more common in men than in women? It is now accepted that epigenetic alterations play a part in the appearance of cancer, and that they are often far more important than the alteration of the genes themselves. Certain genes are activated or deactivated by living conditions. Cigarettes, for example, not only cause genetic mutations, but also epigenetic alterations, by activating certain genes. Yet another example: researchers have seen more than 220 harmful genes being activated in cancerous cells in severely depressed women with poor emotional support networks; while these same disruptive genes remained inactive in women who were well integrated socially.

These discoveries will have major repercussions on cancer therapy; as epigenetic alterations are reversible, it may not be necessary to systematically kill cancer cells. Restoring the proper activation or repression of certain genes could be essential.

If everything is working properly, our cells regularly renew themselves throughout our life. Some die, others divide, producing two new cells, and this cycle is continually perpetuated. Unfortunately, environmental aggressions can bring about epigenetic alterations which will accumulate with time. Today we can bring these alterations to light at the cellular level and we indeed find that the elderly have more epigenetic alterations than younger individuals. It is even possible to guess someone's biological age simply by analyzing their epigenetic diagram. The good news is that our epigenetic configuration is not unalterable, we only need to modify our living conditions (diet, breathing, physical exercise, stress levels) for it to improve. Rachel Yehuda, of the Mount Sinai School of Medicine in New-York, studied stress in pregnant women who were in or near New York's World Trade Center during the events of September 11th 2001. She measured cortisol levels, which indicate stress, in the children once they were born, and these turned out to be quite high. The mothers' stress had been transmitted to their children. She also tested WWII concentration camp survivors, as well as their children, born much later. She also discovered that cortisol levels in these children were much (up to three times) higher than in the general public. Yet these children, now adults, never experienced the camps beyond what they had been told about them. And they were no more exposed to traumatic events than the rest of the population. Could this effect be due to their parents speaking about this trauma in front of them? Although this could be a partial answer, it cannot explain every case, as even babies less than one year old, to whom these events have not yet been described, have high cortisol levels. Stress levels in these individuals are therefore directly linked to past psychological trauma which their parents underwent. They were transmitted to them epigenetically, in the absence of any other traumatic event. Even more surprising; research shows that parents will 'anticipate' their children's genetic characteristics in the months leading up to conception (Alain Boudet).

In the final stages of sperm and egg maturation, a process called 'genomic imprinting' adjusts the activity of specific groups of genes which will shape the identity of the yet to be conceived child (Surani, 2001; Reik& Walter, 2001). Research suggests that events taking place in parents' lives when genomic imprinting occurs have a profound influence on their child's body and mind. Being the product of love or of indifference makes a difference; being in the womb of a mother who wishes to be pregnant or one who does not matters (Bruce Lipton).The quality of our intrauterine life will program our vulnerability to cardiovascular disease, heart attacks, diabetes, obesity and myriad other future conditions. Mounting evidence is showing that our intrauterine living conditions are just as influential as our genes on our long-term health and therefore on our longevity. This intrauterine life will determine our future behavior, both psychologically and physiologically, and will continue to influence us throughout our lives.

When speaking about the component parts of our lifestyle, we should not forget to include our thought patterns. Our fears, our anxieties, our inhibitions, are the product of our reactions to the events we live through. They influence our DNA epigenetically. The more questions we ask, the more curious we are, the more we enjoy life, and the more our neurons activate, the more connections are established, the more our brain stays in shape. Aging is best fought off by staying active, intellectually and physically.

Aging as we see it today is the result of all of these disruptive phenomena coming together to increasingly upset our cellular world. We can certainly focus on aggravating factors and reduce risk. Some risks we choose to subject ourselves to: sun exposure, smoking, drinking too much coffee, too much alcohol, taking drugs, eating too much fat etc. This is all the more significant when we combine several of these behaviors. Other risks we endure: extended exposure to low doses of radiation, to pollutants – air pollution from nitrogen oxide and asbestos, dust, rug and carpeting adhesives, cleaning products. All of these disturb our body's metabolisms. We have good reasons to be optimistic, however, as our lifespan and health are continually improving despite all of this. A girl born in France today has a one in two chance of living to be 100. Today, 90% of women reach their 80s. In 2004 life expectancy was 76.7 for men and 83.8 for women, or an average of 80 years of age for both genders. We could extend lifespan by an extra thirty years for most people, and especially ensure that these extra years be lived in good health. Although we can't have much influence on our genetic heritage or the environment we live in, we can control our lifestyle, our diet, how we maintain our body, our sleep, our tolerance to stress. The challenge today is not to become immortal, but rather to thrive throughout our expanded longevity.

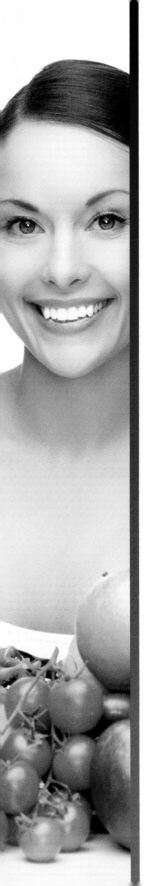

Chapter 1

Nutrition and Longevity

« Food, our third medicine »

- Dr Jean Seignalet -

Healthier eating boosts our longevity. This is no longer cause for debate in scientific circles. But how can it be explained? Our health, and therefore our longevity, depend on the speed with which our organism is able to return to a state of balance (what we call homeostasis) after undergoing any sort of change or stress. This return to equilibrium requires the triggering of thousands of chemical reactions in a matter of seconds. In order to accomplish this, our organism uses specific proteins, called enzymes, which will initiate, catalyze or repress certain chemical reactions depending on the situation. Our organism will acquire these proteins by activating certain genes which will in turn order their production. This is where our diet matters: it will influence the activation of certain genes and the repression of others depending on the specific demands for homeostasis.

June 1944, the allied forces land in Normandy, determined to rid Europe of the Nazi occupier. In September 1944, in the Netherlands, the British lead operation «Market Garden», in an attempt to reclaim bridges crossing the main Dutch rivers, including the Rhine, in Arnhem. The local Dutch seize upon this operation to rebel against the Nazi regime. Unfortunately, the operation fails, and the Dutch citizenry is punished for having taken part. Their food rations are cut to absurdly small portions. One adult ration is shrunk to 580 calories per day (about one quarter of the minimum requirement for a human being).On top of this, the winter of 1944-1945 is particularly harsh, and makes the little available food even less accessible. This period was later called the Dutch famine (or «winter of hunger»).Pregnant women found themselves among the undernourished adults. As they were starving, their newborns were in poor health and smaller than average. Horrific, but not surprising, given the circumstances. What is surprising is that the girls born in these conditions, adults by the 1960s, also gave birth to scrawny children! And these girls, once grown up in the 1980s, gave birth to small babies, and so on... This terrible famine which *pregnant women suffered in 1944, led to permanent changes in their gene pool, which were then inherited from generation to generation.*

1.1 - Too Many Calories

We eat too much! The calorie content of our diet is an ordeal for our digestive system, and this excess impacts on our organism all the way down to the cellular level. It leads to inflammatory and oxidative spikes which precipitate telomere shortening. Our billions of cells depend on proper nutrition to accomplish their work eliminating toxic substances, repairing DNA damage and keeping us healthy. Think about your last really big meal, for Thanksgiving for example. How did you feel right after? Lethargic, tired? Ready to go for a run? Certainly not! Maybe you were beginning to regret drinking too much, or taking too much of that delicious chocolate. Learning to eat less is not that hard, though.

The impact of the ever-increasing availability of hyper caloric industrial food is catastrophic for our health. People have become accustomed to eating excessively, says Bärbel Knäuper, assistant professor at McGill University's Health Psychology Laboratory (Montreal). *Perhaps they ate a bit too much the day before, and the day before that; actually, they probably have been eating a bit too much for a while.* Many people are not aware that they are eating more calories than they are burning; simply because they don't know how many they burn when they exercise, how many there are in the foods they eat, and how many they should eat every day. In addition to this, *when we eat too fast, our brain doesn't have the time to register the message the body is sending it, telling it it's full* (Béliveau). We think we are still hungry when that is not necessarily the case; the organism takes some time to tell the brain that it has eaten enough. Therefore, if we accumulate too many calories and we are sedentary, we can be sure that we will gain weight, and especially abdominal fat. Eating less would solve one part of the equation. The example of calorie restriction is striking. There is considerable evidence that calorie restriction in the range of 50%, while respecting essential nutrient requirements, leads to a substantial increase in longevity, at least in monkeys and mice. For humans, experiments are more difficult to carry out; but we have noticed that most people over 100 practice some form of calorie restriction. We still do not know why calorie restriction would increase longevity, however…

1.2 - Calorie restriction and Longevity

« If we eat less, we age less! »

Yes, you read that right! If we eat less (in terms of calories), we considerably improve our chances of living longer…and in good health.
Calorie restriction has remained the most scientifically researched method for the past eighty years. Everything started in 1930, when scientists at Cornell University discovered that rodents subjected to a nearly starvation diet lived up to 50% longer than average; and that during this period of hyper-longevity they maintained the activity levels of young adults while demonstrating a significant delay in the appearance of age-related diseases.

In 1989, researchers began a very important study on rhesus monkeys. These animals were chosen because they exhibit biological characteristics and an aging process which are very close to those of human beings. The monkeys were divided into two groups. One could feed itself normally, unhindered. The other's diet was 30% smaller than it would normally have been. After twenty years, 30% of the control subjects had died of age-related causes, compared to only 13% of the calorie-restricted group .In other words, calorie restriction divided the risk of degenerative diseases by three. Cardiovascular risk indicators, such as blood pressure and triglyceride levels, were lowered, glycemic control was improved, and cancer rates diminished. Cardiovascular disease rates were halved. The animals undergoing calorie restriction lost fat and not muscle mass, contrary to the other group. No primate in this group showed any symptoms of loss of glycemic control or diabetes, whereas 40% of the monkeys which had eaten as much as they wanted were pre-diabetic. Calorie restriction also inhibited brain volume reduction, in particular in the areas controlling motor and cognitive function. The primates undergoing calorie restriction were therefore more alert and in better health than their freely-feeding kin. The question all of the researchers asked themselves was of course: why?

Why does calorie restriction lead to all of these beneficial outcomes, not only for rhesus monkeys, but also for human beings, as can be seen in Okinawa, an island where many live to be 100, or in certain villages in Sardinia, Greece, and even California?

To understand this, we must once more return to our genes. Certain genes can remain inactive our entire lives… unless some kind of danger comes along and threatens the life of an individual or of the species. That is when a specific type of gene will be activated: survival genes. Their mission is to protect the animal species they inhabit.

Researchers have identified a gene family called sirtuins, which are present in the tissues of almost every life form, from single-cell organisms to plants and mammals. Aging is a highly regulated mechanism which is genetically controlled by these genes, whose task is to activate the production of a specific enzyme protein called SIRT. This enzyme, a deacetylase, improves DNA stability and inhibits the assembly of abnormal DNA.

Increasingly extensive data suggest that sirtuins regulate energy metabolism and endocrine signaling. Sirtuin genes are also activated by a wide range of signals, in response to stresses such as periods of famine or caloric restriction. This suggests that they play an important role in mammalian physiology. They are known to act as guardian genes, protecting cells and improving their chances of survival. They become active when external signals indicate the deterioration of environmental conditions. These longevity genes then wake up in order to induce defensive modifications at the cellular level, such as slowing down our metabolism and increasing cellular respiration, to help the organism adapt to a better survival program. It has also been shown that a second Sirtuin, SIRT2, which is found in yeast, activates when subjected to stress: it increases DNA stability and accelerates cell repair, all while increasing overall cell lifespan. More generally, Sirtuin activation may increase insulin and lipolysis sensitivity, decrease inflammation and play a preventive role in neurodegenerative diseases and cancer formation.

Even short periods of calorie restriction can improve our health and longevity. Walter Breuning, an American citizen from Montana, died when he was 114 years old: his secret to long life? He fasted one day a week nearly his entire life.

Ever since the publication, in February 2012, of an experimental study which evaluated the effect of fasting on cancerous tumors in mice (Lee, 2012. *Fasting cycles retard growth of tumors and sensitize a range of cancer cell types to chemotherapy*), many people have been enquiring about the value of this practice for cancer patients.

Results have shown that:

- Two cycles of fasting slowed the growth of some cancer cells - breast, melanoma, and glioma - just as effectively as chemotherapy.

- Combining fasting and chemotherapy increases DNA breakage in cancer cells, which potentiates the effects of chemotherapy, that is, increases its effectiveness.

Even better: multiple fasting cycles may increase the sensitivity of cancer cells to chemotherapy treatments, which would increase overall survival, as well as survival without disease progression in mice. Fasting may increase the regulation of genes involved in normal as well as cancerous cell growth. Thus, reduction in cancer cell numbers has been observed *in vitro*.

Researchers at the University of California, Los Angeles (UCLA) have shown that intermittent but prolonged fasting - between three and four consecutive days -not only protects our immune system from environmental damage, but also boosts the regeneration of the damaged immune system, by recycling old immune cells and stimulating stem cell production. This study is particularly relevant not only for immunosuppressed subjects but also for subjects suffering from autoimmune diseases.

1.3 - Too Much Sugar

We eat too much sugar! In 1830, we ate 5 kg per year on average. In the year 2000, France reached a record of 35kg per year per person, whereas the United States reached 70 kg: a family of four eats nearly 300 kg per year!

When we eat sugar, our blood glucose levels rapidly increase; our pancreas immediately releases insulin in order to allow the glucose to penetrate into the cell. This secretion is accompanied by the release of IGF (*Insulin-like growth factor-1*), a molecule which stimulates cell growth. Insulin and IGF will also cause an increase in inflammation. Today, we know that these insulin and IGF spikes not only promote the growth of cancer cells, but also their ability to invade neighboring tissue.

Too much sugar is bad for your health, this won't be news to you. We add sugar to food in the form of sucrose (table sugar) or high-fructose corn syrup. In both cases, the sugar is produced by assembling a glucose and a fructose molecule. If we eat too much table sugar, a large portion of it will be turned into fat. Fructose syrup is more complicated, as our metabolism is helpless when faced with this substance, which accumulates as fat in our liver. This ingredient is used when producing foie gras, by force-feeding geese or ducks corn, a source of fructose.

Eating too much fructose may also have a negative impact on blood pressure. A study made up of 4 528 participants showed that consuming 74 g of fructose per day, the equivalent of about four cans of soft drink, would increase the risk of high blood pressure by 28% to 87%.

Soft drinks, as well as their more recent derivatives (energy drinks, vitamin water, and fruit juice cocktails) are calorie 'bombs', sometimes containing more than 40 g of sugar per can. These calories, which do not trigger any feeling of fullness, are added on top of those provided by our food. Several scientific studies have clearly shown that these drinks lead to weight gain, the appearance of type 2 diabetes, cardiovascular disease and potentially an increased frequency of cancer. A review of recent epidemiological studies found that drinking one or two cans per day significantly increases the risk of developing type 2 diabetes and cardiovascular diseases.

According to a study published in the American Journal of Public Health, the regular consumption of sugary drinks is linked with shorter telomeres. During this study, which was carried out on more than 5 000 healthy adults, those who consumed sugary drinks daily were found to have prematurely short telomeres. Drinking 25 cl of sugary drink daily leads to a reduction in life expectancy equivalent to 1.9 years, independently of your weight or the presence of certain illnesses. If you drink 60 cl daily, life expectancy decreases by 4.6 years. Another American study examined the link between the amount of sugar available per person and the prevalence of diabetes in the populations of 175 countries. The higher the amount of available sugar, the more cases of diabetes the country had. For every 150 available calories per person and per day (the equivalent of one 355 ml can of soft drink), the prevalence of diabetes went up by 1.1%.

The ubiquity of sugar in industrial food is the main culprit in this human catastrophe. Sugar used to be an ingredient almost exclusively found in desserts. Today, it is estimated that eight out of ten of 600 000 available food products contain added sugar! This is even worse when these products are offered in 'fat-free' versions. Fat-free vanilla-flavored yogurt may contain as much as five teaspoons of sugar, which is equivalent to half a can of soft drink.

Sweeteners such as aspartame or sucralose have made it possible for manufacturers to offer sugar-free products, which are in theory healthier. This is an illusion, however, as several studies have shown that they lead to an increased risk of obesity and type 2 diabetes. Indeed, our brain doesn't like fake sugars, which contain no calories and lead to dietary dissatisfaction; our brain reacts by stimulating our appetite when confronted with other sweet foods, in order to compensate for the absence of calories in sweeteners.

Recommendations

Agave syrup is extracted from the sap of a type of cactus. Its flavor is similar to that of honey, but with a glycemic index three to four times lower than honey (between 15 and 21, compared to 70 for honey).Among honeys, acacia honey also had a low glycemic index (30).

We don't need to wait for clinical trials to confirm the dangers of sugar to lower our consumption of it. It is already clear that high sugar consumption leads to a higher risk of becoming overweight or obese. This is why a number of organisms and governments are suggesting we limit our consumption of added sugar and of foods containing them. The World Health Organization recommends that less than 10% of our total energy intake should come from added sugar. For a single individual consuming 2 000 calories per day, this would correspond to a maximum of 50 grams of added sugar, the equivalent of a can and a half of an ordinary soft drink (don't forget to take into account the added sugar in cookies, flavored coffee, desserts, ice cream, chocolate etc.)

The American Heart Association, for its part, recommends women consume a maximum of 100 calories from added sugar and for men a maximum of 150 calories. This corresponds to a maximum of 25 g of added sugar for women and 38 g for men.

1.4 - Too Much Red Meat

Most people love meat, simply because it tastes good. Cooking it leads to a series of chemical reactions which generate thousands of scent molecules produced by the reactions between sugars and proteins in the meat. These molecules are registered by our brain and give rise to a new smell: that of cooked meat (Béliveau). Cooking meat also releases glutamate and inosinate; these two molecules are detected on our tongue by taste receptors which tell the brain that a protein-rich food is there. This activates the brain's pleasure centers. Yet we are not carnivorous. We do enjoy and are able to digest meat, but we have neither the anatomy (the teeth and jaw) of a carnivorous animal, nor their ability to metabolize uric acid (the waste from animal protein). According to Béliveau, *we are omnivores biologically designed to eat plant matter, but which adapted culturally to diversify this diet by adding animal products to it.*

All meat has a nearly identical structure: it is made of muscle, fat and collagen. The amount of fat varies a lot depending on the animal: it can go from 1% in certain birds to 30% in beef. Meats are also distinguished by their color. Contrary to popular belief, red meat doesn't derive its color from blood, but rather its high levels of myoglobin, a protein which captures oxygen in the presence of iron, and makes it possible to stock this oxygen inside the muscle and then release it during muscular effort. When it is cooked, the iron is oxidized and the myoglobin loses its ability to capture oxygen, which explains the brown color of cooked meat. White meat is white because it contains very little myoglobin, as its muscle fibers need very little oxygen during muscular effort.

Meat consumption has literally exploded in most places around the world. This despite the fact that we know that red meat-rich diets are linked to high rates of colorectal cancer. The United States, as well as Europe, have rates of colon cancer five to thirty times higher than in India. The Japanese, who formerly did not eat meat, increased their red meat consumption by 700% since 1945. This has led to a 400% increase in colorectal cancer.

> *A major study, carried out on 500,000 individuals, has shown that red meat and processed meat consumption is linked with a linear increase in mortality: the risk of dying prematurely for those who eat 160 g of meat per day is increased by 50%*

Red and processed meat seem to be carcinogenic because of their high calorie content, and especially due to the major biochemical transformations they undergo during cooking. Iron, when oxidized, generates free radicals which can cause DNA mutations. Processed meat contains nitrites which can be carcinogenic. Creatine, which is present in large quantities in muscle cells, bonds to proteins' amino acids when they reach 200 °C, forming heterocyclic amines (HCAs), which are highly carcinogenic. The more the meat is charred, the more HCAs it contains. When you ask for your meat to be 'well done', know that it contains three times as much of this carcinogen.

Almost all of these molecules can be eliminated however, if we marinate the meat in virgin olive oil, along with garlic and lemon juice or herbs (thyme or rosemary). This process also decreases the production of an animal fat derivative, malondialdehyde, by 70%. Malondialdehyde also increases the risk of cardiovascular disease. You can also use Teriyaki sauce or 0.2% concentration turmeric (Béliveau).

Cows are ruminants, and feed on grasses, like clover or alfalfa. Yet today we feed them corn and soya beans. Corn, being a source of sugar, is converted into fat. Because of this, the meat from an animal which was fed corn contains twice as much fat as that of a cow which was fed grass. Corn contains no omega 3. The meat of corn-fed animals contains three times less omega 3, which is anti-inflammatory, and three times more omega 6, which promotes inflammation. The extensive use of antibiotics is even more shocking. It could have serious implications for our health. In the United States, nearly 80% of all antibiotics used are given to livestock (Béliveau).

Quorn

Developing effective and innocuous protein sources: this is what some in the agri-food business have set out to do. Have you ever heard of Quorn? Quorn is a meat substitute made from mycoprotein. It is made out of a fungus, Fusarium venenatum, which is naturally present in soil. Quorn contains no cholesterol and is very lean. It only has 3.2 g of fat, 0.6 g of which is saturated fat, per 100 g of product. It is 12% protein and 5% fiber; meat and poultry contain none. Quorn is low-calorie (95 calories per 100 g), but rich in B vitamins. It comes in several different forms: cubed, ground, as sticks, breaded or plain fillets, or burger patties. It's easy to cook, as you would cook chicken: simmered, steamed, grilled, marinated etc. It has a tender consistency and a neutral flavor, so it will need to be seasoned with spices and herbs, whose flavors it will readily soak up.

In short, there are several reasons for the negative impact of excessive red meat and processed meat consumption on health and longevity. The first is simple; red meat contains too many calories. The second is the production of carcinogenic compounds through cooking or preservation methods. The third is their very low omega 3 content, which promotes silent inflammation. Big red meat eaters generally eat fewer vegetables, and thereby miss out on precious cancer-fighting elements. The solution could be to replace red meat by white meat, but especially it could be to diversify our protein sources, by eating eggs, nuts, and above all fish.

1.5 - Too Much Fat

All scientists agree, excessive fat (not just obesity) indirectly leads to premature aging, which will lead to chronic illnesses, which are often deadly. Fats or lipids are the most energy-rich nutrients. They are found in many types of food: oil seeds and oleaginous fruits in particular. Dairy products, such as cheese or cream, also contain large quantities of lipids, and vegetable oils and animal fat are almost 100% lipid. One gram of lipids contains around 9 kcal, almost double what is found in proteins or carbohydrates (around 4 kcal per gram). This is why fat is our main energy source. But excessive lipid consumption promotes weight gain and related illnesses. Fat and oil do however also provide our body with essential fatty acids, which are vital, and with vitamin E. Fat also has important functions, such as insulation (thin people tend to be sensitive to cold weather) and protecting sensitive organs (the kidneys, for example). It is also an effective vehicle for aromatics and flavors. It is required, at the intestinal level, for the absorption of fat-soluble vitamins, vitamins A, D, E and K. A healthy man of average weight (70 kg) has 7 to 10 kg of body fat, and a woman with of average weight (60 kg) has 12 to 15 kg of body fat.

In order to get thinner, you should eat fat! This may seem shocking, but it's partly true; some fats are necessary for you to stay healthy. And yet haven't we been saying for years that fat is bad for you, and responsible for numerous illnesses, such as obesity, cancer, cardiovascular disease? In fact, moderate amounts of certain types of fat are essential to our health.

1.6 - Obesity, Inflammation and Aging

Weight gain causes diabetes through insulin resistance; prolonged obesity causes the pancreas to decrease insulin production, which forces patients to inject themselves with insulin every day. Obesity is also the main cause of cardiovascular disease. In the United States, an official report published in 2009 estimated that more than 100 000 cancer cases per year could be attributed to patients' excess weight. Current research confirms the fact that excess weight is not only a risk factor for cancer, but that it also undermines the effectiveness of anti-cancer treatments and therefore lowers the chances of survival.

A number of studies have in the past claimed to show that we could be both obese and healthy! A 'fat and fit' theory, which some recent publications still assert. Being overweight therefore wouldn't necessarily be synonymous with cardiovascular disease, hypertension, or diabetes. But an epidemiological study by Inserm, the French Institute of Health and Medical Research, has revealed a link between obesity and the acceleration of age-related cognitive decline. These results are indisputable;all obese subjects underwent accelerated age-related cognitive decline. In ten years, the scores of obese individuals suffering from metabolic abnormalities on a number of cognitive tests decreased almost 25% faster than those of normal-weight individuals. This decline also affects the other subgroup of obese subjects, those without any metabolic abnormalities, but to a lesser extent. 'Healthy' obese people are therefore not exempt either. The message is clear, and confirms that prevention of obesity is necessary.

1.7 - Obesity and Smoking Accelerate Aging

We must now add a new item to the already long list of problems linked to cigarettes and obesity: premature aging. According to a study recently published in the scientific journal The Lancet, the genetic code of smokers and obese people shows signs of premature aging. For example, a woman smoking one pack of cigarettes a day for 40 years accelerates the biological aging of her genetic code by 7.4 years, which is far from negligible.

In order to assess this phenomenon in the studied subjects, researchers examined a biological marker which matures at a constant rate over time: telomeres, which shorten as the years go by.

This study was carried out on 1,122 women, aged 18 to 76. 119 of them were clinically obese, 203 were smokers and 369 ex-smokers. As predicted, researchers found that they all had shortened telomeres, which is linked to aging. These results became worrisome once they saw that obese women, and those who smoked, had significantly shorter telomeres than those who did not smoke and had a normal body weight. The researchers found that each 'pack-year', an indicator derived by multiplying the number of packs of cigarettes smoked daily by the number of years spent smoking, represented an 18% increase in the rate of telomere shortening. Any increase in the number of cigarettes smoked, or in the number of years spent smoking, accelerates aging as well as the risk of contracting cancer and lung or heart disease. This study is an important warning signal, and provides further tangible evidence of the devastating consequences of our bad habits for our entire metabolism.

Cardiovascular disease, diabetes, certain forms of cancer… although it is already extensive, the list of known harmful effects of obesity has just gotten longer. According to work carried out by researchers at the Center for Research in Epidemiology and Population Health (CESP, Paul Brousse Hospital, Villejuif, France) and University College London, cognitive decline may be higher in obese individuals who also suffer from metabolic disorders, such as hypertension, hyperglycemia, hypercholesterolemia, or hypertriglyceridemia.

The fat which we consume through our diet has two functions .It is an energy source, and a vehicle for certain nutrients which are essential to our proper function. Fatty tissue, made of adipose cells, has the responsibility of assembling the great majority of our energy stores. The input and output of fat, as triglycerides, is strictly monitored by a series of hormones and enzymes, the most important of which are leptin, adiponectin and insulin. Fat also provides us with many nutrients such as polyunsaturated oils and fats. Among these we find the essential fatty acids, omega 3 and omega 6, which play a key role in the inflammatory process. Excessive levels of omega 6 in our diet will lead to chronic or silent inflammation, which cause chronic illness and accelerated aging. Omega 3 consumption has the opposite effect, counteracting this pro-inflammatory action and thereby improving our health. Excessive carbohydrate consumption, as it raises insulin levels, will trigger a wave of pro-inflammatory compounds. Obesity is an important factor in premature aging and the early onset of age-related diseases. 'Globesity', a worldwide disease, is reaching unprecedented numbers. And it shows no signs of leveling off. Obesity, and especially abdominal obesity, causes, among other things, accelerated cognitive decline and much faster telomere shortening; when combined with smoking, which is often the case, it further accelerates aging.

1.8 - Too Much Alcohol

The good news! A meta-analysis of studies, involving more than one million individuals, shows that daily alcohol consumption – two glasses of red wine for men, one glass for women is linked to a 20% reduction in the risk of death. This protective effect is due to increased levels of good cholesterol (HDL), which makes it possible to lower bad cholesterol (LDL) levels in the blood, and therefore reduce the amount of atheromatous plaques produced. Alcohol improves glycemic control – blood sugar levels and has anticoagulant and anti-inflammatory properties. All of these factors help in decreasing the risk of cardiovascular disease.

Agnes Fenton, a 110-year-old American, says she drinks three bottles of beer and a glass of whisky every day. She says her doctor told her to consider doing so seventy years ago. He had at that time advised her to drink three bottles of beer daily. This New Jersey woman added the glass of whisky to her diet herself and finds herself no worse for wear...

The bad news! In larger quantities, this protective effect disappears, replaced by a significant increase in the risk of mortality, especially in women (Béliveau).

But that isn't all, excessive alcohol consumption increases the rates of certain types of cancers (mouth, larynx, esophagus, colon, liver, and breast). The carcinogenic agent isn't alcohol but rather a product of its metabolism: acetaldehyde. Individuals who mix tobacco and alcohol may have increased levels, up to 700%, of this carcinogenic metabolite.

A study, carried out on one million women, indicates that alcohol consumption, excluding wine, increases the risk of mouth cancer by 18%. For those who only drink red wine, the risk is brought down to 7%. The dietary context must be taken into account, however, as it significantly alters the organism's reaction to alcohol. For example, an omega 3 deficiency along with excess quantities of omega 6 multiplies carcinogenic free radical levels which are produced by alcohol five to ten times.

Red Wine

Red wine may protect us from cancer. A very large-scale study, carried out on one million women, who were followed during ten years, has shown that red wine may play a beneficial role in preventing several types of cancers. Resveratrol, a molecule which is synthesized by grape vines to fight off microscopic fungi, has one of the strongest anticarcinogenic effects in the plant world. Moderate red wine consumption (from the pinot noir variety in particular) could be enough to stop cancer growth. But the most significant health benefit we derive from red wine remains a considerable reduction (30%) in cardiovascular disease.

Could red wine be all we need to live longer? This is what some studies carried out in the United States tend to show. They highlight the role resveratrol plays in activating 'longevity genes'. The Sirt2 gene controls the secretion of sirtuins, proteins which help increase the lifespan of worms by 40%, according to an experiment carried out by Leonard Guarente, a researcher at MIT, in 2001, and which was repeated in 2009. Its results were published in the journal Nature. Resveratrol, a substance which is found in abundance in red wine, is known to activate Sirtuin secretion. Ingesting large amounts of it could be a very simple and effective way of living longer.

1.9 - Too Much Salt

Table salt is actually sodium chloride (NaCl). The amount of sodium is the crucial factor as regards our health. Food labels therefore indicate sodium content rather than salt content. Since salt is 40% sodium and 60% chlorine, when we absorb 10 g of salt, we are actually ingesting 4 g of sodium. Sodium plays a key role in blood pH control, muscle contraction, and nerve impulse transmission. A daily intake of 500 mg of salt, that is, 200 mg of sodium, is deemed necessary to replace daily losses, which are mainly due to sweating. Today we consume 10 g of salt every day on average, 75% of which comes from industrial food products. Three quarters of our consumption is therefore involuntary and often overlooked.

Most of the food which we eat already contains sodium. Salt is water-soluble and is therefore also in our blood, where it is present as sodium and chloride. Any movement of sodium within the organism is necessarily connected to water; when we ingest sodium, we retain water, when we eliminate sodium, we lose water. An increase in salt consumption therefore leads to an increase in the volume of blood circulating in our arteries, and to a consequent increase in blood pressure. Sodium also plays an important role at the level of each individual cell. Blood, which travels in our arteries, distributes oxygen and nutrients to our cells. In order to supply cells with nutrients, a mechanism which utilizes sodium among other products gives the cell the ability to allow the elements it needs to function to enter it. Once in the cell, the sodium has done its job and must leave, as a cell filled with sodium and water could not function. Another mechanism allows the sodium to exit the cell, but requires the presence of potassium to replace it, through a cleverly arranged network of 'pumps'. The proper distribution of sodium and potassium in the organism is therefore an essential condition for cellular life, particularly in terms of nerve and muscular function: there is about 15 times more sodium in our blood than in our cells, and about 28 times more potassium in our cells than in our blood. Sodium and potassium are an essential team for proper blood pressure control. Consuming moderate quantities of sodium and enough potassium, is a dietary challenge which we must face daily.

A study following 12,267 individuals over nearly 15 years, which examined the relationship between mortality and sodium and potassium intake, was published in the journal Archives of Internal Medicine. Its results show that high sodium intake is associated with a 20% increase in mortality, and conversely, that high potassium intake is associated with a 20% decrease in mortality. Furthermore, high sodium intake, along with low potassium intake, is associated with a significant increase in mortality, particularly cardiovascular mortality.

Ever since salt entered our diet, sodium/potassium ratios have been unbalanced: we consume two to four times more sodium than potassium. It is therefore important for us to correct this ratio, since too much sodium chloride and not enough potassium leads to the risk of hypertension. Many studies have shown that, in hypertensive subjects, a potassium-enriched diet lowers blood pressure. Furthermore, we believe that excess salt may be responsible for nearly 80 000 cardiovascular events each year in France. How can we restore balance?

By avoiding industrially prepared dishes, bread, processed meat, and favoring potassium-rich fruits and vegetables: tubers, legumes, pulses (900 to 1,200 mg of potassium in 100 g), but also mushrooms and algae, and our diet can also be complemented with potassium citrate.

1.10 - Too Much Dairy?

After World War 2, everyone considered milk to be the main staple food along with bread. But today, we now find ourselves wondering whether drinking large quantities of milk may be dangerous...

In terms of longevity and the prevention of osteoporosis, this remained an open question. Swedish studies carried out with large samples, which examined the impact of milk and dairy products on life expectancy, and the risk of bone fracture related to osteoporosis, were therefore very important.

Karl Michaëlsson and his team followed 61,433 women, aged 39 to 74 years old when they were recruited between 1987 and 1990, and 45,339 men, between 45 and 79 years old in 1997. During this 20-year study, researchers recorded 15,541 deaths and 4,259 hip fractures among women, and 10,112 deaths and 1,166 hip fractures for men. These numbers, along with very meticulous dietary surveys, would make it possible to finally understand the impact of milk consumption on lifespan and the prevention of fractures linked to osteoporosis. Compared to women drinking less than one glass of milk per day, women drinking more than three glasses per day have almost doubled all-cause mortality; a 93% increase! Simply put, each extra glass of milk drunk daily, on top of the first, increases mortality by 15%. Even worse, women who drink more milk suffer from more hip fractures than those who drink very little. The results are similar in men, although the rates are lower. According to the researchers, fresh milk is very rich in D-galactose, an inflammatory factor. This is why those who consume more milk have more 8-iso-PGF2α in their urine, and more interleukin 6 in their serum, both of which are markers for oxidative stress, and increase cardiovascular risk (hypertension, cholesterol, insulin resistance) and accelerate calcium loss in bones. The opposite can be seen with products made with fermented milk, which are more cardioprotective.

Lactose and Casein

Lactose is the only carbohydrate in milk. Each lactose molecule is made of glucose and galactose. There are 5 g of lactose in 100 ml of cow's milk.

It plays many roles in our organism: it is first and foremost an energy source, but it also helps to properly absorb the calcium in milk, as well as to promote toddlers' neuro-sensory development. Indeed, galactose, which is released when we digest lactose, is a component in the brain's structure (this is why breast milk, or infant formula, is our only source of nutrition during the first five months of our lives). Lactose also contributes to proper lactic acid bacteria development in the intestinal flora, which are essential to proper bowel function and strong local and general immune defenses. In order to carry out all of these useful functions, lactose must first be digested in the small intestine (right after it exits the stomach) by an enzyme which is secreted by the cells of the intestinal lining: lactase. This enzyme digests lactose and releases its constituent glucose and galactose molecules. They then go into the blood where they are distributed throughout the body. Lactase is 100% active in toddlers, as galactose is vital to their development, and is then genetically programmed to progressively decline with age. We then enter hypolactasia. Hypolactasia is nevertheless not synonymous with lactose intolerance. It is estimated that only 10 to 20% of hypolactasic individuals are lactose intolerant, and that 90% of the French population can digest milk well; even with low lactasic activity, most adults can digest a glass of milk just fine.

Casein is the main milk protein, the other being whey. Casein has two forms: calcium caseinate (traditionally called casein) and micellar casein. Calcium caseinate, or casein, is a protein which the body assimilates slowly. Casein is naturally found in cheese, yogurt, and cottage cheese. It is also in many dietary supplements such as infant formula, high-protein meal replacements or protein supplements for athletes and body-builders. Casein may irritate the immune system and thereby promote mucus production, which can worsen allergies, asthma, eczema or bronchitis among others, or lead to sinusitis and ear infections in young children.

Should We Keep Consuming Milk and Dairy?

Yes, but we should remember that they aren't essential. Everything we find in dairy we can get from other food sources. Our ancestors didn't drink milk, for that matter: it was introduced to us during the Neolithic period by farmers. Today, three out of every four people don't tolerate it, and consume little to none. Yet osteoporosis isn't present in these populations, just as it wasn't present in our ancestors.

In conclusion, drinking milk in adulthood is somewhat bad for your health, whereas fermented dairy, like yogurt, cottage cheese, sour milk and cheese is better for you, both in terms of lifespan and for preventing bone fractures, and protecting your heart.

And What About Goat's Milk?

Goat's milk contains many nutrients, like casein, which make it similar to breast milk. But it contains less alpha 1 casein, which is responsible for most allergies to cow's milk. This effectively makes it hypoallergenic. Another benefit is due to the quantity and nature of its oligosaccharides. The oligosaccharides in goat's milk are closer to those found in breast milk. These compounds reach the large intestine undigested, where they act as prebiotics, and contribute to the development of a probiotic flora which is capable of eliminating any pathogenic bacterial flora. Goat's milk already contains less lactose than cow's milk, about 1% less, and as it is more digestible, it can be tolerated by some individuals who are intolerant of this milk sugar. But careful, this doesn't mean that allergic reactions to goat's milk are impossible. Some people can be allergic to the casein in milk.

The main difference between cow's milk and goat's milk is in their fat: not only are the fat globules in goat's milk smaller, but their fatty acid content is also different. Goat's milk contains more essential fatty acids (linoleic and arachidonic) than cow's milk.

Both are part of the omega 6 series of fatty acids. Goats' milk is also composed of 30 to 35% of medium chain fatty acids, compared to 15 to 20% for cow's milk. These fatty acids represent a quick energy source and aren't stored as fatty tissue. Furthermore, the fat in goat's milk lowers total cholesterol levels and maintains proper triglyceride and transaminase (GOT and GPT) levels. This makes it an ideal food for preventing cardiovascular disease.

And Soya Milk?

Soya milk has almost identical properties to cow's milk, apart from being a plant milk, which means it contains no calcium or lactose, making it an excellent alternative for those who are intolerant or allergic to this sugar present in cow's milk, among others.

1.11 - Too Many Food Allergies

Everyone understands this situation: we all know someone who has lived through, or we have ourselves experienced 'allergies' to one or more types of food.

We all understand this because that type of experience isn't easily forgotten; you eat some shrimp and suddenly you don't feel well, you turn red, maybe you're out of breath. Red patches appear on your whole body, and are extremely itchy. If the link to the shrimp isn't immediately apparent to you, it will be the second time you eat some. At this point, you don't need any clinical tests, you've already figured out what's going on. But if you were to have your blood tested, you would find that your IgE (Immunoglobulin E) levels have gone up, what specialists call type I or immediate hypersensitivity.

This type of allergic reaction, although it is the most visible, is not the most common. Another, more insidious type of reaction, manifests itself long after the food is eaten, and causes symptoms which often have nothing to do with the digestive system or the symptoms of type I allergies. For example, you will feel joint pain without any visible injury, or a persistent migraine or eczema for which the usual treatments will have no effect. If you are overweight, you will be unable to lose weight, despite your best efforts. Your doctor will prescribe a series of clinical tests and medication to treat the symptoms, but so long as the root cause isn't unmasked, the symptoms will persist.

This type of allergy is called type III hypersensitivity, and is the one we will focus on. In this case, another type of 'immunoglobulin' appears: immunoglobulin G, (IgG).

The Culprit:
The Small Intestine

In order to understand what happens, we first need to understand the relationship between the small intestine and the immune system. The digestive system is one of the few organs which communicate directly with the outside world, and is therefore in direct contact with all potential invaders. In order to protect itself, it has a very sophisticated defense system which lines the entire intestinal mucosa.

Normally the small intestine is impermeable; theoretically, no macromolecule can go through it without first having been decomposed into simple molecules. This impermeability is possible thanks to the tight connections between the cells of the intestinal lining.

But there is one exception: foods which should normally be seen as alien may receive a 'permanent entry visa' as long as they cross the intestinal barrier at the appropriate 'checkpoints'! This is called 'dietary tolerance'. Tolerance in the sense that, as food is essential to life, the immune system lowers its guard and lets these intruders through.

But the small intestine is often weakened by bacteria or certain types of treatments, such as anti-inflammatory drugs, antibiotics or aspirin. These modifications cause the impermeability of the cells to weaken: this is called 'Leaky Gut Syndrome'. Certain improperly digested foods may cross the intestinal wall 'illegally', and find themselves in the bloodstream, without a permanent visa. The immune system doesn't recognize them and will call its defenses into action: it will send out immunoglobulins specific to the given food, made especially to neutralize it and no other type of food or dietary component. This component is an 'antigen', the immunoglobulin being an 'antibody'. Their struggle is called an 'antigen-antibody reaction'. For example: improperly digested radish molecules have illegally traveled between two cells of the digestive mucosa. The immune system sends out 'anti-radish' antibodies (anti-radish IgGs), and these IgGs will attack the radish antigen, by latching onto it like a praying mantis; this is a suicide attack, and both will die from it, forming an 'immune complex' which will have to be eliminated. Each suicide attack is accompanied by a local inflammatory reaction, causing collateral damage. This specific reaction is usually trivial and fully manageable, causing no clinical symptoms, but the absence of symptoms is precisely what will complicate things for our organism. Indeed, the repeated ingestion of the antigen will lead to the overproduction of anti-radish IgG antibodies, and cause an inflammatory reaction which will quickly become pathological. Our immune complex disposal system will also become overwhelmed (clogging disease), and no longer know how to eliminate these immune complexes, storing them wherever it can; e.g., under the skin or in our joints.

This immune reaction will have two clinical consequences: a pathology due to immune complex deposits on the one hand, and, on the other hand, a pathology linked to the presence of a chronic inflammatory reaction. Unfortunately, the symptoms related to these pathologies often have nothing to do with those which food would normally produce. This makes it difficult for a doctor to establish a causal link.

There are different biological tests which can be used to find out what foods cause this type of allergic reaction. These tests have been the subject of much debate among scientists however, and have not yet received approval from the authorities. These tests detect the presence of IgG-type 'anti-nutrient' antibodies. Some scientists, allergists in particular, affirm that the presence of IgG-type antibodies does not prove anything!!

Should We Eat Gluten-Free?

Gluten-free diets have recently gained immense popularity among consumers. So-called gluten-free products are multiplying on supermarket shelves. Apart from those suffering from celiac disease– gluten intolerance, for whom this type of diet is completely justified, since it is the only existing treatment, it is reasonable to ask ourselves if other consumers, who don't suffer from this illness, would actually derive any benefit from removing gluten from their diet.

Gluten is made of two protein fractions: glutenins and prolamins. Prolamins are the more toxic of gluten's protein fractions. Wheat contains glutenin and gliadin (prolamin), which together constitute gluten. Wheat gliadin is among the most researched prolamins. These two protein fractions are essential to the elasticity of bread, as they capture air bubbles. Many grains contain gluten, but their prolamin levels will actually determine whether gluten intolerant or allergic individuals will be able to eat them or not.

Wheat grains contain a sugar, wheat starch, and a complex mix of proteins. Gluten is the protein mass which remains after the wheat starch has been extracted. This is the component in flour which gives bread all of its elasticity and fluffiness. Wheat gluten also makes it possible for the bread to rise. Wheat flour is normally made up of 10 to 12% of protein; if it doesn't have enough, the bread won't have enough volume and its texture will be uneven. Gluten is also used to enhance the resistance of puff pastry and frozen dough. It limits crumbling, and even the cohesiveness of meat-based preparations and of some types of processed meats.

Celiac disease is due to an allergy to the prolamin in gluten, which leads to the destruction of the small intestine's lining. Indeed, when gluten is ingested, it causes an inflammatory reaction and causes the destruction of the intestinal villi. Ingested nutrients will no longer be correctly absorbed by the organism, which may lead to malabsorption, weight loss, and potentially serious consequences.

There are other types of gluten intolerance, which do not lead to celiac disease, but are due to gluten hypersensitivity, causing extra-intestinal diseases, arthritis, type 2 diabetes, fibromyalgia, migraines etc. How can this phenomenon be explained? Cereals which contain gluten (wheat, barley, oats, rye, spelt, Khorasan wheat…) when heated at high temperatures, develop glycotoxins, (called acrylamides). These glycotoxins can penetrate tissue, in small intestines which have become permeable, and let undigested proteins through. These then contribute to inflammation, and the deterioration of tissues and joints. We are naturally equipped with mechanisms which inhibit a certain amount of these glycotoxins; but they are more or less effective from one individual to the next, depending, among other factors, on our epigenome. In this way, certain people will only sustain tissue damage after having consumed a lot of glycotoxin during a long period of time, while other, more sensitive subjects, will rapidly undergo damage, even with small quantities. But cereal-based products containing gluten are not the only ones which may contain glycotoxins; they can also be found in grilled meat, dairy products, corn, French fries, heated oil and many other foods.

If you believe you are not allergic to gluten, but only intolerant, it is nevertheless recommended that you have a blood test to search for anti-gluten antibodies. If test results are positive, you would need to go on a gluten-free diet.

If the results are negative, you won't need to avoid gluten. Many testimonies have confirmed, however, that, even without an outright intolerance, a gluten-free diet may improve many symptoms, going from chronic migraines to rheumatic pain. If you want to follow a gluten-free diet, then you will have to learn to choose your food carefully, to avoid any deficits; eating gluten-free is tricky. The food industry offers many 'gluten-free' products in health food stores, and now even in supermarkets. This food is most often made out of rice or corn flour instead of wheat: corn flour spaghetti, puffed rice cakes, corn starch baguettes, rice crackers etc. You may sometimes even find potato starch. But are these alternatives good for us? The answer is no. All of these ingredients have high glycemic indexes: they can lead to weight gain, *as they disrupt blood sugar regulation mechanisms*, says Christine Calvet.

> *In a recent study, researchers analyzed the characteristics of several gluten-free breads. They found that these foods are high in fat, low in protein, have very uneven fiber content and are very carbohydrate-rich. These carbohydrates are mostly starch, which is very quickly digested, representing 75.5 to 92.5 g of 100 g of product. The authors conclude that these foods - and this is the case of most of the alternatives to traditional bread products - have a high glycemic index, which is incompatible with healthy habits for a sedentary lifestyle. Fats are also often imbalanced, favoring polyunsaturated fatty acids and omega 6, which are pro-inflammatory.*

On top of their high glycemic load, many of these foods also contain far too much sugar or agave syrup. They also contain a wide array of additives, such as phosphates, among others. A number of these products may lead to weight gain, due to insulin and leptin resistance, especially as the absence of gluten in the intestine makes it easier for it to assimilate carbohydrates, fats, proteins, and their energy.

An Alternative to Gluten: Buckwheat

Buckwheat is particularly popular in Japan, Russia and Eastern and Central Europe. Buckwheat grain can be eaten whole, roasted or crushed, as well as in flours of varying coarseness, used in crepes, bread and noodles. 10 to 12% of buckwheat's dry weight is made up of protein. The protein content of buckwheat is similar to that of oats, rye, wheat and quinoa, but it is higher than other cereals, such as barley and rice. The proteins in buckwheat contain all of the essential amino acids and therefore have high biological value. Dark buckwheat flour contains around twice as much protein as lighter colored buckwheat flour. And of course, buckwheat contains no gluten.

The total amount of fiber in buckwheat is similar to that in other grains. However, it contains a higher percentage of soluble fiber– pectin and other polysaccharides –, than of insoluble fiber – cellulose or lignin. Soluble fiber is known for slowing down gastric emptying and increasing transit time through the small intestine. This kind of fiber-rich diet therefore contributes to normalizing blood cholesterol, glucose and insulin levels, and thereby helps treat cardiovascular disease and type 2 diabetes. An insoluble-fiber-rich diet, for its part, helps maintain adequate intestinal function.

In a study comparing the composition of buckwheat to that of four other grains (wheat, oats, barley and rye), whole buckwheat grain topped the list, due to its antioxidant properties, as well as its phenolic compound content, a family of antioxidants including, among others, flavonoids and phenolic acids.

Buckwheat is an excellent source of copper, magnesium, manganese, phosphorus, zinc, as well as vitamins (B1, B2, B3, B5, B6).

A recent study, carried out on human subjects, has shown that the consumption of buckwheat lasagna led to a stronger feeling of fullness, compared to wheat pasta. An additional reason to integrate buckwheat-based foods into our diet!

A small note of caution, however: allergic reactions caused by buckwheat and its flour aren't common, but they can be severe; they may cause asthma, urticaria, and anaphylactic reactions. The allergens found in buckwheat are heat-stable, which means they won't be deactivated through cooking. A cross-reaction may take place in individuals who are allergic to latex: they may experience allergic symptoms when they eat buckwheat. Buckwheat may also be contaminated by gluten-containing grains, either in the field, during transport or manipulation, or even during the milling process. It is therefore important to choose flour and food products which are certified gluten-free, as they are the safest. Unfortunately, however, not all gluten-free foods display this symbol, and you will therefore have to learn to read through labels carefully in order to detect potential gluten sources. People allergic to gluten must make sure that the buckwheat products they buy are truly wheat-free (e.g., Soba noodles are often made of a mix of the two flours). Some manufacturers go to extraordinary lengths to ensure the purity of their grain, for example by setting aside some of their equipment, or even their entire factory, for buckwheat processing, excluding all other grains.

Finally, it is recommended that you store your whole buckwheat flour in the refrigerator, or even in your freezer.

1.12 - Not Enough Fish

Fish and other fishery products have extraordinary nutritional value. Along with omega 3, they contain a wide range of minerals which are essential to the proper function of our organism. They simultaneously cover a large proportion of our needs in essential fatty acids, omega 3, vitamins, (in particular vitamins B12 and D), iodine and selenium. Seafood is also very rich in manganese, copper and zinc. The most omega 3-rich species are herring, mackerel, sardines, salmon, red tuna, hake and trout. But all seafood contains some.

Many studies suggest that regularly eating fish diminishes the risk of cancer. The best documented data concerns prostate and colorectal cancer. But fish products may also be beneficial for rheumatoid polyarthritis, psoriasis, age-related macular degeneration (ARD) and Alzheimer's disease. All of these effects may be linked to omega 3 fatty acids, or more specifically to omega 6 to omega 3 ratios.

As they are rich in vitamin D, fish products also help improve ossification and therefore combat osteoporosis. The fish which contain the most of it are salmon, herring, bass, flounder, sardines, mackerel and striped mullet, but it is also found in fish eggs and oysters.

All fish products are an excellent good-quality protein source. Tuna, skate and anchovies are among the most protein-rich species.

Iodine is essential to the production of thyroid hormones, which are extremely important during fetal growth, especially for the development of the nervous system. Fish products cover our needs exceptionally well. Among the best phosphorus-rich foods - phosphorus being essential to proper neuron function, and therefore brain function - we find fishery products, which also offer a very bioavailable form of selenium. Oysters and mussels are particularly rich in selenium, as well as manganese, copper, zinc and other minerals which participate in antioxidant production. Unless you are allergic to them, you should eat fish and fishery products as much as possible.

1.13 - Not Enough Fruits and Vegetables

We have always had a privileged relationship with plant foods. We have been able to identify over 7,000 plants which are used as foods, out of the 500,000 plant species which exist on earth. Thanks to this relationship with the plant world, we now have access to thousands of fruits and vegetables, from all over the world; and even if we have gradually integrated animal products into our diet, our organism remains fundamentally dependent on plants in order to function smoothly.

We know very well the fundamental impact of fruits and vegetables on our health. And these foods are available fresh all year-round. Why then do these foods continue to be neglected by our modern dietary habits? Health authorities around the world agree that a minimum of five servings (400 g) of fruits and vegetables daily are essential to our health and longevity. In the United States, 68% of adults eat less than two fruits a day, and

74% eat less than three servings of vegetables a day. Not only are these quantities too small, but the plants which we do eat have very little variety. For example, in the United States, most of the vegetable consumption comes from potatoes, eaten as French fries, and tomatoes, found in pizzas. This leads, on the one hand, to overabundance of calories, and on the other hand, and in terms of dietary balance, to a severe deficiency in plant foods.

According to the World Health Organization (WHO), fruit and vegetable deficiencies are directly responsible for three million deaths every year around the world; 20% of stomach cancers and 12% of lung cancers could be prevented with a higher consumption of certain fruits and vegetables. Individuals who never eat fruits and vegetables are 53% more likely to die prematurely and live three years less on average than those who eat at least five servings every day. Life expectancy is also likely extended further for individuals who eat a lot of polyphenol-rich fruits and vegetables.

Fruits and vegetables are not only good sources of vitamins and minerals, they also have, in order to defend themselves from a harsh environment, an impressive array of weapons, made up of at least 10,000 distinct molecules, belonging to three phytochemical compound families: polyphenols, terpenes and sulfur compounds. The beneficial action of these molecules is not limited to plant defense, as they also have surprising pharmacological properties, which help in combating chronic illnesses, including cancer, and help to lengthen life expectancy.

Fiber and Longevity

Dietary fiber is made of carbohydrates we cannot digest, which go through our entire digestive system, remaining virtually intact, finally ending up in our stools! They correspond to the plant matter which goes undigested and unabsorbed by the digestive tract, and yet they are essential to our health and longevity. Their specific characteristics make them beneficial for our organism, particularly by improving our intestinal transit. In this way, fiber facilitates the elimination of toxic and carcinogenic substances, and lowers cholesterol levels and glucose absorption. Dietary fiber has many beneficial effects for our health, reducing the risk of cancer, diabetes, obesity and cardiovascular disease.

A study conducted at Harvard University has shown that the risk of colon cancer is lowered by 40% in people who ingest 20 to 30 g of fiber a day. Another study carried out on 32 208 subjects, compared people who eat white bread to those who eat whole grain bread–which contains three times as much fiber. According to this study, the risk of cardiovascular disease in those eating whole grain bread is lowered by 50%.

Finally, another study, which involved 220,000 men and 170,000 women, over nearly 10 years, has shown the beneficial action of fiber on mortality. The amount of dietary fiber which each subject ingested was estimated through surveys. It ranged from 13 to 29 g per day for men and from 11 to 26 g per day for women. The 20% of participants who ingested the most dietary fiber (29 g for men, 26 g for women) had an overall mortality risk 22% lower than those eating the least fiber. As for mortality risk due to cardiovascular, infectious or respiratory illness, this was lowered by 24 to 56% in men and 34 to 59 % in women.

What's the Best Way to Make Sure You Eat Plenty of Dietary Fiber?

Eat whole grains (bread, rice, rolled oats, oat or wheat bran). But dietary fiber is also found in large amounts in fruits (apples, coconut, figs, prunes, redcurrants, blackcurrants), vegetables (cabbage, celery, fennel, onions, mushrooms), pulses (white beans, lentils, green peas). You can also eat nutritional yeast, and almonds.

1.14 - We Don't Drink Enough Water!

Your body is 60 to 70% water, depending on your morphology. After oxygen, water is the most important element for life. It is essential to all vital processes; we can find fluids in nearly every part of our body, both inside and outside of our cells; water keeps our blood and lymph volume stable and regulates body temperature. It makes it possible for chemical reactions to take place in our cells, enables the absorption and transport of ingested nutrients, as well as the brain's neural activity. It also ensures skin hydration, provides us with the saliva which makes it possible for us to swallow food, is used as a lubricant in our joints and our eyes, eliminates the waste remaining after digestion and other metabolic processes.

In temperate climates, an average size person uses up more than two liters of body water per day. The body eliminates more than a liter a day as urine, and an equal amount as sweat, in stools and during breathing. More water is lost in warm weather, during physical activity, while breastfeeding or if we are sick. Everyone therefore has specific hydration needs, depending on our height, lifestyle and the climate we live in.

In order to know how much you should drink, estimate how much urine you eliminate each day (approximately one liter for adults) and add one and a half liters of body water, which will be spent by your metabolism (moderately active person). You have a net loss of two and a half liters. Since diet generally provides us with 20% of our hydration needs on average, we still have to make up for two liters of water. They can be found in broths, hot or cold drinks, and of course, in drinking water.

You shouldn't wait to feel thirsty to drink; when you are active, you can lose a lot of water before feeling thirsty. You should therefore get used to drinking throughout the day. Athletes are prone to dehydration due to sweating. They may suffer from hyponatremia (low sodium levels), which is a sign of an electrolyte imbalance in the bloodstream.

A few suggestions: drink half a liter of water approximately two hours before physical activity; drink throughout the activity, enough to replace the water lost through sweating; remember that you can lose over one liter of water as sweat in one hour during intense aerobic activity; if this kind of strenuous activity lasts for more than one hour, you should have an isotonic drink (which contain carbohydrates, sodium and potassium), also called sports drinks.

During one study carried out in 2011 at the Institute of Psychiatry at King's College London, scientists realized that teenagers who drank no water had more trouble solving problems and concentrating than when they were properly hydrated. Therefore, in order for your brain to be more efficient when you are studying or working, remember to drink lots of water. Water also seems to affect our mood. A study carried out in 2009 at Tufts University, on a group of men and women in similar physical condition, proved that, during physical activity, subjects who drank no water quickly became tired, tense and aggressive. In less extreme cases, such as the daily routine of an active individual, the absence of water during the day may also give you a bad mood and make you easily annoyed.

1.15 - Eggs: They're Good for Your Health!

Emma Morano is an Italian woman with remarkable longevity; born in 1899, she is the second oldest woman in the world. The first may be Luo Meizhen, 127 years old in 2016, and the oldest person on earth; she lives in the south of China, in the Guangxi region, but her birthdate has not been reliably confirmed. Along with Susannah Mushatt Jones, an American woman, they are the only three women whom we know were born in the 19th century, and are still alive today, two decades into the 21st.

When she was 20, Emma suffered from anemia, and her doctor suggested she ate eggs. She followed this advice her entire life. She says that for a long time she ate two raw eggs and one cooked egg every morning. She stopped this diet on her 110th birthday. In total, this woman ate nearly 100,000 eggs!

The nutritional value of eggs mainly resides in their protein content, which has high biological value. An average (60 g) egg has about 7 g of protein, rich in essential amino acids; the balance between these amino acids is very good, to the point that egg protein can be regarded as a reference protein. In terms of nutritional equivalents, two eggs offer as much protein as 100 g of meat or 100 g of fish. The energy content of an average (60 g) egg is approximately 376 kJ (90 kcal). Fat content is 7 g, which is mostly found in the yolk, and two thirds of its fatty acids are unsaturated. One egg also has 180 mg of cholesterol. Eggs have plenty of vitamins (A, D, E) and minerals (iron and zinc). Along with spirulina, it is one of the best muscle-building foods, as its proteins enable you to maintain existing tissue and rapidly gain more muscle mass. The digestibility of eggs depends on how they are cooked, the best option being soft boiled, with well-cooked whites and a yolk which has just begun to firm up.

They say hard-boiled eggs help you lose weight: that isn't entirely accurate. This rumor is based on the fact that digesting hard-boiled eggs takes more time and energy than eggs which are less cooked. Digesting a hard-boiled egg takes far less energy than the calories it provides, however. It is actually a good appetite suppressant, and cooking them doesn't require any added fats. These are the only reasons why hard-boiled eggs could be considered as a weight-loss option.

It is also said that eggs could help us lengthen our life expectancy; that, on the other hand, is true! A study published in The American Journal of Clinical Nutrition has shown that an egg-rich diet lowers inflammation biomarker values by 20%. And we know that inflammation is a major cause of DNA damage and plays a key role in rapid telomere shortening.

Researchers at the University of Connecticut have shown that eating three eggs a day doesn't increase the risk of cardiovascular disease in healthy subjects. Another study from the University of Michigan, carried out on 27,000 volunteers, has not only confirmed these results, but also showed that those who eat three to four eggs per day have even lower risks!

But what about cholesterol? Everyone knows eggs have a lot of cholesterol, which can clog our arteries. It's true that egg yolks contain 180 mg of cholesterol, but its absorption is strongly restricted by another compound found in the yolk: lecithin.

So don't hesitate! You can eat a dozen eggs a week, so long as they come from trustworthy farms.

1.16 - The Intestine, Our Second Brain

Our body is colonized by billions of microorganisms, which cover it on the outside as well as the inside. Up until now, researchers have identified more than 10,000 species of microbes; these include bacteria, fungi and viruses, although the majority are bacteria. We are constantly interacting with these organisms and their genetic material. This complex internal ecosystem is called our 'microbiome'. At the intestinal level, it includes intestinal bacteria, which we categorize as the 'microbiota' or 'gut flora'. It is now accepted that the health of our microbiome is crucial to our own and that it should be considered as an organ in and of itself, which can, to some extent, modify how our genes are expressed. The microbiome's importance convinced the United States' National Institute of Health, to launch the 'human microbiome' project in 2008, an extension of the human genome project.

There is no doubt today that our gut flora plays a part in many of our functions. It contributes, for example, to proper immune function, detoxification, fighting inflammation, neurotransmitter and vitamin production, nutrient absorption, feelings of hunger or fullness, and the use of sugar and fat. Our gut flora affects our mood, our libido, our clarity of thought and even how we perceive the world. Some bacteria are permanent residents; they form long-lasting colonies. Others are only passing through, and travel along the digestive tract, forming small colonies which are essential to certain tasks.

The nervous system is most sensitive to changes in our gut flora, as it is very sensitive to chronic inflammation and free radical activity. And it has been established that our microbial flora is directly linked to this activity. Better still, the intimate connection between our intestine and our brain is a two-way relationship: just as anxiety or fear can cause a stomach ache, the intestine can send out calming or anxiety-provoking signals to our brain. 85% of serotonin, the happiness molecule, is produced by the intestine's nerve cells, and the intestine's neurons are so numerous that we now call them our 'second brain'.

Our intestine has its own immune system: GALT (*gut-associated lymphatic tissue*).It alone represents 70% of our entire immune system. The reason is simple: our intestinal lining is in direct contact with the outside world. And yet it is very fragile, as it is made up of a single layer. This means maintaining its integrity is critically important. The gut flora is there to ensure that the intestinal wall remains healthy. Did you know that the cells in the intestine are renewed every 24 to 36 hours? They regenerate so often that 50% of our stools is made up of intestinal cells. If cell abrasion becomes too important, the intestinal barrier doesn't function as well, and toxic substances are not eliminated as efficiently. This is referred to as 'leaky gut syndrome'. The toxins the intestine doesn't manage to eliminate enter the organism, which triggers our immune functions, and may be responsible for certain auto-immune diseases, or event generated inflammation.

Every large group of intestinal bacteria is made up of many strains, and each one of these strains can have different effects; the two most important groups are the firmicutes and the bacteroidetes. The firmicutes excel in extracting energy from food, and they are also necessary for fat absorption. Obese individuals have high concentrations of firmicutes in their gut flora compared to thin people who, for their part, have high concentrations of bacteroidetes. High concentrations of firmicutes activate genes linked to obesity, diabetes, and cardiovascular disease. In practice, the firmicutes/bacteroidetes ratio is a very good measure of a subject's health and potential for longevity, as this value can modify genetic expression.

The gut flora suffers from three types of damage:

    1 - exposure to substances which kill off bacterial colonies or alter their composition. Chemical substances in the environment, dietary substances (sugar and gluten), water treatment agents, drugs (e.g., antibiotics);

2 - a lack of nutrients needed to keep bacterial colonies in good health e.g., a low fiber diet, which diminishes gut flora diversity, to the detriment of good bacteria;

3 - stress, which is one of the most important factors leading to imbalance. It is well known that severe stress often causes diarrhea or other intestinal disorders affecting the microbial flora.

Probiotics or Prebiotics?

Probiotics are living microorganisms which are beneficial for our organism, and are a part of the gut flora. It is sometimes necessary to reseed our probiotics, for example when treated with antibiotics, after having had diarrhea, or during chemotherapy; these circumstances disrupt our ecological balance. But taking probiotics isn't enough, you also need to give them energy. This is where prebiotics come in; they are a selective food source for intestinal bacteria, specifically tailored for good bacteria. Prebiotics are sugars, like cellulose, lactose, galacto-oligosaccharides, and, above all, inulin. They must possess three essential characteristics: they must be non-digestible, that is, pass through the stomach without being degraded; intestinal bacteria must be able to ferment or metabolize them, and they must thereby improve our health. A daily consumption of 12 g of prebiotics is recommended, which are found in food or dietary supplements, or both.

What foods are high in prebiotics? Gum Arabic, raw chicory root, raw Jerusalem artichoke, raw dandelion greens, raw garlic and leeks, raw or cooked onion, raw asparagus. Artichoke is an excellent source of inulin, a sugar which is prebiotic as it isn't digested but is consumed by good intestinal bacteria in order for them to grow. It also provides large quantities of dietary fiber, both soluble and insoluble.

Probiotic-Rich Foods

Fermented foods contain most probiotic bacteria. The type of fermentation which makes foods probiotic is called lactic fermentation. During this process, good bacteria convert sugar molecules into lactic acid, which allows them to proliferate. In return, this lactic acid protects the food from pathogenic bacteria, as it creates a low-pH, acidic environment, which destroys bad bacteria. Today, we place certain good bacteria strains, such as Lactobacillus Acidophilus, into foods containing sugar in order to trigger this process. Making yogurt, for example, simply requires adding living bacteria strains to milk. Lactic fermentation is also used to preserve food and prolong its shelf life. Here are a few examples of probiotics.

Yogurt made with live cultures, (watch out for added sugar, sweeteners and artificial flavors). For those who are lactose intolerant, coconut yogurt is recommended, as it contains many enzymes and probiotics. Kefir: this is a mix of kefir 'grains' (yeast and bacteria) and goat's milk. It has high levels of lactobacillus, bifidobacteria, and antioxidants. There is also a version made from coconut, Kombucha, a fermented black tea which is served cold. Tempeh: made out of fermented soy. Kimchi, which mixes bacteria and spices. Fermented cabbage. Marinades: a simple and enjoyable probiotic. Fruits and vegetables marinated in brine. Fermented condiments, made with mayonnaise, mustard, spicy or hot sauces, or vinaigrette. Fermented meat, eggs and fish.

Probiotic Dietary Supplements:

There are five types of readily available probiotics: *Lactobacillus plantarum, Lactobacillus acidophilus, Lactobacillus brevis, Bifidobacterium lactis, Bifidobacterium longum.*

Each one has particular advantages. You should eat 12 g of probiotics every day, and eat probiotic foods twice per day. There are 'symbiotic' formulas which combine prebiotics and probiotics. They must be consumed with filtered water. Doing otherwise may negate the desired effects, as chlorine kills all bacteria, including the good ones!

☐ REMEMBER ☐

Our diet influences our gene expression, and therefore our health and our longevity. Having a healthy and balanced diet is a necessary precondition to having a long life. Avoiding fast carbs, with high glycemic indexes, is by far the highest priority; sugar is a serial killer, and we must learn not to get anywhere near it. The second priority is fighting silent inflammation, another serial killer, but far more insidious than sugar. You will need to hunt out all pro-inflammatory foods, and favor anti-inflammatory foods. The third priority is to avoid foods which cause chronic illnesses and cancer and to favor foods which protect us from these diseases: less fat, less salt, less red meat, more fruits and vegetables, more fish, more spices.

SOURCES

Barry Sears.
The Anti-inflammation Zone. New York : HarperCollins ; 2005.

David Perlmutter.
L'intestin au secours du cerveau. Paris : Hachette Livres (Marabout) ; 2016.

Michael Fossel, Greta Blackburn, Dave Woynarowski.
The Immortality Edge. Hoboken (New Jersey) : John Wiley & Sons, Inc. ; 2011.

Paul McGlothin & Meredith Averill.
The CR Way. New York : Harper-Collins ; 2008.

Richard Béliveau, Denis Gingras.
Les aliments contre le cancer. Québec : Trécarré ; 2005.

Richard Béliveau, Denis Gingras.
La méthode anti cancer. Québec : Trécarré ; 2014.

Walter Wahli, Nathalie Constantin.
La nutrigénomique dans votre assiette. Bruxelles : Éditions De Boeck ; 2011.

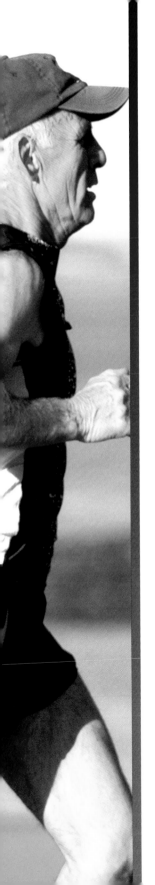

Chapter 2

Physical Activity and Longevity

*« Immobility could kill, physical
activity can change everything »*

- Anonymous -

R obert Marchland, 104 years old in 2016, still bikes for miles. This retired Frenchman celebrated his one hundred and fourth birthday by riding through 22 km of the time trial circuit planned for that year's Tour de France. He had previously set several world records in his age bracket. In particular, the one for distance covered in one hour on track, in 2012 and 2014; nearly 27 km. The Japanese Hidekichi Miyazakiwas listed in the Guinness Book of Records for running 100 m in 42 sec. and 22/100, in Kyoto (Japan).With this score, he beat the record set for this distance for those aged 105 and older. These examples, along with many others, support the view that having a long and healthy life will require regular physical activity. In fact, physical activity is such an important factor for longevity that it is only logical to conclude that its absence will lead to accelerated aging and mortality.

Jeremy Morris, a British scientist, studied the rate of cardiovascular disease in the drivers and conductors of London's famous double-decker buses. Rates of cardiovascular disease in conductors, who go up and down nearly 750 stairs every day, are 50% lower than drivers, who are sitting all day. The same was shown for postal workers: those delivering mail on foot, or by bike, have far lower rates of cardiovascular disease than those working at the front desk.

We know today that the positive impact of exercise is due to a series of metabolic adaptations which generally improve oxygen consumption and energy production. Physical activity targets several processes which are essential to maintaining good cardiovascular health. Furthermore, many studies demonstrate the positive impact of exercise in treating depression; others have proven that regular physical activity - at least three times a week - boosts the brain's metabolism and diminishes the risk of Alzheimer's by 40% in seniors .It also increases bone mass, thereby helping to prevent osteoporosis. And that's not all; physical activity reduces stress, improves sleep and keeps immune function in good working order, heightens libido and self-confidence, by releasing endorphins into the brain, which 'reward' physical activity by triggering a feeling of euphoria. On top of increasing tissue sensitivity to insulin and improving carbohydrate metabolism, regular physical exercise helps avoid, or reduce, the effects of aging on reaction time– the time required to react to any given situation. 65-year-old subjects who exercise regularly have identical, or sometimes even better reaction times than 20 year-olds who don't exercise. They also improve their 'fluid intelligence', that is, their problem-solving skills.

A study carried out at Stanford University on 6,000 men with an average age of 59 years and which lasted six years, showed that those practicing no physical activity had four times the risk of dying than those who regularly exercised; this substantial difference was also applicable for those suffering from cardiovascular disease. Studies carried out on women showed similar results.

2.1 - Physical Activity and Cancer

A large number of studies have clearly shown that very active individuals considerably reduce their chances of developing cancer compared to sedentary people. This is especially true for colon, prostate and breast cancer, potentially reducing the risk by 25%. This is due to several combined factors which together create an environment which isn't conducive to the transformation of precancerous cells into cancerous ones. Physical activity considerably reduces chronic inflammation, thereby eradicating the environment which they require to grow. Reducing abdominal fat, in particular, reduces inflammation and the release of certain cancer-promoting hormones.

According to the French National Cancer Institute, physical activity is linked with a decreased risk of several types of cancer; the level of evidence is «convincing» for colon cancer and «probable» for breast, uterus and lung cancer. Several randomized controlled trials have shown that an appropriate physical activity regimen, during and after cancer treatment, improves patients' quality of life. It lessens anxiety and depression and improves sleep, body image and well-being. Physical exercise also reduces the subjects' fatigue.

Furthermore, these studies show lower overall and specific mortality rates for patients who maintain their physical activity before and after a (breast, colon or prostate) cancer diagnosis. A reduction in the rates of cancer recurrence is also linked to physical activity post-diagnosis.

Several scientific studies have concluded that regular physical activity begun after a breast cancer diagnosis, significantly reduces overall mortality, breast cancer mortality and the rates of recurrence of this cancer. An American study carried out on 121,700 nurses, has shown that the risk of death from breast cancer or of breast cancer recurrence, is lowered by 20 to 50% for women who walk between three to five hours per week, compared to those who walk less than three hours per week (Holmes, 2005). These results were corroborated by the WHEL study (Women's Healthy Eating and Living) which reports that the risk of relapse is 44% lower for women who walk 30 minutes per day, six days a week (Saquib, 2007).

2.2 - Physical Activity and Genetic Expression

Physical activity modifies how fatty tissue genes are regulated: when sedentary people begin exercising, they can modify their epigenome. Charlotte Ling and her colleagues at Lund University in Sweden focused on what was happening inside fat, an energy-hoarding tissue. Their study shows that physical activity influences genes involved in obesity and type 2 diabetes. Physical activity therefore triggers epigenetic changes, at this specific level, in fatty tissue.

Swedish researchers tried to find out if it was possible to modify fatty tissue gene expression for the better, through regular exercise. To this end, they recruited thirty men who were initially not very active, and nearing their forties. Half of them had a family history of diabetes, since researchers wanted to find out if physical activity could, on top of its effect on obesity genes, also modify the expression of genes linked to this illness. To accomplish this, abdominal fat biopsies were performed at the start of the study and six months later. Gene expression rates were measured via DNA methylation, which reflects activity levels. The results, published in the online journal PLOS Genetics, confirm the expected improvement. «This is the first time it has been shown that physical exercise, practiced twice a week for six months, can alter the methylation of more than 7,000 genes found in adipose tissue from healthy, middle aged men», says Charlotte Ling. This improvement can also be seen in more conventional parameters, she adds: «decreased waist/hip ratio, diastolic blood pressure and resting heart rate.»

Why focus on fat cells? Because they have a very active role, at the crossroads of our organism's different metabolisms. Fat, once considered a passive energy store, is now seen as a fully-fledged endocrine organ, capable of releasing hormones, just like the thyroid gland or the pancreas.

Swedish researchers in Carl Johan Sundberg's team resorted to a novel method: 23 young men and women spent 45 minutes pedaling, four times a week, during three months, with only one leg. Each volunteer's unused leg therefore acted as a control, as it had undergone the same amount of methylation as the exercised leg, whether due to age or dietary habits. The differences between the two legs, however, could only have been due to the physical exercise. Although the leg's strength increased with training in all participants, of course, the changes within the muscle cells themselves were far more impressive. Differences were seen in more than 5,000 DNA sites, linked for example to muscle formation, energy supply, inflammatory mechanisms and immune processes. These sites were modified by physical activity in an identical manner in all volunteers.

2.3 - Telomeres and Physical Activity

Physical activity slows down the biological clock which triggers cell death. The telomeres of 50-year-old runners were observed to be as long as those of 40 year old sedentary subjects. In other words, we have proof that physical activity can modify the rhythm of the biological clock found in our genes. And we know how it does this.

A study carried out at King's College London, on 2,401 identical twins, showed a direct relationship between telomere length and regular physical activity. The researchers first precisely determined what kind of physical activity each volunteer practiced, for 12 consecutive months. The tests showed that the intensity and consistency of the physical activity of these volunteers directly influenced the length of their white blood cells' telomeres. These tests also confirmed that, even for twins sharing exactly the same genes, telomere length was indeed influenced by physical activity. The study also confirmed that the volunteers who worked out vigorously for three hours per week were, biologically speaking, nine years younger than those who only worked out for 15 minutes per week. Moderate physical activity, for 90 minutes per week, will give you an extra four years!

But one Swedish study goes even further. It shows that sitting less may be more important, at least in terms of telomere preservation, than exercising more. The authors stress that, although physical activity is on the rise in many countries, time spent sitting is also going up (working on computers, for example). They also mention a study which has shown that standing briefly during periods of sitting significantly affects glucose and insulin metabolism. They conclude that, in order to fight the harmful effects of a sedentary lifestyle in the elderly, stretching our legs for a few minutes may be more effective than exercising, at least as concerns telomere length, since the cardiovascular and cognitive benefits of exercise for senior citizens have been abundantly demonstrated.

Excessive physical exertion is counter-productive, however; certain violent sports, or extreme workouts, will damage your tendons and joints. This damage leads to aggravated oxidation and, more importantly, excessive cortisol production; this hormone provokes very significant increases in cell divisions, and therefore accelerated telomere shortening. Top athletes, who continually strive to stretch their limits during competitions, don't realize that they are shortening their life expectancy!

2.4 - Stem Cells and Physical Activity

Under normal conditions, our muscles are at rest and our skeletal muscles' stem cells are therefore 'quiescent', or at rest. Only after physical activity or some form of trauma do they wake up and get to work regenerating the damaged muscle. Researchers at the University of Illinois have shown that adult stem cells, which are present in muscle tissue, respond quickly to physical activity. They saw stem cells accumulate in mice's muscle tissue after intense exercise. They then tried to find out if this accumulation led to the production of new muscle fibers. They saw that the stem cells had released large quantities of growth factors, which created favorable conditions for the production of new muscle fibers. The good news is that researchers believe they can develop new therapeutic strategies to help handicapped patients recover their muscle mass.

A new study, the results of which have just been announced by researchers at the National Cheng Kung University (NCKU), confirms that physical exercise helps reverse the age-related reduction in neural stem cell production in the hippocampus in mice. According to the researchers, physical exercise promotes the production of a chemical substance in the brain which fosters the production and maturation of new stem cells.

In 2015, researchers brought the Sprouty1 gene to light, which is responsible for maintaining stem cell stores in muscle tissue. It becomes inhibited as we age, and older subjects may have less than half as many stem cells in reserve compared to younger individuals. Scientists are therefore looking for a way to reactivate Sprouty1, in order to combat the loss of muscle mass due to aging or certain illnesses.

2.5 - Sedentary Lifestyle

You can walk for thirty minutes per day, but if you don't move for the rest of the day, your inactivity will cancel out the benefits of walking regularly. People who spend seven hours a day in front of the TV (yes, that happens!), are 85% more likely to die prematurely from myocardial infarction than those who watch it for less than one hour a day. This remains a challenge for 85% of city-dwellers who go to work by car, sit for eight hours in front of their computers, maybe go jogging for half an hour, then go home, sit in front of the TV and only get up to eat dinner! The people who will benefit the most from the effects of exercise are those who will find a way to stay as active as possible for the rest of the day.

After having spent only 20 minutes sitting down, the spine's ligaments relax. This is a bad thing for runners, says Stuart McGill, the director of the Biomechanics Lab of the University of Waterloo (Canada), as the muscles and ligaments no longer offer any support. The spine needs about half an hour to become fully 'rigid' again, which matters a lot when we need to move. The gluteal muscles, in particular the gluteus medius, tend to elongate when we sit for too long, which makes it impossible to properly stabilize the pelvic floor when we run. Other muscles and tendons end up straining more to compensate, which may lead to a range of issues which runners know all too well: pulled muscles, knee pain etc.

2.6 - Too Much Rest Isn't Good for Our Health!

Rest is the opposite of what seniors need! The most dangerous thing we can say to someone who is retired is: «*So you're retired? You deserve it, after everything you've done! You should rest now.*»

Staying still may kill them prematurely.

Swedish researchers asked five volunteers, including two athletes, to stay in bed 24 hours a day for three weeks...Once the results came in, the researchers concluded that these five volunteers had, in those three weeks, lost twenty years of life expectancy! The good news is that resuming regular activity got rid of this loss.

> *A study carried out by researchers at the University of Sydney, between 2006 and 2010, concluded that the more we sit, the more likely we are to die young, and that people who sit for more than 11 hours a day are 40% more at risk of dying within the next three years than people who sit for less than four hours a day. This confirms a study by the American Cancer Society, which showed that the mortality rate of people who sit for more than six hours a day is 20% higher for men, and 40% higher for women, compared to employees who spend less than three hours a day sitting.*

2.7 - The Science of Physical and Sporting Activities

Physical activity has become the subject of an entire scientific field, whose primary goal was to optimize athletic performance. But the colossal financial investment which was poured into this research, justified by the sports industry, has also made it possible to prove the collateral benefits of physical activity on health and longevity. Today, not only are these benefits wholly accepted, but we even allow it to be prescribed, which is the first step to having social agencies take responsibility for this practice. The math is simple: generalizing physical activity, even subsidizing it, leads to lower health costs. The principle of homeostasis also applies to physical activity, insofar as, in order to stay young, we constantly have to rebuild muscle, whereas we naturally tend to lose muscle with age. Every time we exercise, our muscles get stronger, our enzymes and our proteins move more easily through our bloodstream, thereby curbing inflammation, which causes scarring. Our heart gets stronger, our brain draws more blood, our arteries are more flexible, our organs receive more nutrients, and, above all, our immune system is vastly improved.

2.8 - Physical Activity, to Conserve Muscle Mass

Sarcopenia

This is the name given to the gradual decline, as we age, in muscle fiber numbers, which are replaced, little by little, by fatty tissue. We lose about 150 g of muscle a year past the age of 50. Muscle loss is seen in men, more so than in women, starting at around 25 to 30 years of age, and even more after 50. At first it goes unnoticed, as part of the muscle is gradually replaced by fat, which will keep total volume more or less constant, but its function worsens and, of course, it becomes weaker. This is one of the major signs of aging, visible on the body and our silhouette, but it isn't inevitable. This phenomenon is neither inescapable nor irreversible. We can preserve our muscle over time.

One week of uninterrupted rest leads to a 10 to 15% reduction in muscle strength. In order to maintain our muscles, the math is really quite simple: *protein-rich food + physical activity = increase in muscle mass* (RVH Foundation; Canada).

Protein-Rich Foods and Amino Acids

Protein intake is crucial to muscle building, but the balance of essential amino acids is also important. According to studies, lean meat is most effective: poultry, fish and shellfish. Egg protein (which is found in the whites) has the best amino acid balance. It is the most easily assimilated protein for human beings. This can be supplemented by the protein found in cheese, chia seeds (which are also high in omega 3), whey, hemp or spirulina. Whole grains along with pulses also represent a good, balanced plant protein source. You may also supplement your leucine intake, as it is an essential amino acid, and among the most involved in muscle metabolism. It is found in higher concentrations (in descending order) in pulses: lentils, peas, beans; but also in fish, shellfish, lamb, beef, pork, poultry, cheese and eggs.

Vitamin D promotes muscle building (as well as boosting bone strength).

Citrulline: watermelon has high concentrations of this amino acid which promotes muscle protein synthesis and increases growth hormone levels. Citrulline seems to be the best amino acid for muscle gain past 50 years old. Indeed, ingested amino acids are increasingly quickly captured by the digestive organs, at the expense of our muscles which they have more trouble reaching. But this doesn't apply to citrulline.

Creatinine: according to some studies, creatinine intake may promote the development of lean body mass, rather than body fat, but only when following an exercise regime involving short, intense bursts of energy, or resistance training (e.g., weight training). This doesn't work for endurance sports such as running, biking, walking etc. The effects observed by these studies are not miraculous either, but creatinine remains one of the products most frequently used by athletes, as it may also increase muscle performance (5 to 15% according to studies). A dosage of around three grams per day seems to be reasonable.

And What About Growth Hormone?

It isn't necessarily recommendable to inject yourself with growth hormone to gain muscle, as its side-effects are hard to control; this can make it dangerous. Some amino acids promote its production, e.g., arginine, betaine or citrulline. You should also remember that muscular exercise (interval training in particular) causes your body to produce equivalent amounts of growth hormones (and they're free!)

2.9 - Other Physical Activities

Sports are the best way to gain muscle, at any age. Many studies show this, and it has recently been demonstrated that similar levels of exertion can be carried out whether we are 25 or 75. Some types of exercise build more muscle than others, however. We thought for a long time that light endurance training (running, biking, swimming) was the best way to maintain our musculature as we age. In fact, studies show that alternating between endurance and high intensity exercise works best. Resistance exercise (first with your own body weight, then with free weights) is a good way to begin training. Interval training, in which short bursts of intense effort are alternated with longer endurance periods (no matter the sport), are also very effective, as they promote growth hormone production. The one to two percent of muscle mass lost on average each year past 40 can therefore be almost entirely recovered in three weeks of training, with three or four sessions a week.

High Intensity Interval Training (HIIT)

This is a powerful tool, both for beginners and athletes. In the past only practiced by experienced athletes, interval training has become easily accessible to all, even a beginner sportsman.

Interval training simply consists of alternating periods of intense activity with periods of more moderate activity. In the case of walking, you may, if you are in good shape, incorporate short periods of running into your usual brisk walks; but if you are not feeling up to it, you could also alternate, as feels comfortable, regular walking and intervals where you walk faster. The key to HIIT is to make sure that the high intensity intervals are at maximum effort, not just a faster heart rate.

During intense physical exercise, our muscles produce waste which may cause muscle soreness. Too much of this waste may therefore make exercise painful or tiring. But by alternating intervals of intense physical exercise with more relaxed periods, you will help limit the accumulation of waste in your muscles. If you simply wish to increase your exercise routine, set specific times and speeds for each intense interval, depending on how you feel that day. After warming up, you may increase the intensity for 30 seconds and then go back to your usual pace. The next intense interval may last two or three minutes. You may increase the speed, time and frequency of these periods of more intense exercise in any configuration you like.

Interval training isn't for everyone, however. If you have a health problem or don't exercise regularly, talk to your doctor before trying interval training. This type of physical exercise helps burn more calories, but you should remember that too much of it may hurt you.

How does HIIT work?

HIIT exercises and conditions both the aerobic and anaerobic energy systems. Aerobic activity includes low intensity activities which last longer, such as walking, cardio, step, or treadmill exercises. They are called aerobic as they involve oxygen heavily. Your aerobic exercise capacity is therefore limited by your lung and heart capacities.

Anaerobic activity involves short bursts or high intensity effort, such as a 100 m speed run, for example. Anaerobic means without oxygen, and this type of metabolism depends on energy which is stored in our muscles as glycogen or creatine. This activity leads to the production of lactic acid, which will cause the burning sensation, or even cramps, we feel during short, intense effort. During this intense activity, we accumulate a sort of 'oxygen debt', which will be redeemed by our heart and lungs during the recovery phase, as well as neutralizing the lactic acid. During this phase, the aerobic system takes control once more, by converting carbohydrates into usable energy.

HIIT causes metabolic changes which will enable you to improve your cardiovascular capacity, will produce new blood capillaries, and deliver more blood to your muscles, which will therefore develop a greater lactate tolerance. More importantly, these alternating sets cause you to use all three types of muscle fiber, and this will enable you to practice all kinds of physical activity.

Warm up and always take the time to recover, for at least five minutes, before and after every HIIT session. Warm up with the same activity you planned for your HIIT session: run slowly if you are planning to run, or pedal more slowly if you have decided to go biking. Exercise as hard as you can during the high intensity intervals, until you can feel a burning sensation in your muscles: this means you've used all of your anaerobic resources.

No matter how you feel when starting the exercise, you should always respect the intervals. If you have already gone through the entire session you have planned and feel like you can do more, increase the duration or intensity of every interval the next time.

If you experience chest pain or trouble breathing during HIIT, stop doing the high intensity intervals, briefly recover by walking, and stop exercising for the day. If these symptoms persist, you should immediately ask for medical assistance. If you feel weak, take the time to gently recover, then lie down on your back and keep your legs high, by laying them on a chair or against a wall, for example. This will stop your blood from pooling in your legs.

Researchers at Newcastle University in the UK released the results of a randomized clinical trial which studied the impact of high intensity interval training on hepatic fat, glycemic control and heart function in patients suffering from type 2 diabetes. The results of this study showed that patients performing HIIT had significant improvement in glycemic control (without modifying their diet or drug regimen), improved heart function, and 39% less hepatic fat.

Growth hormone secretion is strongly stimulated by physical exercise, in proportion to the intensity of the exercise. Furthermore, increased growth hormone secretion can be seen during exercise, but also during recovery after muscular exercise, the time when anabolism is most active. The effects of strength training on growth hormone secretion are due to the training sessions in and of themselves. For healthy athletes who do not have a restricted diet, HIIT significantly increases growth hormone, catecholamines and adrenalin. All of these hormones are involved in fat burning. This means that the more you produce these hormones, the more you burn fat. And they also inhibit the production of an enzyme which promotes the storage of fatty tissue.

In terms of longevity, some Italian studies have recently shown that very high growth hormone levels foster telomere lengthening. This study was carried out on 476 healthy individuals between 16 and 104 years of age. The results of telomere measurements showed that high levels of growth hormone were correlated with 10% longer telomeres.

Excess Post-Exercise Oxygen Consumption

What happens to your engine after a long car ride? Once you've reached your destination, the engine, still warm after you've turned it off, will gradually cool down, until it reaches its resting temperature. The same thing happens to our body after physical activity, which means we may continue to burn more calories than usual, even when we are resting.

This phenomenon is called EPOC (Excess Post-Exercise Oxygen Consumption). Our body consumes more oxygen after intense physical exercise, in order to compensate for our oxygen 'debt'.

What About Cardio Training?

Aerobic exercise, such as running on a treadmill for an hour, doesn't lead to similar increases in growth hormone production as intense but brief exercise; furthermore, we quickly reach a plateau in cardio, in terms of fat burning. This is one of the reasons why we tend to 'give up', as results aren't very visible.

A recent study compared long-distance runners, running ten kilometers, to people practicing interval training. The long-distance runners burned twice as many calories, but the others burned nine times more body fat! Why does interval training burn so many fewer calories but more fat? There are two reasons for this: the first is that our metabolism continues to work intensely long after we are done exercising. The second is the rapid and sustained increase in growth hormones.

Free Weights

Resistance training with free weights or your body weight, as is the case with push-ups, for example, is very useful, as it increases your muscle strength by 25 to 100% in one year. It's never too late to start, as long as you choose the right kind of workout; it is best to begin with a specialized coach. Resistance training works by forcing your muscle cells to adapt to this overload, which will make them grow and recruit nerve cells which make them contract. To ensure optimal function, your muscles should undergo maximum contraction, for a very short period of time.

Stretching

Stretching is a gentle exercise, whose objective is to stretch out and relax the entire organism. The suggested set of exercises will relax different parts of your body. Stretching mixes different fitness methods; movements from classical gymnastics and others from eastern disciplines such as yoga. Despite their simple appearance, these movements are quite complex. This is why they must be performed carefully, to avoid any pain or accidents (in the tendons in particular). For them to be as effective as possible, they must be performed with proper breathing technique, stretching your muscles when you exhale. This is why classes are strongly recommended at first. Wait a few months before performing exercises on your own, as you should first properly understand the point, and purpose, of each movement.

Anyone can stretch. This gymnastics method is recommended for anyone, whether you are completely stiff or are as limber as a championship gymnast. Many people improve rapidly. Don't give up if this isn't your case, however, you are guaranteed to see results in due time. Be patient, tangible results may often take several months to show. The more you stretch regularly, holding poses for as long as possible, the more you will see rapid change, and the more your fitness will improve.

The basic principle is passive stretching. Every exercise is done gently. It isn't useful, as was formerly taught in school gym classes, to briefly and repeatedly push through movements, in the belief that this will make you go further. When you push your torso down to touch the ground with your fingers, for example, it won't help to repeatedly jerk your torso downwards. It is better to remain still while you lean over, concentrate on your pose, and exhale gently, slowly and deeply, trying to go down a little further each time you exhale. Your breathing should dictate your movement, and it should always be done gently. If you concentrate on your breathing, you will quickly feel the muscle tension in your neck, your shoulders, your back and your lower limbs fade away. You will also manage to extend surprisingly far, so long as you take your time. For best results, you should stretch every week, or every day if you can. Stretching will improve your quality of life, and will make you enjoy your favorite activities more, no matter your age. Stretching reduces the risk of muscular injury and slows joint degeneration.

Testosterone

Testosterone is very involved in muscle building and, as you would expect, its levels in the blood also decrease with age. You can increase the body's sensitivity to the effects of testosterone with certain plants like *Tribulus terrestris* (which has many common names, including goat's head), Maca, Ginseng or *Ashwaganda*. These plants may also boost testosterone production. You should also pay attention to your zinc and vitamin E levels (which are often too low).

If your testosterone levels are grossly insufficient, substitution treatments can be considered; but only with natural, bio-identical testosterone, and in the lowest possible doses, making sure to avoid all contraindications, and especially under the supervision of a competent anti-aging doctor.

▢ R E M E M B E R ▢

Physical activity is, quite simply, the key to longevity. It can change everything, as it mobilizes thousands of genes whose expression will be beneficially altered. Through regular, weekly or daily physical activity, we lengthen our telomeres, trigger stem cell production, protect our DNA, our heart and our blood vessels, get rid of diabetes, protect ourselves against cancer, lose abdominal fat, reinforce our immune system, increase our libido, improve our mood, think more clearly... the list goes on!

Physical activity is a must, we shouldn't live without it!

S O U R C E S

David A. Kekich. Smart,
Strong and Sexy at 100? New-port Beach, (Californie) : Maximum Life Foundation ; 2012.
Michael Fossel, Greta Blackburn, Dave Woynarowski.
The Immortality Edge. Hoboken (New Jersey) : John Wiley & Sons, Inc. ; 2011.
Michael Roizen, Mehmet Oz.
YOU: The Owner's manual. New York : William Morrow ; 2005.
Stretching:
Docteur Catherine Aubé, chiropraticienne.
Centre chiropratique, Les Portes du Fontainebleau, Blainville,
Québec (Canada) http://www.centreevoluetre.com

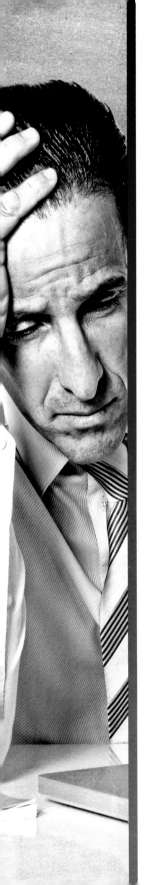

- Part 4 -

Chapter 3

Stress and Longevity

« Stress is life! »

- Hans Selye -

S tress influences our genetic expression, both positively and negatively. Stress is a part of life. All change leads, in all of us, to an adaptation reaction, the objective of which is to maintain homeostasis; this is a non-specific phenomenon, which applies to all animal species. A small cat, when it sees a big dog, will react: its heart will start beating faster, which means it will take in more oxygen and produce more energy, which will give it a better chance of survival. It will quickly choose a strategy: either confront the dog, or retreat ('fight or flight'). It will generally choose to run away, and once the danger is gone, its body will slowly calm down and recover its energy. This is an example of well-managed stress, where energy expenditure was adjusted for an immediate, ideally suited action. But if that little cat had decided to confront the dog, or taken too long to decide, its response would not have been appropriate; its energy expenditure would have been too large or lasted for too long, and it would have led to exhaustion, eliminating any chances of survival. Stress response therefore depends on two factors: the stress itself, on the one hand, and the stressed subject, on the other hand. Once the brain has interpreted a situation as stressful, the stress response is triggered.

3.1 - Stress and Cellular Aging

Although we have long known that stress affects both behavior and health, recent research has shown that it also directly attacks our DNA. There is a definite cause and effect relationship between stress and cellular aging. Elizabeth Blackburn (Nobel Prize in Physiology or Medicine in 2009) demonstrated this in a monumental study, in 2004, carried out on a group of sixty-two premenopausal mothers.

Every participant in the control group was the mother of a physically and mentally healthy child, while in the other group, they all had a child suffering from a chronic disease. For years, these mothers were subjected to tests which measured their stress levels and how their white blood cells were aging, as well as oxidation (oxidative stress), and the length of their telomeres .In order to quantify this effect, the researchers measured telomere length in both groups. They noticed that, age being equal, telomere length in women caring for a sick child was much shorter than in women with healthy children. On average the length of these women's telomeres seemed ten years older than that of women in the control group. Accelerated cellular aging is therefore one of the significant effects of stress.

3.2 - Stress and Genetic Expression

Recent research in epigenetics has shown that everything in our environment, including our emotions, affects whether millions of switches in our DNA will be turned on or off. Emotions in particular are at the heart of this interaction. We know that emotional imprinting during fetal development, from conception all the way to birth, will influence the development of the child's personality and identity. It has been discovered that a second phase of epigenetic reprogramming takes place after fertilization, just before the cellular differentiation process is triggered (for embryonic stem cells).This second reprogramming phase makes it possible for the fetus's genes to adapt to its environment.

Epigenetics opens up new possibilities, in terms of treatment, as hundreds of these epigenetic markers can be reversed. If a baby rat has an inattentive mother, it can be given to a more affectionate adoptive mother, who grooms it often, and it will develop normally. It is now accepted that disease-causing disorders may be reversible, even when they originate before birth. This phenomenon is known as 'neuroplasticity', a mechanism which allows the brain to alter itself, through experience. Underused connections tend to disappear, while other connections which are more solicited are reinforced. Neuronal networks are activated or deactivated as needed.

Neurologist Hunter Hoffman (University of Washington Harborview Burn Center) had the idea of showing burn victims movies taking place in an icy universe while they were being treated. Once the treatment has been performed, he asks one severely burned patient to assess the severity of his pain on a scale going from 0 to 100. The patient points at 38. With painkillers alone, the pain is estimated to be between 90 and 100.

A recent study shows that our prenatal environment can alter our epigenome. Researchers analyzed the DNA in the blood of teenagers whose mothers smoked and continued to do so during pregnancy. These teenagers had significant epigenetic markers in their blood cells concerning a gene involved in brain development, the BDNF gene. These results suggest that prenatal exposure to tobacco may have an impact on brain development via epigenetic mechanisms.

3.3 - Managing Stress and Emotions

How we manage our emotions is a key factor in stress. It is the primary source of pathological complications. The stronger the emotions, the less reasoning becomes possible: too much emotion impairs effective thinking. Exercising control over our emotions is therefore the primary objective of stress management techniques. « *First I calm down, then I think and act.* »

Meditation

"Meditation is life experienced and perceived" (David O'Hare)

Our homeostasis, our vital balance, is controlled by our autonomic (or vegetative) nervous system. Our health depends on it, as it regulates everything. Every one of our vital functions depends on it (breathing, temperature, alertness, heart rate, hormonal regulation etc.); they are beyond our conscious control. Furthermore, all of these functions are interdependent. This means that if one variable is altered, all of the others will immediately and automatically adapt to it. The only function we can consciously alter, to some extent, is breathing: we can amplify, slow, and even stop it for some time, but there is a limit (asphyxiation) past which we lose that ability. We are nevertheless able to influence our autonomic nervous system through our breathing. This is what all of the different meditative practices do. Among other things, they balance and harmonize our sympathetic and parasympathetic nervous systems, by supplying us with very high cortisol levels in the morning (which is essential to waking up), and as much melatonin as possible at night (which is just as desirable for quality sleep).

Meditation has been the subject of more than 2,500 articles, published in the most prestigious scientific journals. Today, more than seventy of the one hundred and twenty-five medical schools in the United States offer meditation classes; this is because, since 1958, many studies have shown that this practice has highly beneficial effects for our health. The first significant experiment was carried out at Harvard University by cardiologist Herbert Benson, who did not believe that meditation could reduce hypertension. A few weeks after having begun testing, he saw not only a significant reduction in blood pressure, but also decreases in cholesterol levels, chronic pain, drug dependence and anxiety.

Another study led by Dr. David Orme-Johnson and published in the journal Psychosomatic Medicine in 1987, showed that those who meditate have 44% fewer medical consultations, 87% less cardiovascular disease, 30% fewer infectious illnesses. The latest research in psycho-immunology, published in late 2003, was carried out by Prof. Richard Davidson, the director of the Medical Imaging Lab at the University of Wisconsin, and Jon Kabat-Zinn, with groups of students. It shows that a meditation training program, even a short one, has a positive influence on the immune system, as it helps regulate the brain's emotional center.

Meditation techniques can also slow down telomere shortening, by reducing cognitive (mental) stress. Other researchers have produced similarly positive results concerning cognitive performance and the ability to concentrate.

In a recent study carried out at the University of California, Los Angeles (UCLA), psychologists selected two groups of students whom they monitored with a particular type of scanner (MRI) which allowed them to examine their brain activity. The first group practiced so-called mindfulness meditation, while the other did not. The scans made of the meditating group registered high activity in the right prefrontal cortex as well as a calming effect on the amygdala (a part of the brain which controls emotion), showing how meditation can help deal with emotions in a more detached manner.

Another study, which was presented at a conference of the American Heart Association, has shown that patients with narrowing coronary arteries who meditate are half as likely to have a heart attack, a stroke, or dying due to these causes, compared to those who don't meditate.

Mindfulness-Based Cognitive Therapy (MBCT)

Mindfulness meditation is seeing things as they are rather than how we would like them to be, says David O'Hare. You concentrate entirely on the present moment, and examine what you feel. How long you meditate or where doesn't matter: you can do it while walking, running, before going to sleep etc. The only thing that matters is that you do it regularly. The practice of mindfulness meditation is very open. You can focus on a specific object, on an activity, on your own breathing, on your body. You will focus on this (physical or spiritual) object and gradually become conscious of your connection with this object, how you envision it, how it makes you feel, what sensations it generates. You will observe, perceive, without becoming attached to any mental states. Any pleasant emotions which may appear should not be held onto or prolonged, just as unpleasant ones should not be avoided. You simply move along, through concentric circles, out from the center of your attention. While working on sharpening your perception, both spiritually and physically, you will let the subjects you meditate upon come and go. Thus you will focus on the meditation itself, your own breathing, the way in which your muscles work to maintain your posture, holding your focus etc.

Your body will also benefit from mindfulness meditation. By concentrating on the smallest of sensations, of motions, on the tiniest muscle movements, you will learn to relax. Tension will become an anomaly, and will no longer correspond to your ordinary state, but to that which the accumulation of stress had led to. Your attitude will become synonymous with tranquility, will inspire others to relax. You will learn to move more delicately, by realizing that your formerly sweeping movements were unnecessary.

This of course requires regular practice, with proper attention given to the smallest of sensations. You will also have to be patient. These changes sometimes take a while to appear, and the people around you will often notice them before you do.

Walking Meditation
(David O'Hare)

Whereas other meditation techniques are static, this is the simplest form of moving meditation, where your eyes are open in order to avoid obstacles. Your attention is no longer exclusively focused inward, you also pay attention to your environment. You pay attention to elements usually ignored by classical meditation, like the wind, the cold, the sun, the rain, and especially sounds and smells. You also learn about your posture, and balancing walking and breathing. You have to pay attention to how you stand, examining all of your joints one by one, and then, once you start walking, paying attention to the signals sent out by all of your senses. Observe, acknowledge and then move on, without any judgment, whether these feelings and images are pleasant or not.

3.4 - Speaking to Our Cells

Guy Corneau is a famous Canadian psychotherapist. A few years ago, he was diagnosed with stage IV cancer, the most advanced stage. Against all odds, he was diagnosed as cured one year later. He talks us through this journey in a book, *Rebirth*. It is a message of hope and an invitation to think about the meaning of illness.

How did Guy Corneau decide to be healthy? By speaking to his cells!

Does this mean we now live in an esoteric universe, where everything is decided in our inner world? Perhaps... Some scientific evidence does however support the idea that speaking to our cells, using our everyday language, may influence the activation (or repression) of hundreds of genes. Our DNA may very well understand our language. Russian scientists say our DNA may understand our language, or at the very least be sensitive to the frequencies we produce when we speak.

Here is an example of the dialectic process which Guy Corneau uses to speak to his cells:

Step 1: *First, focus on your heart, then call upon your body's master cell... and ask it to reach one of the affected organs.*

Step 2: *Concentrate on the stomach. Listen to what the cancer cells have to say. Let whatever happens happen... Then thank the sick cells, and tell them that their tenure is over... Tell them that they can die.*

Step 3: *Ask the master cell to call on the stem cells in the stomach and ask them to produce plenty more stomach stem cells... Then move on to the spleen... And so on...*

Step 4: *Finally, witness your whole being, in perfect health...*

You can find the full audio version of this exercise, in French, on www.guycorneau.com.

The most important aspect of this dialog is, once he has listened to the struggling cells, that he tells them that they can die. This makes complete sense once we know that the key characteristic of cancer cells is their immortality, as they suppress apoptosis (programmed cell death).

The second fundamental aspect is invoking the power of stem cells. Christian Drapeau, a Canadian neurophysiologist, supports this method: « *It would therefore be possible, via visualization exercises, to stimulate nerve endings in certain parts of the body, which would thereby encourage stem cell migration towards tissue in need of repair.* »

Guy Corneau speaks to his cells once a day, for about 20 minutes. He tries to reprogram cancer cells thanks to his imagination!

Guided imagery: researchers used a positron camera (scanner) to show that the same areas of the brain are activated whether we imagine an event or we actually live through it. This technique is risk-free and is a very useful tool for solving health issues, including combating aging.

3.5 - Don't Worry, Be Happy!

Or : « *Medicine heals and love cures!* »

We could all lend ourselves a hand if we were willing to see our own bodies in a holistic manner, that is, if we took our psychological and social environments into account. Visualization reinforces self-regulatory mechanisms and the immune system. We refer in this case to 'self-healing emotions' (Liliane Reuter). Since we are able to see it, visualizing ourselves in good health gives the cellular process a sort of direction, directs cells towards homeostasis. But for this we must first be aware of what good health can accomplish; the strength of our will to live is most effective in arousing self-healing mechanisms.

3.6 - Sleep and Meditation

Hundreds of thousands of people die every year because of undiagnosed, and therefore untreated sleep disorders. Meditation could be the answer! Scientists discovered that people who meditate regularly sleep for longer and more deeply than those who don't meditate. The reason is simple: they are far more relaxed!

You don't even need to meditate just before bed, since regular meditation leads to higher levels of two very important hormones: serotonin (the happiness hormone) and melatonin (the sleep hormone), while causing cortisol levels (the stress and waking hormone) to diminish. It is truly beneficial, as sleeping well means we feel well-rested during the day, which improves our chances of sleeping longer and deeper the next night, with less cellular stress, longer telomeres and a longer lifespan.

Sleep and Longevity

It is difficult to scientifically demonstrate the correlation between sleep and longevity.

New studies indicate that our metabolism is negatively influenced by the loss of sleep. Jonathan Cedernaes (Uppsala University, Sweden) and his colleagues monitored 15 healthy average-weight men, whom they forced into insomnia. Analysis of sampled tissue showed that the regulation and activity of the genes constituting their biological clock had been altered, after only a single sleep-deprived night. «Our findings demonstrate that a single night of wakefulness can alter the epigenetic and transcriptional profile of core circadian clock genes in key metabolic tissues.»

Naps and Longevity

Cardiovascular risk is significantly lowered in nap takers. You could not begin to imagine the influence such a small daily break has on cardiovascular mortality, according to a recent study carried out in Greece in 2007 on 24,000 individuals who took naps and were monitored for six years. They all began the study without any cases of cardiovascular disease, cancer or other illnesses. Compared to subjects who never took naps in the afternoon, those who did so for half an hour a day were 37%

less likely of dying of cardiovascular disease.

Even those who only occasionally napped also benefited, to a lesser, but still significant extent, their risk being 12% lower. As the value of napping was higher in men, the authors suggested reductions in working hours were more likely to be responsible for this effect rather than the sleep itself.

3.7 - Sex and Longevity

Here we must rig the game in our favor! In the hierarchy of nature, reproductive ability gives us higher priority, and sexual activity, even if it isn't necessarily geared towards reproduction, is useful as a type of 'anti-aging mimicry'.

Making love may not only be good for our mental health, but also for our physical health and our longevity. Our entire organism may benefit from a healthy sexuality. In 2007 a study led by the British neuropsychologist David Weeks at the Royal Edinburgh Hospital showed that an active sex life allows us to delay the aging process. The 3,500 men and women aged 20 to 104 years old who participated had two things in common: a relatively intense sex life and *seeming much younger than they actually were.*

Frederic Saldmann confirms this: there is a link between sexuality, longevity and health. Sex brings about well-being, which improves happiness and delays the aging process. More specifically: *having sexual intercourse twelve times per month increases life expectancy by ten years!*

An explanation? Oxytocin, a hormone released during orgasm, relaxes and energizes us, and gives us a feeling of fulfillment. Serotonin and dopamine, for their part, are produced by the brain after sex, and are the messengers of pleasure and euphoria. Pleasure then releases endorphins: this natural sedative gets rid of anxiety and stress!

Blood pressure increases at the same time, which provides more oxygenated blood and hormones to the cells, and gets rid of carbon dioxide and toxins. This cardiovascular stimulation then activates the heart and the lungs, lowers cholesterol levels and burns calories; during orgasm, we may reach a peak of 180 beats per minute. This is excellent exercise for the heart muscle, which needs it in order to work properly, barring certain contraindications. But that isn't all. According to Doctor Saldmann, *regular sexual intercourse protects against many illnesses, in particular prostate cancer in men, and breast cancer in women, as well as cardiovascular disease. This is all the more important, he says, as the latter becomes more frequent with age, just as sexual activity declines.*

An American study carried out on 30,000 men concludes that frequent ejaculation protects men from prostate cancer. «We found that 21 ejaculations a month reduce the risk of prostate cancer by a third», says Frédéric Saldmann. The study states that the cancer-prevention benefit becomes significant starting at 12 ejaculations per month. And from a medical point of view? Frequent ejaculation allows the prostate gland to evacuate carcinogens which accumulate in the prostate. «Releasing semen contributes to the regular cleaning of the prostate», says Frederic Saldmann. For men just as for women, making love three times a week will make you gain ten years of life expectancy.

Stress is an integral part of our life, of our adaptation system, and therefore of our homeostasis. Too much stress is bad for us, and too little stress isn't good either. Emotions positively or negatively influence genetic expression, depending on how they are handled. It's possible, and even fairly easy, to manage stress and emotions, by using proven relaxation methods. Relaxation is very useful, of course. It improves concentration, optimizes reasoning, improves performance and our longevity.

S O U R C E S

Christian Drapeau.
Le pouvoir insoupçonné des cellules souches. Québec : Les Éditions de l'Homme ; 2010.

Fréderic Saldmann.
La vie et le temps. Paris : Flammarion ; 2011.

Guy Corneau.
Revivre ! Québec : Les Éditions de l'Homme ; 2010.

Liliane Reuter.
Votre esprit est votre meilleur médecin. Paris : Robert Laffont ; 1999.

Marie Lise Labonté, Nicolas Bornemisza.
Guérir grâce à nos images intérieures. Québec : Les Editions de l'Homme ; 2006.

Nathalie Zammatteo.
L'impact des émotions sur l'ADN. Aubagne : Éditions Quintessence ; 2014.

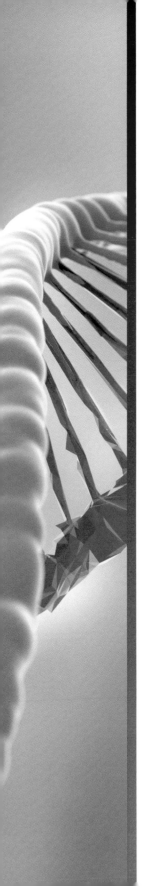

- Part 3 -
Conclusions

« The better we understand, the better we heal »

- Françoise Dolto -

Leading a healthy lifestyle is all in a day's work. We must always get back to it, as attacks are constant, seven days a week, 24 hours a day, all year long, every year of our life. The method is simple but achieving it regularly, no matter how simple, is difficult.

So how can it be done?

We need about six months for healthy habits to stick; during this period, strength of will must constantly be tended, as temptations run strong. If we happen to falter, we must know how to manage our mistakes. The first step is knowledge: learn about the best ways of eating well, moving well, effectively managing our stress and our emotions. Today it is undeniable that a healthy lifestyle is an essential prerequisite for a long and healthy life. The second step is to gradually apply the ingredients of a healthy lifestyle, by working simultaneously on all three of its components: improving our diet, our physical activity and our meditative practice, every day. The third step is to maintain these practices indefinitely; this is a difficult step, as once the positive effects of a healthy lifestyle begin to appear, we tend to let go and satisfy our desires: small pleasures, slacking off on exercise etc. Social support or having a coach will be particularly important during this phase.

In order to help you to execute these steps, we wanted a program which would take into account all of the essential elements for hyper-longevity, lived in optimal health. And we designed it, just for you.

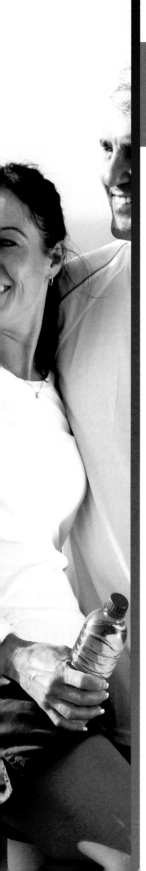

Part 5

THE JLIFE PLAN

Chapter 1 : Taking stock

Chapter 2 : JLife Nutrition

Chapter 3 : JLife Fitness

Chapter 4 : JLife Stress

Conclusion

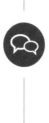

Introduction

« The things we have to learn before we can do,
we learn by doing »

- Aristotle -

When you buy a computer, it is most often shipped with a sizeable, and sometimes intimidating, instruction manual. In fact, not a single one of the accessories which populate our daily lives is free from some kind of detailed instruction booklet. But what about our life? Did we ever receive its instruction manual?

We have spent millennia searching for it. Whether we call it well-being, harmony, happiness or the fountain of youth, it remains hidden, and through our work, we are slowly uncovering just a few of its pages. Today we can offer you a few more, thanks to our JLife program, which is designed to squeeze even more life into your life.

By reading this book, you have acquired enough knowledge to understand why we age and what we can do to delay, or even 'reverse' aging. You now have all the necessary elements to consider undergoing a *cellular revitalization* protocol, but you may still have some reservations.

Some are absolutely convinced that what they have already read is credible enough for them to take immediate action, but they don't know where to start, due to the wealth of available information, which can also be quite complex. They would like an instruction manual. We are there to help them. Others have properly assimilated the information contained in this book. Yet they are not entirely confident that these hyperlongevity methods are effective. They may be convinced that death is not only inevitable, but even essential to the survival of the species. To those who believe this we say: « *Be patient, keep reading the final section of this book, and see for yourself if we can convince you... at least try it out!* »

Others simply don't believe it. They think that all of these theories are only hypotheses and that scientists are clearly getting too convinced too soon. If this is the case, they should try to apply the lifestyle modification protocols to themselves, as described below. We are certain that they will improve their health.

In order to know in which category you belong and to help you evaluate whether you are ready to go through this extraordinary adventure, we suggest that you fill out the following questionnaire.

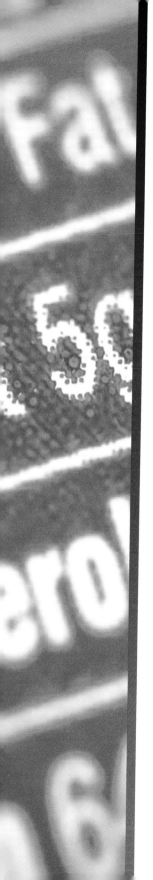

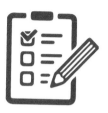

Questionnaire

on your readiness for change

Questionnaire on your readiness for change

Are you ready to alter your habits? Your attitude when faced with a hyperlongevity protocol will either hinder or accelerate your success. Take this short test in order to know if you might need a little help before getting started. Be honest with yourself! It is important that these answers reflect who you really are and not who you would like to be!

		TRUE	FALSE
1	I have thought long and hard about my future, my age, my current lifestyle, and I have come to the conclusion that something needs to be changed.	TRUE ☐ +1	FALSE ☐ 0
2	I have accepted that I need to make PERMANENT rather than temporary changes to the way I live in order to experience a successful rejuvenation protocol.	TRUE ☐ +1	FALSE ☐ 0
3	I will only feel completely satisfied if I see rapid and noticeable changes.	TRUE ☐ 0	FALSE ☐ +1
5	I am seriously considering undergoing a cellular regeneration program because I want to, and not because someone else suggested it to me.	TRUE ☐ +1	FALSE ☐ 0
6	I believe taking part in this program will solve other problems in my life.	TRUE ☐ 0	FALSE ☐ +1

| 10 | As soon as I perceive any results, I inevitably lose my motivation to continue. | TRUE ☐ 0 | FALSE ☐ +1 |

Score and results

Score total

_____

Recommendations

There is no single answer which can determine on its own whether you are ready for change.

1 - *If your total is 8 or higher, you likely have good reasons to take on a rejuvenation protocol right away, and you have an appropriate outlook on the continued efforts you will have to make. You will still be able to learn more about the areas in which your score was 0.*

2 - *If your total is between 5 and 7, you should examine your motivations for taking on this kind of program and accompanying methods. Reconsider those questions for which you got a score of 0.*

3 - *If your total is 4 or less, this means that it may not be the right time to begin this change. Your answers suggest that you may not be ready to make the necessary efforts to succeed in this challenge. You should reconsider your motivations and perhaps advantages and disadvantages. Go deeper, and familiarize yourself with the method, answers will come little by little.*

JLife is an ambitious program, which stems from a logical observation: any death which takes place earlier than after 122 years, 5 months and 14 days should be considered premature. This is of course referring to the woman still holding the world longevity record: Jeanne Calment. This program has two objectives: the first is to help repair damage and slow down the process of cellular aging, the second is to trigger a process of cell regeneration. This is a simple, non-aggressive protocol, which does however require continued vigilance, as damage is repetitive; this is therefore a constant, daily battle.

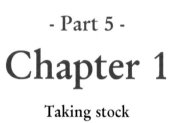

- Part 5 -

Chapter 1

Taking stock

Before taking on a cellular regeneration protocol, you should undergo physical, mental and emotional exams, in order to assess your biological age. The goal is to estimate the condition of your DNA, your telomeres and your stock of stem cells, as well as your general health and any possible issues linked to aging.

1.1 - Where should you start?

It all depends on how determined you are to know more, as well as on your budget...The exams can go from a basic protocol to the very best comprehensive exam.

The basic protocol

Here is a very simple protocol with which to start off: it includes an anthropometric and morphological exam, a functional assessment, then a questionnaire to evaluate your cellular age, and finally, a simple biological exam which you can ask for when seeing your doctor.

Your morphological and anthropomorphic data

Photos

The first thing you need to do is to have some pictures taken of your face and body (do not take 'selfies' of yourself). Take these pictures with proper lighting and without any makeup or glasses. Take several different attitudes (smiling, not smiling). Keep these pictures in order to compare six months later (under the same conditions).

Self-examination

Hair

Gray hair is entirely independent of aging. Graying can however suggest certain nutritional deficiencies which could have an incidental effect on how you age.

The aspect, loss, and sometimes even the coloration of your hair may be influenced by deficiencies in proteins, minerals, sulfur amino acid (cysteine), group B vitamins or polyunsaturated fats.

Skin

Is it too dry? This may indicate dehydration. The more we age, the more water we need, but dry skin may also suggest a lack of polyunsaturated fats (omega-3 and 6).

Dark, geometrical spots, commonly called age or liver spots, reflect the accumulation of a pigment called lipofuscin in your tissue. Count the number of brown spots on the back of your hands, and repeat this every six months.

Nails

Are they soft, brittle, ridged with white spots? These alterations can indicate deficiencies: in proteins; minerals (iron, sulfur, calcium, silica and often zinc); sulfur amino acids (cysteine); group B vitamins or polyunsaturated fats.

Your morphological data

Height (in meters). For example: 1.83 m.

Weight (in kilograms). In the morning, on an empty stomach, without any clothes.

Waist size (in centimeters). Use your navel as a marker.

Hips (in centimeters). Measure the circumference of your hips, using your iliac spines (the bony tips you can feel on both sides of your pelvis).

With these four measurements, you will be able to calculate four fundamental parameters.

1 - Your Body Mass Index (BMI)
which lets you assess your corpulence

Perform the following calculation: **weight (kilos) divided by height (meters) squared = BMI** (Kg per m2)

$$BMI = \frac{\text{weight (kg)}}{\text{size}^2 \text{ (m)}}$$

Results:

If your BMI is below 18 kg/m2, you are too thin;

If your BMI is between 18.1 and 25 kg/m2, you have a normal weight;

If your BMI is between 25.1 and 30 kg/m2, you are overweight;

If your BMI is over 30 kg/m2, you are classified as obese.

Note that these values do not apply to those who are very short or very tall; likewise, children should refer to age-specific tables.

2 - Waist size

Today, all specialists agree that abdominal fat is the most detrimental to your health. Measuring your waist circumference allows us to quantify it. The distribution of fatty (or adipose) tissue is of particular relevance. Excess weight may be evenly distributed or concentrated in one part of the body. Android fat distribution mainly affects the upper body (torso, abdomen). Gynoid fat distribution mainly affects the lower body (buttocks, hips, legs). The former mostly affects men, the latter, women. As for severe obesity, it is generally mixed.

Waist size accounts for two types of fatty tissue: subcutaneous fat (under the skin) and visceral fat (located deeper, surrounding the inner organs).

The latter is most significant when it comes to cardiovascular risk.
A simple tape measure is all you need: measure the circumference of your waist starting at your belly button.

For women

If your waist size is less than **88 cm**,
you do not have any particular risk factors;

If your waist size is between **88 and 95 cm**,
you have increased cardiovascular risk to be taken seriously.

If your waist is larger than **95 cm**,
you have substantial cardiovascular risk factors.

For men

If your waist size is less than **100 cm**,
you do not have any particular risk factors;

If your waist size is between **100 and 110 cm**,
you have increased cardiovascular risk to be taken seriously.

If your waist is larger than **110 cm**,
you have substantial cardiovascular risk factors.

3 - Waist/hip ratio

This ratio lets us assess your morphology.

A ratio between 0.85 and 1.00 suggests an android morphology, meaning that your body fat is concentrated around your abdomen, which can be dangerous to your health.

A ratio between 0.80 and 0.85 indicates that you have a gynoid morphology, meaning, among other things, that your body fat is mainly found in your hips and buttocks.

4 - Body fat measurement

This represents the percentage of fat in your body. If you weigh 80 kg and have a body fat percentage of 20%, that means that you are 'carrying' 16 kg of fat, distributed throughout your body. In general, to be in good health, men should not go over 15-20 %, whereas women should not exceed 25-30%.

Most of the time, it is measured via bioelectrical impedance, but the results are only estimates. Easy to use and not that hard to understand! You put both feet on the scales. A harmless electrical current travels from one leg to the other. The scales measure the speed at which this electrical current travels. It will be faster if you have more muscle and slower if you have more fat. Body water content and your bones also have an effect. In short, we are measuring your body's electrical resistance. A mathematical formula then allows us to deduce what percentage of your body is made up of fat.

A bioelectrical impedance scale can therefore estimate your weight and how it is distributed as fat, muscle, water and bone. A huge number of factors come into play (body type, temperature, whether your feet are wet, whether you worked out recently, etc.), which means results can vary a lot... Bioelectrical impedance scales do not offer very precise information (this means they cannot, for example, be used in scientific studies). They cannot allow you to compare your body fat to your neighbor's, either.

Functional assessments

Skin elasticity test

This reveals the deterioration of the subcutaneous connective tissue, which is linked to wrinkle formation. The loss of skin elasticity occurs around the age of forty-five, although variability in the range of plus or minus 10% is not unusual. In order to perform this test, you pinch the skin on the back of your hand, between your thumb and index finger, and count how long it takes for the fold to disappear. It should take:

- Less than 5 seconds for a functional age between 45 and 50 years old;
- Between 10 and 15 around 60 years old;
- Between 35 and 60 seconds beyond 70 years old.

The ruler catching test

This test assesses your reaction time to an external stimulus. It is essential, as this factor can determine your capacity for 'survival' in case of an aggression or accident, and we know that it is affected by age. In order to perform it, ask someone to hold a flat, 50 cm graduated wood ruler vertically, by its upper extremity. Place your thumb and index finger, 8 to 10 cm apart, at equal distance from the 50 cm mark, at the bottom of the ruler. Ask the person holding the ruler to let go of it without warning you, and attempt to grab the ruler as soon as they have done so. Your score is determined by the mark at which you were able to grab the ruler. Perform the test three times and determine the average of the three scores: it should be around 28-30 at 20 years old and reach about 15 at 60 years old. A 20 year-old will therefore take 20 cm to react whereas a 60 year-old will need 35!

The static balance test

This test is useful to examine the condition of the central and peripheral nervous system. This test must be performed barefoot or with flat-heeled slippers, on your left leg if you are right-handed and your right leg if you are left-handed. On a hard surface (no carpets or rugs), join both feet, close your eyes and lift one foot about 15 centimeters off the ground, bending your knee 45 degrees. Then attempt to balance on the other foot, without moving it and while keeping your eyes closed. Ask someone to record how long you are able to stay in this position. Perform the test three times and calculate the average.

For someone 20-25 years old, you should be able to stay balanced for more than thirty seconds. At forty years old, the average duration should only be fifteen seconds, between 65 and 70, it is reduced to around five seconds.

Measurement of vital capacity (VC)

Today, this is very easy to achieve, thanks to spirometers –or peak flow meters–, which can be found in specialized shops or medical centers. It is performed by measuring the amount of air which is expelled after having breathed deeply and will assess both the proper function of the respiratory system (muscles, bronchi, lung tissue) and that of the central nervous system's control. Furthermore, and this is absolutely essential, this test is not affected by physical training.

Until 30 years of age, VC should reach five liters. At 40 years old, it should be between four and five liters. It is only, on average, between three and four liters at 50 years old, three liters at 60 and below three liters at 70 and beyond.

The Ruffier test

This test assesses cardiovascular adaptation to effort. However, it has the drawback of being both affected by physical training and representing a (slight) risk for elderly or fragile individuals, for whom the required intensity will be lowered. It is therefore strongly recommended that this test be performed in a clinical setting.

1 - Measure your pulse at rest for 15 seconds and write it down (P0).

2 - Then perform 30full squats in 45 to 60 seconds.

3 - Write down your pulse (measured for 15 seconds) as soon as you have finished the exercise (P1).

4 - Measure your pulse once more, one minute after having finished the exercise (P2).

5 - Multiply the sum of the three numbers, P0+P1+P2, by 4. The Ruffier index is produced by the formula:

$$(P0 + P1 + P2)x4 - 200/ 10$$

It should be inferior to 3 for subjects in very good physical condition, between 5 and 10 for those in good physical condition, between 10 and 15 for those in average physical condition. Furthermore, your pulse at the end of the exercise should not be above 150 beats/minute and after one minute you should have recovered more than 70% of the way to your resting heart rate.

Those with an index higher than 15 should be monitored: they may be fatigued and/or sedentary. For elderly individuals, or those in poor physical condition, 20 squats in 45 to 60 seconds will suffice. The same protocol should be kept for later measurements.

Biological age assessment questionnaire (annex 1)

We have so far found no specific markers for our biological age, that is, the exact condition of our DNA. We therefore suggest that you evaluate your biological age with a questionnaire which focuses on your lifestyle, your heredity and your present state of health. This evaluation will, by its own nature, be subjective and imprecise, but it will serve as a reference point to assess your progress. Go to annex 1 (page 399) and follow the instructions.

Cardiovascular evaluation

Simple evaluation

This consists of a clinical exam during which a doctor takes your pulse, your blood pressure, and listens to your heart. This exam is generally followed by an electrocardiogram. In certain cases, particularly if the doctor suspects a possible risk of angina or heart attack, they will ask for cardiac enzyme levels to be assessed.

Further exams

These are generally part of a continued exam, performed by a cardiologist, but not necessarily at the same time: they consist of echocardiography, a Doppler ultrasound, a stress test, and a Holter monitor, in order to monitor your heart rate and blood pressure, and finally a scintigraphy, which allows measurement of the heart's contractile function and the search for the presence of coronary disease.

Specialized exams

These are basically radiology and heart rhythm exams, in particular coronary angiograms and His bundle measurements.

Biological measurements

Lipid profile

A lipid profile allows us to measure the levels of the different lipid compounds present in our blood, in order to evaluate the risk of cardiovascular disease. These are measured from a blood sample taken with an empty stomach. This profile allows us to monitor blood lipid levels, in particular cholesterol (including LDL and HDL cholesterol) and triglycerides.

High LDL cholesterol ('bad cholesterol') and triglyceride levels, as well as excessively low HDL cholesterol levels ('good cholesterol') are lipid abnormalities, and considered to be cardiovascular risk factors.

Lipid abnormalities, as well as high blood sugar levels, promote the growth of atheromatous plaques on the arterial walls. This is called atherosclerosis, which can lead to the complete obstruction of an artery.

Cholesterol, which is mainly produced by the liver, is also supplied by our diet. It travels into the organism's cells as LDL cholesterol. When there are excessive amounts of LDL cholesterol in the blood, it deposits itself onto the arterial walls and obstructs blood flow. This is why LDL cholesterol is nicknamed' bad cholesterol'. HDL cholesterol collects the excess cholesterol in the blood and brings it to the liver, which eliminates it. It therefore has a protective effect, and is nicknamed 'good cholesterol'. Triglycerides, which are supplied by our diet, are stored in fat cells, and are used as an energy reserve by our organism. High levels of LDL cholesterol and triglycerides, along with low HDL cholesterol levels, are the main lipid abnormalities.

Each one of these increases the risk of developing a cardiovascular disease. On the other hand, high levels of HDL cholesterol have a protective effect. HDL cholesterol levels higher than 0.4 g/L (>1.0 mmol/L) along with triglyceride levels below 1.5 g/L (<1.7 mmol/L) are considered ideal.

Blood sugar levels

Blood sugar levels with an empty stomach (after eight hours without eating) are a good indicator of our capacity to regulate a number of key hormones (insulin, glucagon, cortisol). Excessively high blood sugar levels can point to the risk of diabetes, and be a source of many illnesses (in the kidneys, eyes, nervous system) leading, among other issues, to the formation of sugar/protein bonds, also called Maillard reactions or glycation, which accelerate aging. Normal blood sugar levels are between 0.7 g/l and 1.1 g/l, (4.03 to 6 mmol/l).If you have high levels, we suggest you see your doctor, who will be able to recommend further testing.

Blood C-reactive protein (CRP) levels

C-reactive proteins, abbreviated as CRP, are produced by our liver and released into the blood during inflammation or infection. Blood levels of this protein increase quickly, in less than 24 hours, and remain as such until recovery. Normal CRP levels should be below 6 mg/L. They can be significantly increased in smokers, obese individuals and those who regularly drink alcohol.

Erythrocyte sedimentation rate (ESR)

The erythrocyte sedimentation rate, abbreviated as ESR, is a non-specific test which is easy to perform and useful for the early diagnosis and monitoring of inflammatory or infectious phenomena, such as rheumatism. Along with CRP levels, this test allows us to better target inflammatory states, which are the main cause of DNA damage.

Normal erythrocyte sedimentation rate values:

ESR in the 1st hour < 7 mm

ESR in the 2nd hour < 20 mm

These values may vary depending on the technique used by the given medical analysis lab. It will be specified next to the results.

Complete blood count

A complete blood count or full blood count, most commonly abbreviated FBC, is an exam which is essential to properly diagnose any potential bone marrow problems, or detect so-called peripheral abnormalities. It offers valuable insight into the organs which produce blood cells, blood lines, defense processes and hemostasis (coagulation). It allows us to detect many pathologies: anemia, increased white blood cell counts in reaction to an attack, issues with coagulation and platelet consumption, etc.

Homocysteine levels

Homocysteine levels indirectly indicate how well methylation– the process which activates or deactivates genes - is working. Homocysteine is a pro-inflammatory molecule which is produced when abnormal proteins are metabolized. The methylation process is responsible for the elimination of homocysteine when it reaches toxic levels; if high levels persist, this means that methylation is not doing its job properly. High levels of homocysteine also indicate a high risk of cardiovascular disease.

Functional intestinal flora exam

This is one of the key elements for the assessment of the health of your immune system. Ask your doctor for a functional analysis of your microbial flora.

This basic protocol - morphological data, functional tests, cardiovascular exam, biological tests- is more than adequate to properly respond to aging. Nevertheless, if you want to know more, there are a number of more sophisticated biomarkers.

Biomarkers of aging

For decades now, biogerontologists have been searching for a biomarker of aging which could measure our true biological age. This would be a better indicator of life expectancy than our chronological age. Such a biomarker would be a powerful tool, allowing us to assess the effectiveness of actions meant to modify our lifespan, without having to embark on large studies, which take many years, and are nearly impossible to carry out on human beings. Unfortunately, aging is a complex issue, as it involves many organs and functions. Due to this, we have no choice but to depend on a large array of biomarkers, which are specific to each function.

Biomarkers of oxidative stress

Oxidative stress is the result of an imbalance between, on the one hand, the production of free radicals and reactive oxygen species (ROS), and on the other hand, the capacity of the organism's protective mechanisms to neutralize these two types of toxic compounds before they cause any damage.

A blood test focusing on oxidative stress requires the selection of suitable biomarkers, a solid knowledge of the field and strong interpretative skills.

High MDA levels

Plasma malondialdehyde, abbreviated as MDA, is a marker of lipid oxidation, and is considered to be an end-product of polyunsaturated fat oxidation. High MDA levels therefore indicate oxidative stress, in particular lipid oxidation, which is a scientifically proven cardiovascular risk factor, but they are also evidence of more general oxidative stress in the organism (our brain, for example, is particularly lipid-rich).

Thiol proteins

Thiol protein levels are without doubt one of the most significant markers of oxidative stress. Only low thiol levels are significant. Thiol proteins, which contain a sulfur atom, act as exceptionally potent 'buffers' in the blood .During periods of significant oxidative stress, thiols restore 'redox' (reduction-oxidation) balance by eliminating free radicals .Thiols oxidize and are then eliminated; lowered thiol levels are therefore a marker of oxidative stress. Extremely low thiol levels are most often evidence of past and/or chronic oxidative stress. Low thiol levels are also considered an indirect marker of protein oxidation.

Urinary 8-hydroxydeoxyguanosine (8OHdG) levels

8OHdG is a molecule which is eliminated in our urine. It is specific to oxidative attacks, and is easy to detect. A major European study has shown a strong correlation between lymphocyte 8OHdG levels and cardiovascular mortality in young men.

1.2 - Other biomarkers

Urinary hormonal profile

From 30 to 70 years old, cortisol secretion increases by 50% while DHEA secretion decreases by 90%. The ratio of cortisol to DHEA is very useful.

Urinary pentosidine and furosine levels

Urinary levels increase with age and indicate glycation.

1.3 - Detection of food intolerances

Today, we can precisely evaluate your dietary intolerances by using a blood test which will hunt down the IgG (Immunoglobulin G) type antibodies present in your blood. Every kind of food can be tested, and if your body treats it as an 'antigen', it will produce corresponding antibodies. In this way, certain labs can detect your intolerances from a selection of more than 300 foods (Imupro300).

1.4 - Bone density

Bone densitometry, also known as osteodensitometry or dual-energy absorptiometry, is a medical exam which measures bone density, that is, its mineral content. Low bone density is a strong indicator of the risk of fracture, whether for vertebral compression or hip fractures.

Bone mineral density (BMD) is expressed compared to an average of a normal population of the same age and sex, which makes it possible to assess bone condition compared to the given chronological age.

1.5 - Telomere length

Analyzing telomere length is a key step, not only for scientific research, but also for individuals wishing to monitor how their telomeres evolve during a cellular regeneration protocol. Measuring telomeres for research requires very sophisticated, and therefore costly equipment. For individuals, the most important thing is to measure an average length of the shorter telomeres, rather than measure all of them. Why?

So long as telomeres are still present (down to around 5 000 base pairs) the cell continues to do its work and, more importantly, to divide, avoiding apoptosis and senescence. If we calculate the average of all telomeres, the results may be skewed as, on the one hand, certain cells multiply very frequently, meaning that their telomeres shorten more quickly, and on the other hand, within any given cell family, shortening rates are completely different. Only measuring short telomeres allows us to indirectly evaluate the amount of senescent cells. We suggest you perform this test once a year to evaluate your progress. For now, the only lab which offers this test is in Madrid (www.lifelength.com).

Before embarking on a cellular regeneration protocol, it is important that you analyze your current state of health, and, if possible, your biological age, both as precisely as possible. No biomarkers specific to biological age currently exist, but an array of indirect markers can help you establish a baseline and help you evaluate your progress. Among the necessary tests, the most important are CRP and homocysteine levels and, if possible, an analysis of the average length of your short telomeres (from the Life Length lab in Madrid).

S O U R C E S

Leonard Hayflick.
How and Why We Age. New York : Ballantine books ; 1994.

Michael Fossel, Greta Blackburn, Dave Woynarowski.
The Immortality Edge. Hoboken (New Jersey) : John Wiley & Sons, Inc. ; 2011.

Michael Fossel.
The Telomerase Revolution. Dallas : Benbella Books Inc. ; 2015.

William Evans.
Biomarkers. New York : Fireside ; 1992.

www.lifelenght.com

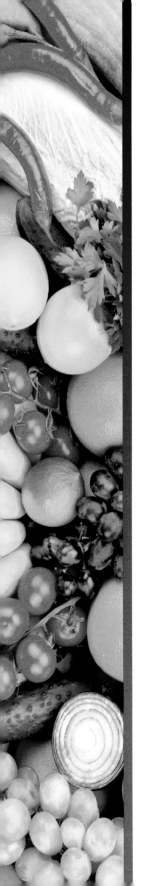

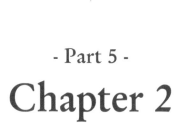

- Part 5 -

Chapter 2

The JLife Nutrition plan

The JLife Nutrition plan combines a nutritional plan with specially tailored dietary supplements.

First, fill out the questionnaire on your dietary profile in annex 2 (page 420).The results will be useful to calibrate your diet.

2.1 - JLife nutrition

Don't expect any recipes or specific menus, there are no miracle foods or diets. Our aim is to focus on the causes of aging, in particular oxidative damage, inflammation, glycation, methylation, telomere shortening and the protection of our stock of stem cells, in order to suggest the most suitable foods and dietary supplements.

Antioxidant nutrition

Oxidation and oxidative stress are mainly responsible for the damage which our DNA undergoes. Fruits and vegetables are essential to our fight against oxidation. Nearly 10 000 different molecules exist which can help us in this fight.

Plums contain the best antioxidants, as well as vitamins C, E, and beta-carotene. The laxative and diuretic properties of plums make them an ideal choice to assist our organism's elimination processes.

Berries, which have high concentrations of vitamins and polyphenols, are the best antioxidant foods after plums to fight free radicals.

Garlic contains quercetin, which belongs to the flavonoid family and lowers 'bad cholesterol' levels, as well as selenium, which helps to block free radicals, thereby protecting cells from aging. The WHO recommends that adults eat two to five grams of fresh garlic a day, or about one clove.

Broccoli and other brassicas: rich in vitamin C, vegetables from the cabbage family, broccoli in particular, act against cardiovascular disease. The best way to benefit from brassicas is to steam or stir-fry them.

Bell peppers contain more vitamin C than oranges, pound for pound. Red bell peppers are best, as they contain nine times more carotenoids, five to eight times more flavonoids and twice as much vitamin C. An excellent source of vitamin A as well, bell peppers boost our immune system, strengthen the body's natural defenses, and prevent cardiovascular disease.

Tomatoes contain lycopene, a powerful antioxidant which prevents cardiovascular disease and cancers, in particular prostate cancer. They should preferably be eaten cooked.

Turmeric: another anti-inflammatory food, this spice helps fight premature cell aging, certain types of cancer and diabetes. Turmeric promotes digestion and strengthens the immune system.

Green tea is a source of polyphenols, promotes mental alertness and lowers the risk of cancer. Regular consumption also ensures proper hydration.

Cacao fights cancer, cardiovascular disease and hypertension. Chocolate owes its antioxidant properties in large part to its high flavonoid content.

Anti-inflammatory nutrition

Fighting inflammation is imperative!

As omega 3 have anti-inflammatory properties, it is recommended that you eat lots of fish and other foods which contain them, such as salmon, anchovies, sardines, walnuts, flax seed and omega 3 enriched eggs. You should favor the use of olive oil and rapeseed oil.

Saturated fats and trans fats should be avoided in an anti-inflammatory diet. Foods such as butter, cream, cheese, fatty meats, skin from poultry, coconut oil and palm oil should be eaten sparingly, while hydrogenated vegetable oil should be avoided entirely.

Foods with high omega 6 content (sunflower oil, soybean oil, corn oil and safflower oil) should be taken in moderation as high doses may be pro-inflammatory. Meat is to be avoided as much as possible, as its saturated fat content is pro-inflammatory. Chicken should also be eaten in moderation, as it contains omega 6 fatty acids. pulses and fish are the best alternatives to meat and poultry.

Anti-inflammatory foods

☐ Fresh fruit :especially berries, blackberries, raspberries, blueberries;

☐ Pulses: lentils, kidney beans, chickpeas, etc.;

☐ Nuts and seeds: walnuts, flaxseed, pumpkin seeds, hemp seeds;

☐ Oils: cold-pressed rapeseed oil, extra-virgin olive oil, walnut oil, pumpkin seed oil, flax seed oil;

☐ Soy products: tofu, tempeh, edamame, miso and plain soy drinks;

☐ Herbs and spices;

☐ Fatty fish: salmon, mackerel, trout, sardines, herring;

☐ Fresh vegetables;

☐ Whole grain: barley, brown rice, quinoa, spelt, cracked wheat, rolled oats, millet, amaranth, rye.

Pro-inflammatory foods

☐ High-fat dairy products: butter, sour cream, whole milk, cream, ice cream;

☐ Deli meat, cold cuts, sausage, pâté;

☐ Red meat: beef, pork, lamb, veal;

☐ Poultry;

☐ Refined grain: white bread, white rice, white dough, chips, baked products made with white flour, bagels, doughnuts, pretzels, crackers, rusks, cookies, cakes, muffins;

☐ Refined sugar: white and brown sugar, soft drinks, soda, pastries, sweetened cereal, glucose-fructose, high-fructose corn syrup, candy;

☐ Trans fat sources: pie crusts, hard margarine, cookies, crackers, pastries.

Antiglycation nutrition

You should avoid overcooked, grilled, browned, broiled or caramelized foods. How you cook your food can multiply the amount of glycation end-products by ten, compared, for example, to boiling your food. The golden skin on poultry or fish which have been grilled, or worse, fried or breaded, is particularly high in glycation end-products. The same goes for bread crust, rusks, cookies, doughnuts, fried food, etc.

All foods with a high glycemic index, that is, which spike your blood sugar, will of course promote glycation. This is the case for sucrose, pastry with added sugar, overly refined grain and flour, jam, potatoes, etc. Among those with the highest glycotoxin content: grilled meat and industrial foods with added protein or milk powder (cookie dough, pizza, fast-food, industrial cheese, etc.)

Cooking in a humid and acidic medium reduces the production of glycotoxins, tomatoes and lemons are therefore recommended, as well as baking soda or baker's yeast, to replace baking powder in bread or pancake dough.

Plants and antiglycation foods

Here are various plants whose antiglycation action has been proven: guava and walnut leaves, allioideae (garlic, onions, leeks), calendula, turmeric, cabbage, rosemary, cinnamon, thyme, clove…

Antiglycation substances

Carnosine: mainly found in our muscles and brain, concentrations of this molecule, which is produced by our body out of amino acids (alanine, histidine), decline with age. It can undergo a glycation reaction with sugars, thereby preserving other proteins. Once glycated, carnosine is not toxic to our organism and can be eliminated. Animal studies have shown lifespans increased by about 20% thanks to carnosine. Finally, it is also chelates toxic heavy metals, and helps to eliminate them.

Aminoguanidine: according to certain studies, it may have a protective effect on the retina, neurons and kidneys in diabetic individuals. Just like carnosine, it can act as a substitute for proteins in glycation reactions. Other studies have shown improved blood flow in those suffering from arteriosclerosis, and decreased levels of bad cholesterol (LDL).

Vitamin B1 and one of its derivatives, Benfotiamine, have been proven to prevent protein glycation in diabetics.

Pro-methylation nutrition

Methylation is one of our body's most important reactions. It is essential to our health but decreases with age. A healthy organism produces large amounts of methyl groups and no particular supplementation is necessary. Certain foods have a high concentration of methyl groups: quinoa, beets, cooked dark green vegetables such as spinach or broccoli, egg yolks, lamb, chicken...

In order to optimize methylation we need:

☐ A diet with sufficient amounts of B vitamins, and especially folate - vitamin B9 - :whole grains, brewer's yeast, beans, nuts, fish, eggs ;

☐ Sufficient sulfur intake: sulfur can be found in garlic, onions, brassica vegetables, egg yolks, fish, etc. Sulfur is required to transfer methyl groups;

☐   To avoid sugar, which reduces your stock of vitamins;

☐   To avoid tobacco, alcohol, caffeine, which limit the activity of B vitamins;

☐   To maintain a healthy intestinal flora, in particular to properly absorb vitamins.

Choosing a cooking oil

If we wish to cook certain foods, we know that they should be not be cooked excessively and always at low temperatures. The oils we cook with should also be carefully chosen so as to not endanger our health.

Virgin oils and refined oils.

Refining oil requires the use of hexane solvents, high temperatures–between 180 and 220 degrees Celsius–,as well as bleaching and deodorizing. None of this is very good for our health, especially hexane residue, trans fats and the destruction of polyunsaturated fatty acids by the heat. Refining oil, although it makes it possible to raise its smoke point, severely denatures polyunsaturated fatty acids. Furthermore, cooking generates oxidative damage, even when oil is heated below its smoke point. This leads to the production of free radicals, which promote inflammation and various degenerative diseases. It is better to use saturated fat, which is heat-stable, especially butter and virgin coconut oil.

All of this anti-aging nutritional advice is applied in a diet known all around the world: the Mediterranean diet.

The Mediterranean diet

Although there are varied dietary habits in the fifteen or so countries which surround the Mediterranean Sea, we can detect at least one constant: the copious use of olive oil. When talking about the Mediterranean diet, we are more specifically referring to the traditional diet of the Greek islands of Crete and Corfu – which is why it is sometimes called the Cretan diet.

The interest in this type of diet comes from the *Seven Countries Study**, produced by Ancel Keys in the 1950s.In it he showed that, despite a high dietary intake of fats and a somewhat rudimentary health care system, the inhabitants of these islands, as well as southern Italy, enjoy not only a high life expectancy, but also very low rates of coronary disease. Later, professor Serge Renaud, who discovered what is referred to in the field of nutrition as the « *French paradox* », published the *Lyon Diet Study*. This study revealed that subjects who had already had a heart attack and subsequently followed a diet similar to the typical Cretan one showed heart attack and stroke rates which were 75% lower, whereas those following a diet which solely restricted fat consumption only showed a 25% decrease*

Since the publication of this study in the highly respected medical journal The Lancet in 1994, the popularity of the Mediterranean diet has spread around the world. Scientific studies have continued to prove its effectiveness in preventing many illnesses.

This diet must be taken as a whole. It combines dietary moderation and a wide variety of foods (and therefore of nutrients), along with an active lifestyle. Its core principles are easy to understand and adhere to: abundant fruits and vegetables, garlic, onions, spices and herbs; the use of olive oil as the main fat; the daily consumption of pulses, nuts and seeds; the daily but moderate consumption of red wine; large amounts of fish (several times a week) but limited use of chicken, eggs and sweet foods (a few times a week); very limited consumption of red meat (a few times a month).

2.2 - Active Nutritional Supplementation

As much as setting up a diet plan can seem easy, making one for nutritional supplementation is much more complex.

If you go online and search for « *anti-aging nutritional supplements* », you will immediately feel lost, as the number of substances which are touted at anti-aging is staggering. Every day new substances are discovered, extracts, flavonoids, carotenes, anthocyanins, and all of them claim to have some exceptional quality

Sarri K, Kafatos A. The Seven Countries Study in Crete: olive oil, Mediterranean diet or fasting? Public Health Nutr. 2005 Sep; 8(6):666.

or activity. To these we can add another significant parameter, their price. It may vary quite a bit for a given product, potentially being multiplied by twenty, even if nothing, or hardly anything, is changed to justify this gap.

Our active nutritional supplementation program is incremental. It is divided into three steps which are essential to its effectiveness. The first step takes care of the groundwork and promotes cellular and extracellular detoxification, as well as intracellular nutritional replenishment. The second step will help you slow the signs of aging and their potential pathological consequences. The third step is dedicated to revitalization and potentially to cellular regeneration.

Step 1

This is an essential, even vital step, as it will help your cells eliminate substances which impede their functions. To this end, we present five supplement categories which will have to be taken for at least six weeks.

Vitamin and mineral supplementation

This is made complicated by the wide array of existing formulas. Which should you choose? The best, of course, would be the most comprehensive and natural one, enriched with ingredients which boost its activity and facilitate absorption (amino acids, enzymes, certain botanical substances) … Alright, so which one should you take?

Vitamins and minerals have official recommended doses, referred to as recommended daily allowances(RDA). They correspond to the amount of vitamins and of certain minerals necessary to avoid suffering from deficiencies and their attendant illnesses, such as scurvy, beriberi or pellagra. This is the absolute minimum amount of nutrients needed to maintain the biological functions and health of already healthy individuals. A great many studies highlight the beneficial effects vitamins and minerals have on our health when taken in much higher doses than those suggested by RDAs. This is what is called the *No Adverse Effect Level* (NOAEL), and it represents a dose which, taken over a long period of time, in the same amount, has no observed negative effects.

In some situations, such as in the event of a premature birth, metabolic disorders, infection, chronic illness, or certain drug therapies, covering essential nutrient needs may require larger quantities. Environmental factors such as stress, pollution, or sun exposure may also increase requirements. As they are only designed to prevent illnesses associated with nutrient deficiencies, RDAs are not designed to indicate what we may need to stay healthy, strong and vigorous, or to prevent age-related disease. All the more so considering the fact that the needs of every one of us are unique.

Inset

Sample formula (Vitamins and Minerals)

Daily dose   3 capsules

Amount per dose

Vitamin A (2 500 IU beta-carotene, 500 IU palmitate)	3 000 IU
Vitamin D3 (cholecalciferol)	1 000 IU
Vitamin K1 (phylloquinone)	140 µg
Vitamin B1 (thiamine hydrochloride)	15 mg
Vitamin B2 (riboflavin)	20 mg
Vitamin B3 (niacinamide)	60 mg
Vitamin B5 (calcium pantothenate)	30 mg
Vitamin B6 (pyridoxine hydrochloride)	30 mg
Vitamin B12 (methylcobalamin)	300 µg
Vitamin C (ascorbic acid, ascorbyl palmitate)	300 mg
Vitamin E (d-alpha tocopheryl succinate, with mixed tocopherols)	40 mg
Folic acid	400 µg
Biotin	500 µg
Boron (calcium borogluconate)	1 mg
Calcium (ascorbate, pantothenate, D-glucarate)	218 mg
Chrome	200 µg

Copper (chelated bisglycinate)	1 mg
Iodine (potassium iodide)	150 µg
Magnesium (magnesium glycinate)	40 mg
Manganese (gluconate)	1 mg
Molybdenum (citrate)	150 µg
Potassium (71.3 mg of potassium chloride)	37.4 mg
Selenium (sodium selenite, or selenomethionine)	200 µg
Zinc (gluconate)	30 mg

Prebiotics and probiotics

Their importance has only been appreciated in the past few years. They are close friends of our intestines, protect our intestinal mucosa ,helping us absorb and digest fats and carbohydrates; they are indispensable allies of our immune system, helping to revive faltering organic defenses, or in the event of allergies, intestinal, cardiovascular or pulmonary infections.

The list has recently been extended with new strains which occasionally have more specific applications:

☐ *Bacillus subtilis* is specific to irritable bowel syndrome;

☐ *Lactobacillus gasseri* helps us better manage our weight;

☐ *Lactobacillus reuteri* takes care of the cardiovascular system;

☐ *Saccharomyces boulardii,* for its part, is the ancestor of anti-diarrheal treatments.

The main obstacle to proper probiotic consumption is their potential destruction by our stomach before they can reach our intestines. Traditional gelatin capsules release their contents almost immediately once they come into contact with stomach acid, and are entirely disintegrated fifteen minutes after ingestion. This rapid dissolution of the active ingredients can damage some nutrients which are particularly sensitive to acidic pH levels. This is not the case, according to a new study, of delayed release capsules (DRcaps™) which only begin to release their contents an average of 52 minutes after ingestion and are fully disintegrated 72 minutes after having been swallowed. Release therefore takes place only after the capsules have moved past the stomach. In this case, one to two capsules a day is enough to ensure proper dosage (30 to 60 billion CFU).

Omega3

Omega3 supplementation is essential, for your health as well as longevity; analyzing your fatty acid profile can help optimize dosage. An average dosage would be around three grams, once or twice daily. Try to take EPA and DHA-rich omega3.

Remember that other fatty acids (omega6, 7, 9) also have anti-aging applications, such as in coconut oil, the omega7 in sea buckthorn, or medium-chain triglycerides, which are made of fatty acids with carbon chains 6 to 12 atoms long; they are however less significant, and less commonly used than omega3, and their anti-aging properties have so far not been sufficiently demonstrated.

Coenzyme Q10 (Ubiquinone)

Coenzyme Q10, found in the form of Ubiquinone or Ubiquinol, is first and foremost a defender of the mitochondria, and therefore an indirect energy source for our body. Coenzyme Q10 is in fact able to help mitochondria convert fats into sugars and adenosine triphosphate (ATP), our body's main energy source. Concentrations significantly decrease with age. For older individuals, its reduced form, Ubiquinol H2, should be favored, as it requires lower doses, and is better absorbed.

Average doses are 200 to 400 mg/d for Ubiquinone, and 100 to 200 mg/d for Ubiquinol H2. Be careful not to take coenzyme Q10 at the same time as fiber, as these will inhibit absorption; it is recommended to combine it with a small amount of fat, however (oil, butter, vitamin D).

Turmeric

Turmeric, curcuma, curcumin, curcuminoids: so many names for this colorful culinary pigment, an essential element of Indian Ayurvedic medicine. Extracted from the turmeric plant, it is sometimes used as a substitute for saffron, which is far more costly.

Turmeric is a first-rate anti-inflammatory agent. It protects us from mutagenic substances, fights osteoarthritis, inhibits the development of cancerous cells (especially colonic adenocarcinomas). Unfortunately, it is not very well absorbed at the intestinal level, therefore it is important to ensure that its active ingredient or curcuminoid concentration not be below 90%. If this is the case, we can suggest an average dose of 300 to 500 mg daily.

Silymarin

Silymarin is a flavonoid complex extracted from milk thistle. It protects the liver from many toxic products, including certain types of medication, is a powerful antioxidant which increases liver glutathione levels by 35 % in healthy subjects, promotes protein synthesis in the liver, making it possible to replace damaged cells with healthy cells more quickly. It inhibits leukotriene synthesis and is therefore anti-inflammatory. The recommended dose is 350 mg daily.

Many other substances could have been included in this list, but we chose to simplify the process and not push you to take too many pills or capsules every day.

Practically speaking.

The essentials: vitamins and minerals, omega3, coenzymeQ10.

Strongly recommended: probiotics, turmeric.

Last but not least: silymarin if you feel the need to detoxify your liver.

This step is meant to delay, or slow down, chronic illness linked to cellular aging. It is important at this stage that you review the aforementioned health assessments and determine which function or organ you wish to strengthen. You will choose among the suggested targets those which best match your current state of health. You may use these ingredients for a short period of time or in a prolonged manner, potentially even for your entire life. These are not drugs, and generally do not exhibit any inherent toxicity. This does not mean, however, that they should be abused. It should also be noted that certain substances are useful for several different pathologies; this is why we may find the same ingredients in several of the systems under consideration.

The heart and blood vessels

If your cardiovascular evaluation, your lipid profile, your homocysteine levels and your CRP levels are not satisfactory, we suggest you continue taking omega3 and coenzyme Q10 and choose, with the help of your doctor, the supplements which best suit your condition.

Magnesium and potassium(as *malate, orotate, pidolate*).As a heartbeat regulator, magnesium probably has a protective effect on the arteries. It may help prevent cardiovascular disease risk factors. Potassium balances the transit of sodium (salt) in and out of cells, and actively participates in cardiovascular protection.

Nattokinase is an enzyme which is extracted from a Japanese food called « *natto* », which is made of fermented soybeans. Fermentation is achieved by adding a probiotic, *Bacillus subtilis*, to soybeans. Nattokinase has a powerful fluidizing effect, so avoid combining it with aspirin. An average dose is 50 mg, twice daily.

Red rice yeast (*Monascus purpureus)* is a type of microscopic fungus which is cultivated on rice. This yeast contains a deep red pigment. It is therefore the yeast which is red, not the rice. Red rice yeast supplements have undergone promising clinical trials, suggesting cholesterol-lowering activity. They are produced from a specific yeast strain (*Monascus purpureus Went*) and normalized, in order for it to contain a certain percentage of monacolins. These monacolins are in fact statins, that is, substances which inhibit cholesterol synthesis. The main monacolin in red rice yeast (monacolin K) is chemically identical to lovastatin, a synthetic drug normally prescribed for hypercholesterolemia. In fact, this drug was originally extracted from yeast (*Monascus ruber*).

Policosanol is generally extracted from the waxy substance found in sugarcane. Researchers have observed that it affects the synthesis of cholesterol in a slightly different way than statins. They also noticed that policosanol reduces low-density lipoprotein (LDL) oxidation and platelet aggregation, and has a vasodilating effect.

If your homocysteine levels are high, we suggest you take the following vitamins together: vitamins B6, B9, B12, and trimethylglycine (TMG). TMG converts homocysteine into methionine, then into SAMe. TMG should be taken with a multivitamin formula with large doses of vitamins B6, B12 and folic acid, as these nutrients are also involved in the methylation cycle. 3nb (3-n-butylphthalide)

If you suffer from arterial hypertension, we recommend taking a new celery seed extract: 3nb. Animal studies have generally demonstrated that it leads to a 14% drop in blood pressure as well as a 7% decrease in cholesterol levels. It acts both as a diuretic and a vasodilator by producing prostaglandins. The recommended dose is 150 mg daily.

Practically speaking

The essentials: magnesium, potassium and a vitamin B6, B9, B12 and TMG complex.

Toreduce cholesterol: red rice yeast (never cease treatment without speaking to a doctor).

To fight hypertension: 3nb (never cease treatment without speaking to a doctor).

The brain, memory and the nervous system

5HTP (5-Hydroxytryptophane)

Nerve cells use 5HTP to produce serotonin, one of the brain's main neurotransmitters. 5HTP occurs naturally in the seeds of *Griffonia simplicifolia*, an *African plant*. 5HTP increases serotonin levels in the brain just as effectively, but without the side effects, of selective serotonin reuptake inhibitors (SSRI) like Prozac®, for which it is a true natural alternative. A Norwegian study has shown that 5HTP improves sleep.

Useful dose:50 to 100 mg daily(do not mix with an antidepressant).

GABA (gamma-Aminobutyric acid)

This amino acid is used by the brain to promote calm and tranquility. Its concentration decreases with age.

Studies show that GABA:

- produces a relaxing effect 60 minutes after being taken, while simultaneously lowering anxiety in healthy, stressed volunteers; at the same time, it strengthens their immunity, which stress has weakened;

- promotes relaxation and sleep; contrary to the many sleep aids which target GABA receptors, taking it directly does not lead to daytime drowsiness or a risk of dependence; by lowering anxiety, it promotes deep and restorative rest;

- improves cognitive performance in elderly subjects.

Dose: 500 to 700 mg daily.

Bacopa monnieri

Bacopa monnieri is a renowned Ayurvedic tonic (nicknamed Brahmi, referring to the creator god of the Hindu pantheon, Brahma) which has been used for more than 3 000 years and the effects of which were the subject of a study carried out over 30 years. Individuals who take it have improved memory and unusually fast reaction times.

Useful dose: about 600 mg daily (of a leaf extract with a bacoside content of 50%).

Phosphatidylserine

This is a particular kind of fat combining glycerol (an alcohol), phosphoric acid and an amino acid, serine. It promotes nerve cell membrane fluidity, thereby maintaining active receptors to transmit nerve signals. Most of the studies which have examined it confirm that it improves short-term memory and most of the cognitive functions altered by aging.

Useful dose: 100 to 300 mg daily.

More supplements which are very valuable for brain function can be seen on the website www.jlife-sciences.com

CDP Choline(cytidine diphosphocholine): the best available form of bio choline.

Magnesium threonate: improves memory in elderly subjects.

Vinpocetine: derived from the lesser periwinkle plant, it improves alertness.

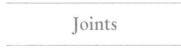

Joints

Bone and joint pathologies become increasingly frequent with age, and the tools we have to combat them grow more and more limited. This makes the discovery of bone morphogenetic proteins (BMPs), which are naturally present in our bones, a major advance.

Cyplexinol® (Bone Morphogenetic Protein – BMP)

Cyplexinol® is a protein which, when combined with a specific stem cell, can activate a group of other cells, leading to bone and cartilage regeneration, and especially the synthesis of osteoblasts and chondrocytes. This protein, which is naturally present in healthy bone and cartilaginous tissue, will activate mesenchymal stem cells which will then differentiate on the one hand into osteoblasts, thereby promoting bone formation, and on the other hand into chondrocytes, making it possible to produce new cartilage.

The useful daily dose of Cyplexinol® is 150 mg, but it can be doubled or tripled without causing issues, depending on the given situation.

Glucosamine, 1 500 mg

Glucosamine is a protein which is extracted from crustaceans (or plants in order to avoid the risk of allergies). In this dose, it has an anti-inflammatory effect which makes it possible to decrease dosages of other drugs such as non-steroidal anti-inflammatory drugs or even cortisone. This molecule slows down cartilage destruction. Men should avoid combining it with chondroitin (which may have a negative impact on the prostate).

MSM

Methyl-sulfonyl-methane (MSM), also called dimethyl sulfone, is a stable, rich, and natural source of organic sulfur. Although some fruits and vegetables naturally contain sulfur, it is destroyed when food is cooked, processed or stored. Studies show very clearly that MSM levels in our organism decrease sharply with age. Supplementation is all the more tempting a solution as it is cheap and without any risk of toxicity, which is remarkable. Sulfur is found in particularly high concentrations in our joints, where it takes part in the production of chondroitin sulfate, glucosamines and hyaluronic acid. It plays a crucial role in maintaining connective tissue and proteins stable and intact.

Several studies have demonstrated the value of MSM supplementation which, as a 'natural lubricant', promotes joint comfort and can relieve the pain of arthritis or rhumatoid polyarthritis. For maximum effectiveness, you should take between two and eight grams daily.

Celadrin®

Celadrin® is a complex of esterified fatty acid carbons (myristic, myristoleic, oleic, palmitoleic, palmitic, lauric, decanoic and stearic acids), specially developed and patented to reduce inflammation and pain in the joints, with no side effects. What distinguishes Celadrin® from other chondroprotective nutrients is the speed with which it acts and the continuous and cumulative benefits it provides. Research has shown that the esterified fatty acids in Celadrin® inhibit inflammation in endothelial cells and significantly reduce the pro-inflammatory effects of arachidonic acid. Celadrin® also decreases production of interleukin-6 (IL-6) and controls other immune factors responsible for inflammation. Celadrin® also acts by restoring the plasticity and elasticity of cell membranes in the fluids which enable the joints to move with ease. Celadrin® demonstrably reduces pain and improves mobility in a range of joint, muscle and tendon pathologies. The usual dose is one gram per day.

SAMe: relieves joint pain, promotes mobility and prevents cartilage degradation.

Boswellia serrata: mainly used for its anti-inflammatory properties, and therefore pain relief.

Uncaria tomentosa: improves inflammatory response, stimulates collagen production and supports the immune system.

Hormones

Entire books would be necessary to describe and convey the role of hormones! The use of anti-aging hormones should however be done under medical supervision and if possible only after a biological test.

Among them:

☐   DHEA;

☐   Pregnenolone;

☐   Melatonin;

☐   Natural progesterone;

☐   Natural testosterone,

☐   Natural thyroid hormone;

☐   Growth hormone;

☐   Thymus extracts.

Whenever possible, use transdermal creams or a compounded formulation.

Eyes

Lutein and zeaxanthin

Lutein, zeaxanthin and meso-zeaxanthin are present in our eyes, which they protect from the risk of macular degeneration and cataracts, two ophthalmic diseases which are responsible for deteriorated vision and blindness in the elderly. They also make it possible for healthy eyes to react better to bright light.

These three carotenoids compose our macular pigment. Studies have shown that supplementation can increase its density, and therefore the effectiveness of the protection it offers. The carotenoid antioxidant lutein is particularly concentrated in the macula which it protects from age and oxidative stress-related degeneration. Meso-zeaxanthin is a xanthophyllic carotenoid; it is most concentrated in the center of the macula, where lutein is least concentrated.

Asthaxanthin

This is a highly protective algae. Asthaxanthin is the red pigment which gives their color to crustaceans, salmon and flamingos. It is an exceptionally powerful antioxidant carotenoid which also has immuno modulating, anticancer, anti-inflammatory, cardio and photo-protective properties. Many *in vitro* and *in vivo* studies, both on animals and humans, demonstrate the antioxidant power of asthaxanthin and its usefulness in preventing and/or treating neurodegenerative diseases linked to oxidative stress and cardiovascular disease, as well as its effectiveness in protecting the eyes and skin from ultra-violet ray damage.

Daily dose: 4 mg, extracted from the *Haematococcus pluvialis algae*

Saffron

Saffron (Crocus sativus) is an age-old spice, very widely used and unfortunately often challenged and replaced by turmeric, the cost of which is much lower. In the past few years, there has been renewed interest in saffron, after a number of studies managed to isolate extracts with powerful concentrations of different active compounds. Among them we find potent antioxidants which are particularly useful for our eyes. These carotenoids provide significant protection from age-related macular degeneration (AMD), and also bolster the antioxidant defenses of our retinal photoreceptors, thereby preventing and treating this illness, even at an advanced stage. It is now accepted that the antioxidant effect of crocin and crocetin protect our retinas from daily oxidative damage caused by an excess of free radicals, exposure to high levels of natural light, and smoking. AMD is one of the main causes of vision loss, especially after sixty, potentially leading to total blindness.

Daily dose: 20 mg.

Type 2 diabetes

Many highly active substances can be used to help combat this very common illness.

Aminoguanidine

Aminoguanidine can prevent the production of advanced glycation end products. Clinical studies have shown that aminoguanidine helps increase collagen density in arterial walls, reduce LDL cholesterol, and improve the health of diabetics and their renal function. It improves insulin sensitivity and tends to lower blood sugar levels, both in healthy and diabetic men.

The daily dose is 300 mg.

Benfotiamine

Benfotiamine inhibits the formation of advanced glycation end products remarkably well, by transforming them into harmless compounds. This makes it a particularly important molecule for diabetics whose nerves, blood vessels, eyes and kidneys are the main target of the advanced glycation end products (AGEs) which they produce in large numbers. Regular intake of benfotiamine can significantly improve quality of life, as has been shown in controlled studies.

The daily dose is 300 mg.

Berberine

The berries of Berberis vulgaris, or barberry, contain a powerful plant alkaloid: berberine. This substance is traditionally used for its immuno stimulating, antifungal and antibacterial properties, and for its capacity to stabilize digestive disorders. It has also turned out to be a new weapon to combat type 2 diabetes and pre-diabetic states. It therefore plays a key role in certain metabolic diseases such as diabetes, insulin resistance, obesity or complications associated with diabetes.

According to the research done on berberine, the average recommended dose varies between 1 000 and 1 500 mg per day, split into two or three doses taken before each meal.

We can also mention:

Carnosine, a powerful anti-aging agent;

Pyridoxamine, a particular, natural form of vitamin B6 which blocks the formation of advanced glycation end products;

Chrome, which readjusts insulin secretion imbalances.

The immune system

Immune system deficiencies will directly affect lifespan by causing auto-immune diseases, or even cancer.

AHCC (Active Hexose Correlated Compound)

This is the most widely used immuno stimulating nutritional supplement in Japan .AHCC is extracted from the mycelium of the shiitake mushroom (*Lentinus edodes*). It contains many active ingredients, some of which are derived from alpha and beta-glucane. AHCC improves immune response through a number of different mechanisms: it induces macrophage and Natural Killer Cell proliferation, the measurable activity of which increases by more than 300%.

The daily dose is 1 000 mg.

Lactoferrin

Lactoferrin, a glycoprotein, is one of the most active components of colostrum (the first form of breast milk) and whey. It is a powerful antioxidant which also has remarkable and unparalleled immuno stimulating, antiviral and antimicrobial properties. It belongs to the cytokine family, which is responsible for coordinating cells' immune response to infections and tumors. In healthy individuals, lactoferrin is concentrated around the body's orifices (mouth, nose, eyes) which it protects from infection. It directly stimulates the immune system.

The daily dose is 500 mg.

The prostate

We mention the prostate here simply because this gland causes disorders which are closely linked with aging, and will affect one out of every two men older than fifty.

The substances which have shown clinical activity are mainly:

Saw palmetto (Serenoa repens)

The berries of the saw palmetto (*Serenoa repens*) are traditionally used by native Americans to decongest the urinary tract and treat genital disorders. Many double-blind, placebo-controlled studies have demonstrated the effectiveness of saw palmetto extract in alleviating the symptoms of benign prostate hypertrophy. Saw palmetto also decreases smooth muscle contraction, thereby relaxing the bladder and sphincter muscles, which cause the sudden urge to urinate. For men over 40, saw palmetto extract is the first line of defense against benign prostate adenoma.

Useful dose: 370 mg daily.

Selenium and methylselenocysteine

Selenium is a micronutrient which is essential to our lives. It is essential to the activation of certain key enzymes such as certain thyroid hormones and glutathione. It is found in Brazil nuts, seafood and certain grains. Certain anticancer studies have recently focused on a particular form of it: methylselenocysteine, which is naturally found in certain plants such as garlic and onions. Methylselenocysteine is easily converted into methylselenol which is the most effective form of selenium as it targets the process of apoptosis in cancer cells.

The daily dose is 200 μg.

We can also mention:

☐ Lycopene, a powerful carotenoid extracted from tomatoes;

☐ Pomegranate extract (with certified levels of ellagic acid and ellagitannin);

☐ Nettle root extract, a powerful anti-inflammatory agent;

☐ A specific pollen extract, which will decrease prostate volume; useful dose: 300 mg daily.

Step 3

We have now drawn up an, admittedly incomplete, catalog of the main functional substances capable of combating the most frequent disorders. Many of these substances, thankfully, do not apply to you, but you will have to choose a few before moving on to the next phase, that is, prolonging your lifespan, which will require you to make use of other kinds of supplements.

Among those which we have already mentioned, some will also be appropriate here: omega3, coenzyme Q10, alpha-lipoic acid

We have also elected to include five more traditional supplements, to which recent literature has not granted the attention we believe they deserve. They do have the advantage of having been very thoroughly scientifically studied and of demonstrating an undeniable level of activity.

1 - **NAC (N Acetylcysteine)**: it contains sulfur and stimulates glutathione levels, contributes to detoxification processes, maintains

cellular integrity and combats telomere shortening. Recommended dose: 500 mg once or twice daily.

2 - **Vitamin D3**: currently under particularly intense study, it decreases the risk of the most aggressive types of cancer such as colon, lung, ovarian and prostate cancer. It is essential to maintaining blood calcium levels.

Useful dose: 3 000 to 5 000 IU/day.

3 - **DMAE (dimethylaminoethanol)**: a nutrient which is crucial to acetylcholine production, an essential factor for memory, which is found in small quantities in brain cells and for which it stimulates all functions; it combats the production of lipofuscin, a brownish pigment which generates liver spots on the skin.

Recommended dose: 200 to 300 mg daily.

4 - **L-carnosine**: comes from the combination of 2 amino acids, alanine and histidine. Studies conducted in Australia have shown that carnosine regenerates cells which have reached the end of their lifespan. Soviet studies on terminally old mice have shown significant increases in lifespan, reaching up to 20%.

Recommended dose:500 to 1 000 mg daily.

5 - **ALCAR (Acetyl-L-carnitine):** essential to mitochondrial integrity, guaranteeing fatty acid penetration. ALCAR improves your mood, slows down cellular, and especially cerebral aging, and may combat Alzheimer's disease. Taking it in combination with alpha-lipoic acid may boost its activity.

Recommended dose: 500 mg to 1g once or twice daily.

New anti-aging molecules

They come from very recent research on the causes of aging: DNA damage, telomere shortening, and a diminished stem cell pool.

Damage repair

Resveratrol (and especially its isomer, trans-resveratrol) extracted from the red grape vine, vitis vinifera, is the ancestor of all anti-aging products. Polydatine is a resveratrol glucoside, that is, a resveratrol molecule bonded to a sugar molecule. When Polydatine enters the bloodstream, the resveratrol molecule separates from the sugar molecule. Resveratrol glucosides are absorbed at a different rate than classical trans-resveratrol, which effectively improves the bio availability, half-life and potency of resveratrol.

Pterostilbene has been used for hundreds of years by Ayurvedic medicine. Many beneficial effects are ascribed to it relating to the prevention and treatment of a whole range of ailments, including cancer, dyslipidemia, diabetes, cardiovascular disease and pain. Its anti-inflammatory and antioxidant effect allows it to efficiently combat certain effects of aging. Pterostilbene can effectively remedy dyslipidemia which otherwise provides a foundation for atherosclerosis and coronary disease. It can also improve your HDL/LDL ratio.

Pterostilbene and resveratrol are both stilbenes, which are closely related structurally. This means they have similar, but not identical functions. Researchers have shown that they act synergistically to activate longevity genes. Pterostilbene also mimics many of the effects of caloric restriction. It beneficially regulates genes involved in the development of cancer, atherosclerosis, diabetes and inflammation, which causes many illnesses. Oxaloacetate mimics and reproduces the known beneficial effects of caloric restriction, without having to actually undergo it. Oxaloacetic acid, or oxaloacetate is naturally found in freshly picked oranges and apples. This molecule is highly unstable however, and cannot be preserved for more than a day at room temperature. It is present in every cell of our organism, and its metabolites are directly involved in the production of mitochondrial energy, as it is an intermediate in the Krebs cycle. In this way, oxaloacetate has properties similar to resveratrol but acts through different mechanisms. It regulates the expression of certain so-called survival genes, which are activated during caloric restriction. Oxaloacetate therefore mimics the cellular conditions brought about by caloric restriction without having to limit our dietary intake. Thanks to a complex process, oxaloacetate can now be stabilized and made completely bioavailable.

Nicotinamide riboside (NR), the 'hidden vitamin', similar to niacin (vitamin B3), is a triple-action molecule: anti-aging, slimming and energizing.

NR makes you burn more calories at rest (by increasing NAD, which is essential to mitochondrial ATP metabolism); increases all metabolic activity by activating Sirtuin enzymes 1 and 3; reduces the activity and toxicity of beta-amyloid peptides in Alzheimer's disease.

We recommend a 250 mg daily dose.

TA-65®, which has been extensively described in this book, is the lead player in work done on telomeres. It is a rare extract of the *Astragalus membranaceus* plant and is difficult to isolate, which might explain why its price has not yet become totally accessible, and that certain companies have chosen to focus on isolating other active ingredients of this ancient Chinese plant as solid extracts, such as astragalosides and cycloastragenols.

Epitalon

The most recent of the ingredients available to us was born from the work of Professor Khavinson, a scientist and researcher who is still active, and the director of the St. Petersburg Institute of Bioregulation and Gerontology (Russia).

Epitalon stems from the combination of low doses of four amino acids: L-alanine, L-alpha-glutamine, L-alpha-aspartyl and glycine. Epithalon is believed to be a telomerase activator, enabling the synthesis and growth of telomeres, as well as cellular DNA repair. The four bio-peptides which make up Epitalon are natural bioregulators, which affect all physiological functions, decrease mortality by nearly 50% by re-establishing homeostatic balance through the interaction of these bio-peptides with DNA.

Epitalon improves immune response as we age by activating lymphocyte production in the thymus and interferon gamma production in T cells. Epithalon inhibits the development of spontaneous mammary tumors through negative regulation, which inhibits certain genes, in particular those of mammary and colonic adenocarcinomas, and by increasing cell apoptosis.

Many other substances with anti-aging properties exist, and would warrant devoting an entire book to them. We only wish here to encourage our readers to explore the subject furtherin order to discover them. We will mention:

☐ **Extracts from Asian mushrooms** such as Reishi or Cordyceps;

☐ **Saikosaponin A,** extracted from Bupleurum Falcatum, which activates the telomerase gene as well as the P16 and P53 genes, which are responsible for its significant anti-tumor effect, triggering apoptosis in cancer cells through the mitochondria;

☐ **PQQ or pyrroloquinolinequinone,** preferably combined with coenzymeQ10, is an incredibly potent antioxidant ,and the only one able to generate new mitochondria, even in senescent cells, up to 20%! Such a synergy could rectify most cognitive deficits.

New substances with undeniable anti-aging characteristics and virtues are discovered every day. Clinical or animal studies are essential to validate their short or long-term effectiveness. So never take supplements based on someone saying « I read that... « or » I was told that...» It would be irresponsible, and possibly even dangerous. Nowadays, it is indeed possible to adjust our nutritional supplementation to our specific needs, as our options are so numerous, but doing so requires scientific knowledge, so ask your doctor or a trained specialist for help.

S O U R C E S

David Servan-Schreiber.
Guérir. Paris : Laffont ; 2003.

Dominique Rueff, Maurice Nahon.
Stratégie longue vie. Archamps : Éditions Jouvence ; 2013.

Richard Béliveau, Denis Gingras.
Les aliments contre le cancer. Québec : Trécarré ; 2005.

Richard Béliveau, Denis Gingras.
La Méthode anti cancer. Québec : Trécarré ; 2014.

Barry Sears.
The Anti-inflammation Zone. New York : HarperCollins ; 2005.

Paul McGlothin & Meredith Averill.
The CR Way. New York : HarperCollins ; 2008.

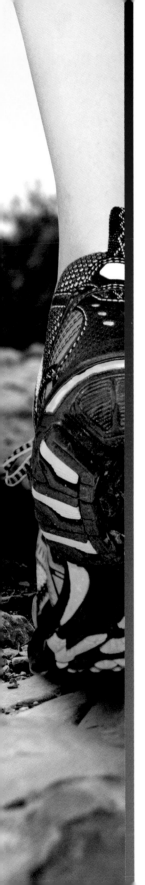

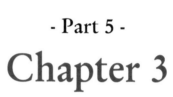

- Part 5 -

Chapter 3

The JLife Fitness plan

As we get older, we run into three obstacles. The first is shortness of breath; we don't have the same respiratory capacity we used to, and we run out of breath quickly, in ever shortening distances. The second concerns our joints: they aren't as flexible as they once were and limit our mobility. The third obstacle is muscle loss; the more we age, the more muscle we lose!

The good news is that these obstacles are far from insurmountable, which means that we can very realistically hope to regain the respiratory capacity of our thirties, the joints of our forties, and the muscle of our youth; so long as we put in the necessary effort and consistency. All we need is:

1 - sufficient protein intake;

2 - regular resistance training;

3 - high intensity exercises;

4 - regular stretching exercises.

Before embarking on the JLife Fitness program, we recommend you fill out the questionnaire in annex 3 (page 436), which will assess your current physical condition. One last thing: before any physical activity, it is essential that you see your doctor to check for any potential contraindication or precautions you should take.

3.1 - Choosing your proteins

During prolonged and/or intense exercise, amino acids, which are part of our muscles' makeup, are used up to supply the energy necessary for the effort we are generating. Even if the use of these amino acids is minimal in terms of quantity, it has a significant impact on our muscles' function. After exercising, our organism automatically goes into a muscle protein rebuilding phase (called 'anabolism') the effectiveness of which largely depends on the availability of amino acids and of different hormonal signals, including insulin. Your protein intake after exercising will therefore boost muscle reconstruction.

Which are the best proteins to improve your muscle mass? There exist two different sources: amino acids, which are the precursors to proteins, and whole proteins which are made of assembled amino acids, and come from a variety of sources. The idea is to combine both sources as wisely as possible. It is important that you favor the use of proteins which have high biological value, such as animal protein (especially eggs, fish, milk and dairy products), whose nutritional value is generally higher than that of plant protein, as they have a better balance of essential amino acids, with higher concentrations of leucine, and are easier to digest.

Proteins are not all digested at the same rate. Ideally, the snack you take after your training sessions should contain both fast-digested and slower-digested proteins. The former are rapidly digested and absorbed, and immediately supply the organism with amino acids for about the next three hours. The latter are digested and absorbed more gradually, and begin supplying amino acids two hours after having been ingested, and for the next six hours. Slow protein therefore continues the work begun by the faster kind, and promotes muscle anabolism for a longer period of time.

Milk naturally contains a mix of fast protein (20% whey) and slow protein (80% casein), which makes it a very good protein source for recovery.

What amount of protein should you consume?

Recommended intake is generally somewhere between 1.2 and 1.5 g for every kilogram of bodyweight daily; and up to 2 g if you wish to increase muscle mass quickly. We need to ensure at least two thirds of our protein intake comes from our diet, and the rest from supplements with high biological value.

When should you consume protein?

The optimal intake period is during the early recovery phase (that is, immediately after exercising) when muscle anabolism is highest and requires high amino acid availability. It is recommended that you take 10 to 20 g within the first thirty minutes after exercising. For example, during the stretching which is usually done for five to ten minutes after exercising. In the case of prolonged and very significant effort, protein metabolism may be affected by the increased use of amino acids as an energy source. In this case, it is recommended that you take a special type of amino acid while exercising: branched-chain amino acids (leucine, isoleucine, valine), as they reduce muscle protein degradation, delay muscle glycogen depletion (our muscles' sugar supply), and may help diminish central nervous system fatigue.

3.2 - Alternate resistance training and high intensity training

Sports are useful at any age for muscle building. Many studies prove it, and it has recently been shown that the same amount of effort can be expended whether we are 25 or 75. Certain types of exercise build more muscle than others, however. For a long time, we believed that light endurance training (jogging, biking, swimming) was the best way to maintain our muscle mass as we aged. In fact, studies show that alternating between endurance and high intensity exercises works best.

Resistance training (first with your bodyweight, and later on with free weights) is a good way to begin training. Interval training, in which short periods of intense effort are alternated with longer endurance periods (no matter the sport), is also very effective as it promotes growth hormone production. The one to two percent of muscle mass which we lose every year on average after 40 can therefore be recovered within a few weeks of training, by training three to four times a week.

3.3 - Stretching

Have you noticed the difference in how men or women who are around sixty year old and young adults walk? It is often obvious, and it can make it easy to differentiate between younger and older individuals, even when just seeing them from behind. This is entirely due to our joints' mobility, which gives young adults a graceful form, allows them to easily climb stairs, and coordinate their muscle groups properly, so that they can rush down them just as easily, without ever tripping. And yet some octogenarians can do just as well, and even better than the young. What is their secret? Daily stretching of the muscles responsible for walking and our gait! Stretching is the key factor for a youthful and slender appearance; it can help you lose fat and reach the limits of your muscular capacity during exercise. Furthermore, when you are able to increase the length of your stride, your center of gravity improves and you are less likely to stumble or lose balance, and can therefore avoid any accidents. Stretching improves your daily life, from walking your dog, to taking out the trash, to a mad dash to catch your plane!

There are different stretching methods, such as yoga or Pilates.

Yoga was developed in India over several millennia, and is a method of self-development, combined with a spiritual practice. It has several dimensions, the main ones being the following: devotion (bhakti yoga), selfless action (*karma yoga*), knowledge (*jnana yoga*), health and concentration through a healthy lifestyle and postures (*hatha-yoga*). Yoga classes are most often based on the latter dimension, hatha-yoga. Its role in the traditional spiritual path is to discipline the mind and maintain the body in optimal health, for the individual to be able to meditate better and longer. The tools of hatha-yoga are breathing exercises and over 1 000 postures. The postures are made up of stretching, bending and twisting motions, which improve spine flexibility and act on every organ and gland. Holding these postures also trains the mind and develops your perseverance and concentration, while also procuring the benefits of meditation.

Pilates (named after its inventor, Joseph Pilates) enables us to restore balance to our body's muscles, by focusing on the core muscles which are involved in posture and support the spine. The goal of its exercises is to strengthen the muscles which are too weak and relax those which are too tight. Movements are executed while taking into account our breathing, proper spinal alignment, as well as more generally maintaining good posture. This method emphasizes properly balanced strength. Tense muscles exert tensile stress on the surrounding joints; as the body's muscles mainly function in antagonist (opposing) pairs, if one muscle is pulling too hard in one direction, it is very likely that its antagonist will, conversely, be stretched out and/or weak. If we want to correct these forces, we therefore need to correct antagonist muscle groups. This also allows us to balance our posture.

3.4 - Practically speaking

The first step is to define your current level, your physical activity profile, which you can do by filling out the questionnaire in annex 3 (page 436).

The second step will be to develop a daily stretching plan which should last five to ten minutes. This stretching program is entirely personal, and has to be tailored to you, based on your muscle structure and level of flexibility.

The goal is to decrease muscle tension and improve your mobility.

The third step will be to design, depending on your fitness level and your cardiovascular condition, a daily program for a period of six weeks.

Here are a few suggestions.

'Sedentary' level

Every day:

☐   5 to 10 mn of stretching,
☐   5 mn of cardio to warm up.

Choose a kind of exercise which you enjoy, and do:

☐   30 seconds of explosive effort, but only at 50% of your maximum;
☐   90 seconds at a very slow pace but without stopping;
☐   30 seconds of explosive effort at 60% of your maximum;
☐   90 seconds at a very slow pace, without stopping.
☐   End with some stretching.

Total: 15 to 20 mn.

Note: progressively increase effort until you reach 100% of your maximum.

'Moderately active' level

Every day:

☐ 5 to 10 mn of stretching,
☐ 5 mn of cardio to warm up.

Choose a kind of exercise which you enjoy, and do:

☐ 30 seconds of explosive effort, but only at 70% of your maximum;
☐ 90 seconds at a very slow pace but without stopping;
☐ 30 seconds of explosive effort at 80% of your maximum;
☐ 90 seconds at a very slow pace, without stopping;
☐ 30 seconds of explosive effort at 100% of your maximum;
☐ 90 seconds at a very slow pace, without stopping.
☐ End with some stretching.

Total: 20 to 25 mn.

'Active' level

☐ Increase the number of explosive effort periods to five while still alternating with 90 second rest periods.

Total: 25 to 30 mn.

3.5 - Physical activity without exercise

Daily goal: don't sit or lie down during the day for more than 30 consecutive minutes.

No matter the space you are in, move your muscles passively or actively. At home, at work, in a train station, a subway station, a bus stop, an airport or a plane. Even if the seatbelt sign is on, you can still mobiliseyour muscles. Target each muscle group, paying special attention to each one, using any gadgets you can find: hand grips, exercise bands, balls, fitness equipment which can be attached to chairs, tables, beds… take the time to search around and you'll be surprised by all the available choices.

Park your car further away from your destination, avoid escalators and elevators (except in skyscrapers!), favor the stairs. Volunteer to take the dog for a walk or take out the trash etc.

Regularity and consistency are the cornerstones of good exercise; sports and physical exercise are relatively easy to accomplish, but doing so six days a week for your entire life is incredibly difficult; and yet it is an essential prerequisite to good health and greater longevity. Yet it is not enough if you spend the rest of your time sitting in front of your computer, so you will have to use your imagination and creativity to keep moving at home, at work and everywhere else.

S O U R C E S

David A. Kekich.

Smart, Strong and Sexy at 100? New-port Beach,
(Californie) : Maximum Life Foundation ; 2012.

Michael Fossel, Greta Blackburn, Dave Woynarowski.

The Immortality Edge. Hoboken (New Jersey) : John Wiley & Sons, Inc. ; 2011.

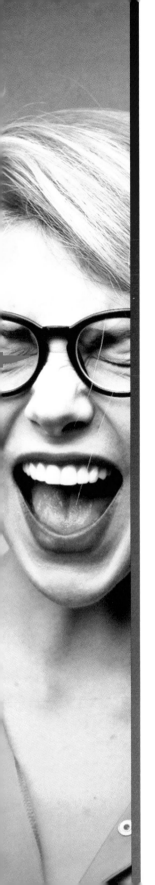

- Part 5 -

Chapter 4

The JLife Stress plan

« To each his own life, to each his own stress »

- Dr Charly Cungi -

Our family, professional, and social lives are constant stressors, and analyzing our reactions to them is crucial. Indeed, if stress lasts, this is because it is constantly being reinforced, and we do not know how to control it.

The first step of the JLife plan is therefore to evaluate the relevant players. On the one hand, the stressors, and on the other, the reactions of the stressed party: you.

The scale on which we rate stressors allows us to quantify the intensity of the stressful situations which you have faced.

4.1 - Stressor rating scale
(as specified by Cungi)

The questionnaire has 8 questions.

For each one, answer yes or no.

If the answer is no: add 1 point.

If the answer is yes: add 2 points.

Answer as soon as you have read the question.
(the first answer which pops into your mind is the right one)

1	Have I in my life endured traumatic situations such as a death, long periods of unemployment, romantic disappointment etc.?	YES ☐	NO ☐

2	Am I currently living through the same traumatic situations (death, long-term unemployment, romantic disappointment, refusal of retirement etc.)?	YES ☐	NO ☐

3	Am I currently suffering from work overload, or is my work environment highly competitive, or am I living in a permanent state of emergency?	YES ☐	NO ☐

4	Does my job not suit me (or does my retirement not suit me), is this a source of frustration, or does this depress me?	YES ☐	NO ☐

5	Do I have substantial family issues (couple, children, parents)?	YES ☐	NO ☐

6	Am I in debt, is my income too low to support my lifestyle, does this worry me?	YES ☐	NO ☐

7	Do I have many non-work-related activities, are they a source of fatigue and stress?	YES ☐	NO ☐

8	Do I suffer from a debilitating disease, or does the fear of death cause me anxiety?	YES ☐	NO ☐

Answers

Total points

_____

If your total is between 8 and 10
you live with few stressors.

If your total is between 11 and 13
you live with an average amount of stressors.

If your total is between 14 and 16
you live with a high amount of stressors.

Go through this test again every 3 months.

Source :

Dr Charles Cungi. Savoir gérer son stress.

Paris : Éditions Retz ; 2003, p 31.

4.2 - Stress rating scale

The stress rating scale evaluates
your general reaction to stressors.

This questionnaire is made
up of 11 questions.

For each one, answer yes or no.

If the answer is no: add 1 point.

If the answer is yes: add2 points.

Answer as soon as you have read the question
(the first answer which pops into your mind is the right one).

1	Am I emotional, sensitive to the comments and criticisms made by others?	YES ☐	NO ☐
2	Am I easily or rapidly angered or irritated?	YES ☐	NO ☐
3	Am I a perfectionist? Do I tend to be dissatisfied by what I or others accomplish?	YES ☐	NO ☐
4	Do I have a fast heartbeat, do I sweat excessively, do I shake, do I have involuntary muscle contractions in my face or eyelids?	YES ☐	NO ☐
5	Do my muscles feel tense, does my jaw feel clenched, does my face feel tense, or my body in general?	YES ☐	NO ☐
6	Do I have trouble sleeping?	YES ☐	NO ☐
7	Am I anxious? Do I often worry?	YES ☐	NO ☐
8	Do I have digestive issues, pains, headaches, allergies, eczema?	YES ☐	NO ☐
9	Am I tired?	YES ☐	NO ☐
10	Do I have more significant health problems?	YES ☐	NO ☐
11	Do I smoke or drink to energize or calm myself? Do I use any other stimulants or sedatives?	YES ☐	NO ☐

379

Answers

Total points

_____

If your total is between 11 and 14
your level of stress is low.

If your total is between 15 and 18
your level of stress is average.

If your total is between 19 and 22
your level of stress is high.

Go through this test again every 6 months.

Source :

Dr Charles Cungi. Savoir gérer son stress.

Paris : Éditions Retz ; 2003, p 31.

These two scales will allow you to properly evaluate and analyze your stress in order to get a personalized solution.

1ˢᵗ case
Your stressor (14/16)
and stress (19/22) scores are high

You are tense and often irritated, you try to accomplish too many things at the same time, which means your performance will tend to diminish and you may settle into a constant state of physical, mental and emotional exhaustion. You must urgently address this.

2ⁿᵈ case
Your stressor score is high (14/16)
whereas your stress score is low (11/14)

This is the ideal case, as it seems you are perfectly capable of handling events and changes which are beyond your control. A note of caution: review you stress score and make sure you are being completely honest. We sometimes under estimate our level of stress.

3ʳᵈ case
Your stressor (8/10)
and stress (11/14) scores are very low

This is certainly possible, but not 'physiological'. We all require constant stimulation in order to test our capacity to return to a state of equilibrium. This permanent 'passivity' opens the door to a large number of health problems. Review your scores.

4th case
A low stressor score (8/10)
whereas your stress reactions are high (19/22)

Your response to minimal stress is disproportionate and you need to take swift action.

5th case
An average stressor (11/13)
and stress score (15/18)

This is the most frequent and common case: you react in a balanced manner to normal situations.

(To evaluate your stress in more detail, fill out the questionnaire in annex 4, page 439)

You now have precise information on how you react to stressful events. In the next step, we will examine why given situations trigger you to be irritated, angry, anxious or discouraged. In particular, we will try to look at your 'automatic thoughts', your internal dialog when you are exposed to triggering situations.

According to Charles Cungi, these internal thoughts (we call them 'cognitions') are generally repeated in the same way. They are classified into three categories: those which relate to ourselves (I am useless!), those which relate to others and our environment (He's always late!), and those which relate to the future (He won't come!). But the important thing is that these thoughts are always closely linked to a specific emotion: « *I am useless* » implies some form of despair; « *He's always late* » implies irritation, and « *He won't come* » implies worry. Every thought is linked to an emotion, and therefore changing our thoughts influences our emotions, and *vice versa*.

In fact, stress is a habit, and to break out of it, we need to change our habits. Many different methods were designed for this, which focus on emotions, thoughts and behaviors.

4.3 - Hypoventilation

Relaxing is often difficult to do when we are stressed, and is only possible in privileged situations: when we are calm, with music playing, for example. But this is clearly not enough if we want to solve these problems. The goal of anti-stress relaxation is for it to function mainly in difficult situations.

Hypoventilation works on the idea that the less we breathe, the more we calm down! This obviously goes against the popular belief that taking a deep breath will help us calm down, and achieves the opposite effect... The explanation: when confronted with lower oxygen intake, the body reduces its activity to consume less of it. Emotions, which consume a lot of energy, then follow this general slow-down.

How to proceed

Step 1

Measure your pulse on your wrist and write down your heart rate (for example, 95 beats per minute).

Step 2

Empty your lungs calmly, then take in a small breath, which you will hold for a brief moment, then breathe out calmly.

Step 3

Check whether your heart rate has slowed down; keep going until the new rate has become clear and constant.

Step 4

After some practice, you will feel your chest relax. This feeling of calm and of releasing tension represents the beginning of relaxation.

Note: measuring your pulse is only necessary while you are learning this technique. Start by practicing this technique in unstressful situations, then gradually apply it to more difficult situations.

Practice hypoventilation in all situations and positions. You can supplement this with a rapid relaxation method which is very easy to learn.

4.4 - Rapid relaxation

Sit down comfortably, and begin by performing hypoventilation. All you need to do is close your eyes and focus on your breathing for a few seconds, and every exhalation will bring you nearer to feeling calm and relaxed. At first, ten or so breaths are necessary, each one relaxing you more and more. Little by little, you will become able to reach deep relaxation after fewer breaths, until only a single one is necessary. Eventually you will be able to achieve the same results with your eyes open!

4.5 - Mindfulness meditation

Or should we say: « *mindful concentration* » (David O'Hare), as this kind of meditation is the result of a harmonious balance between concentration and mindfulness. To concentrate is to uninterruptedly direct all of our attention onto a specific subject, and correcting any distraction as soon as it is noticed. Mindfulness is the unrestricted acknowledgment of everything which occurs while we are concentrated, whether they be negative or positive thoughts. In practice, we first need to develop our ability to concentrate and, little by little, patiently integrate this constant state of attention which mindfulness provides.

4.6 - Walking meditation

This is a mindfulness exercise. Walk (with your eyes open!), and pay attention to everything that surrounds you. Walk slowly, without changing your gait in any way. First, begin by concentrating entirely on your speed, on your legs, your feet, your breathing, on the smells and sounds which surround you. Observe, acknowledge, and... move on! Consider the pleasure it gives you to control your own body, your own legs well enough to attain the constant balance which makes it possible for you to walk. If your attention drifts from walking or your environment, calmly bring it back. Synchronize the rhythm at which you walk with your breathing. When you've decided to end this meditative exercise, simply stop.

4.6 - Mindful eating (David O'Hare)

This is a method of mindfulness meditation in which you concentrate on the act of eating and all of the sensations which come with it. You should only practice this when you are eating alone and your environment isn't distracting. It consists of attentively examining the meal which is in front of you; the goal is to savor, with every one of your senses, each sensation which your meal, its ingredients and your drink provide. Every sense should be involved until the end of the meal.

4.8 - Classics

There are dozens of excellent meditation techniques, here are just a few. Transcendental meditation

This technique is of Indian origin, and has been simplified for a Western audience. This mental relaxation technique is practiced with the help of a 'mantra'. Mantras are words, or sounds, which are spoken out loud during meditation. This technique is practiced by millions of people around the world.

Zen

This word which is now often used very loosely, actually represents a set of ritual practices which go back 2 600 years. These practices were passed down from master to disciple, from generation to generation, up to the present day. It consists of breathing while sitting in the lotus position, in order to slow down, through slow exhalation. Air is expelled slowly and silently through the nose, and once the exhalation has finished, inhalation is brought about naturally.

Qi Gong

This traditional Chinese method combines slow gymnastics, whose movements are broken down, with breathing exercises and concentration, focusing on all of the muscle groups.

4.9 - Sleeping better: learning good habits

Effective stress management can only be achieved through good sleep.

First and foremost, we need to mitigate all forms of mental and physical stimulation. Avoid intense physical exercise and sports two hours before you plan to go to sleep, as well as hot baths just before going to bed. On the contrary, all agitation should be kept to a minimum. Some herbal infusions (e.g. passionflower, valerian) facilitate sleep. Breathing in front of an open window, practicing diaphragmatic breathing, clearing your nose, listening to soothing music, reading a few pages of a book (without any suspense) can help a lot. These activities should, if possible, be repeated at the same time each day; routines cause conditioning which will send your body signals that it is time to fall asleep.

Where we sleep

When we have trouble sleeping, the space in which we sleep can also be a determining factor. Your bedroom should be exclusively dedicated to rest. Why not soundproof it, considering that as we age, we become sensitive to the slightest noise? Window blinds, soundproof glass, carpeting, or a soundproof partition will get rid of any unwanted noise. It's worth the investment. You can't put a price on restful sleep. The quality of your bedding should not be disregarded either: a good frame as well as a good mattress, a warm duvet in the winter and a light blanket in the summer help to improve sleep by making you more comfortable. Bedroom temperatures are often too high 65 ° F (18/19° C) is enough. Too low or too high a temperature will wake you up. Airing out your room daily is always a good thing, but sleeping with the window half-open is even better, if you can. If you do not sleep well, you should avoid napping after 3 p.m., and never for longer than twenty minutes. It is essential to realize that sleeping requires no particular effort but rather demands that you let it wash over you, unrestricted.

How to fall back asleep after waking up?

Waking up in the middle of the night is understandably not a welcome event. If our mind switches on at that moment, there is a high risk that we will stay awake longer than we would like. Mental agitation contributes to worsening this unease. This vicious cycle of obsessive thoughts and ruminations needs to be broken with disengagement techniques: some examples are breathing from your abdomen, counting down, remembering pleasant moments, focusing on sensory impressions.

▫ REMEMBER ▫

Coping with stress is a daily affair. First and foremost, it requires that you know the causes and consequences of this stress. Thanks to the different available test methods, you will be able to find within this arsenal one or several methods which work best for you.

Today, meditation/concentration techniques have proven themselves and their effectiveness is no longer in question. You will be truly surprised by the results.

SOURCES

Charles Cungi.
Savoir gérer son stress. Paris : Éditions Retz ; 2003.

David O'hare.
5 minutes le matin. Vergèze : Thierry Souccar Editions ; 2013.

David Servan-Schreiber.
Guérir le stress, l'anxiété et la dépression sans médicament ni psychanalyse.
Paris : Éditions Robert Laffont ; 2003.

Ronald Siegel.
The Mindfulness Solution. New York : The Guilford Press ; 2010.

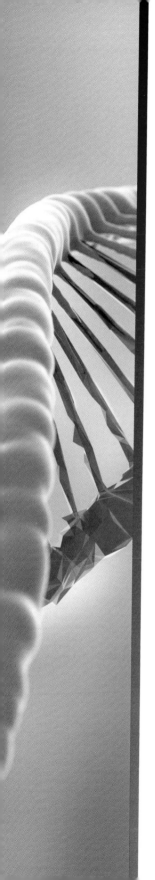

- Part 5 -
Conclusions

« We need a better reason than simple survival to persevere in the struggle to live. »

- David Servan-Schreiber -

In order to live much longer than the average person, you must REALLY want it and truly apply yourself! Methods do exist, but they must be used synergistically. They all have the same goal: to boost cellular homeostasis by tapping into the body's natural energy. It is precisely because they contribute to the body's harmony, balance and coherence that these methods are both effective and generate no side effects. They are mutually reinforcing and tackle aging from different angles, in order to produce a synergy which is more potent than cellular senescence. Even if each of these methods has proven its effectiveness in combating aging factors, their combination, when adapted to each of us, will have the greatest chance of breathing new life into your life. So, where to start? First of all, learn about the causes and consequences of aging as well as the tools which are available to us today to remedy it. Secondly, assess your biological age and use all available biomarkers. Finally, strike on all fronts, with a healthy diet, appropriate nutritional supplements, regular physical activity and a suitable meditation method. And don't forget to learn about the uses of stem cells and certain growth factors. But the most important thing is regularity and consistency in practicing these methods, as our DNA deteriorates every day, and requires our constant dedication.

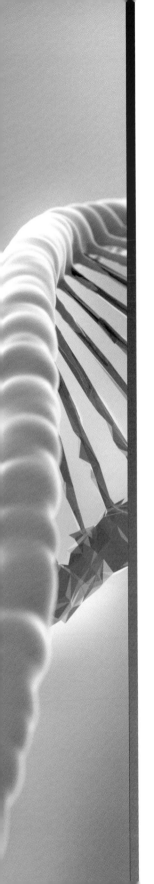

Concluding
Remarks

Work hard, put all the effort in you can:
This wealth we lack the least.
A rich farmer, sensing his impending death,
Called his children, and spoke to them without witnesses.
«Do not sell the inheritance
Left by our forebears, he said.
A treasure is kept inside.
I do not know where; but with a bit of courage
You will find it, you will figure it out.
Go search the field when summer ends.
Dig, scratch, plow, leave no earth unturned
Anywhere your hands can reach.»
After the father's death, the sons worked the field,
Everywhere, over and over again; so that within a year
It produced more than ever before.
There was no money to be found, but the father had been wise
To show them before his death
That work is a treasure.

THE FARMER
& HIS CHILDREN

- Jean de La Fontaine -

I drew inspiration from this fable written by Jean de La Fontaine, and let myself make a promise I knew I would not be able to keep.

Yet beyond this promise, through my hard work, I found another, much more thrilling one: « *To live a life as long and healthy as is possible* »

This flexibility in time comforts me. We are told we will all die one day. Perhaps! But certainly not tomorrow, nor the day after tomorrow! Today we are told that, during all of this additional time, we could live a completely healthy life. We could have a youthful body, a youthful mind, a youthful love life, for as long as possible; what must we do to make this a reality? First we need to understand, and then act accordingly. Understanding alone is a fruitless pursuit if it is not followed by action.

Understanding the secrets of cellular function, while knowing that the past ten years have completely revolutionized our knowledge of cellular biology. The central dogma proclaiming the omnipotence of genes in governing all life has been shattered. The findings of epigenetics have provided scientifically substantiated proof that our environment influences the behavior of our 60 trillion cells without modifying our genetic code. the role of which is strictly limited to acting as a database of blueprints for the assembly of our proteins, but which can be activated or deactivated by our intra and extra-cellular environment, and, especially, by our beliefs and perceptions. The consequences of this for our health are crucial, as it may indeed be possible to treat many illnesses by modifying our environment or the way we think and feel.

Understanding the secrets of aging as well, in order to delay or even reverse it, with the knowledge that aging is due to inadequacies in our DNA repair mechanisms, shortening telomeres and reduced stem cell reserves.

Understanding as well that our life expectancy has continually increased since the start of the 20th century. During the First World War, doctors and surgeons had one solitary goal: for their patients to survive, no matter the collateral damage; to this end, they had no reservations about amputating a leg, without any anesthetics, to the sound of a beating drum which would drown out the patient's screams. During the Second World War, antibiotics appeared, and we were finally able to treat patients and avoid amputating their limbs. Millions of lives were saved and medicine made a spectacular leap forward: we were no longer simply saving lives, we were also treating illnesses. The earlier work of Jenner and Pasteur on vaccination had brought about a new kind of medicine: preventive medicine. In only one hundred years, medical science made more progress than it had since the dawn of humanity, and life expectancy doubled, going from forty to eighty years old, which grants us… six more hours to live each day.

Understanding, finally, that our cells are intelligent, that they can teach us how to live and lead us towards spirituality. Albert Einstein stressed this: mystical experiences inspire all true science. Recognizing our environment as an energetic whole is the basis for science and alternative medicine as well as the spiritual wisdom of religion.

Could everything that exists in the Universe be the product of happenstance and necessity? Random chance, by definition, is constrained by no determinative principle and corresponds to no specific identified cause. Contrary to this, necessity is the essential quality of all that which is necessary, in all of the various meanings of the word. Are we not born by chance, are we not the product of an incredible set of circumstances? Yet if we go back as far as we are able, Science tells us that our universe is as it is thanks to an improbably fine tuning of the fundamental physical constants, and that if this were not the case it would only have led to chaos. So, far from being the product of blind chance, could we be that of an inflexible necessity? This revives the eternal existential question: where do we come from, and what are we?

A human community called Humanity

Bruce Lipton considers that evolution depends on interaction among species. He thinks that the Earth, and all of the species which inhabit it, constitutes a vast, interacting, living organism. « *Imagine a population of trillions of individuals living under one roof in a state of perpetual happiness* ». Such a community exists: it is made up of the cells of a healthy human body. Cell communities clearly function better than human communities. If humans modeled their lifestyle on that of healthy cell communities, our societies and our planet would be more peaceful and vibrant. Lipton asks us to « *harness our cellular intelligence in order to climb another rung of the evolutionary ladder.* »

A modern Western individual seeking to lead a healthy life has an exceptional wealth of possibilities. Recent social, scientific and medical innovations provide more opportunities than ever before in terms of prevention, treatment and rejuvenation. If we manage to live longer, the question of *genetically modified humans*, as Radman calls it, will no longer be relevant, by definition. The question will rather be about what we wish to change: once we rid ourselves of the genetic burden which plagues our lives, and then reinforce our individual genome, we will have a choice to make: either build man for pleasure, or build him for specialization (Radman). We can bet that specialization will attract us, with all of the attendant social consequences that the construction of a human anthill will have, freedom from individuality, freedom from the fear of change, to each their own specialty, to each their own mission. So, would we be willing to accept a human anthill on earth?

Another, much more elegant alternative could see the light of day. A sort of plan B, which could lead to what I have called the *epigenetically modified human*. In fact, we already have the technology needed to identify epigenetic switches (there exist a few million of them); furthermore, we are constantly improving our knowledge of the consequences of activating or deactivating certain genes; finally, we know how to control this activation (or deactivation) by acting on certain systems, e.g. methylation, among others. We can therefore endow the *Epigenetically Healthy Human©* (EHH) with all of the assets which will enable him to live as long as possible and in perfect health!

For one more day

Every year, the US National Academy of Sciences sponsors a large event, to bring together scientists specialized in biological and earth sciences. During one of these conferences, a young scientist asked the following question: « *If a man has lived 32 873 days (90 years), could he have done something more, during his life, which might have made it possible for him to live...one more day?* » The answer was obvious: « *Yes, of course!* » He could have eaten less sugar, or exercised for 30 more minutes, or taken larger doses of antioxidants. And if we managed, in this way, to add one day to his life, why not two? And so on... The moral of this story is not that there are no limits to longevity, the moral is that this longevity does not happen overnight, but rather is planned out, day by day! How many more 'days of life' could we gain if we had more control over our environment? If we invented new biotechnologies? If we had a better lifestyle? The debate on life expectancy is far from over.

For one more day...in good health

The question could be asked in another way: what could we do to be in better health tomorrow compared to today?

The main goal of a sustainably healthy life is to constantly return to a perfect balance between activating and inhibiting forces; this despite the millions of changes which daily life imposes upon us. This perfect balance is called homeostasis. In order to reach it, our human machinery must trigger thousands of chemical reactions every second. These require the presence of tens of thousands of specific proteins which are assembled on demand according to blueprints unique to our genes. Yet to send out the assembly blueprint, its gene must be activated; this is the determining factor: who decides to activate or deactivate this or that gene? This is a fundamental question, considering that the activation or deactivation of a gene can save...or kill us!

So what could we do to be healthier tomorrow than we are today? Activate 'good' genes and deactivate 'bad' ones. How? Through regular physical activity and a healthy diet, through proper management of our stress and our emotions, by avoiding toxic thoughts and speaking to our cells; all while keeping up to date with and harnessing all of the new technologies which allow us to improve our management of our epigenetic switches. Do all this every day, and you will score an extra healthy day; for how long? As long as possible.

And maybe then the promise of immortality will become more than a promise.

Dr. William Amzallag

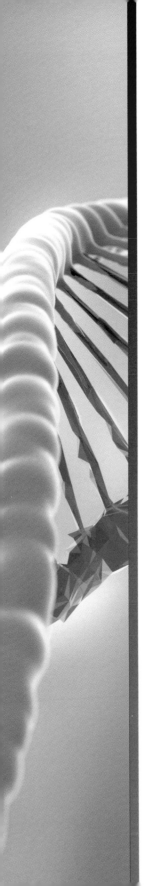

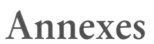

Annexes

- Annex 1 -

Evaluate your biological age

Take 30 minutes of your time to fill out this test and remember: there are no right or wrong answers. If you aren't sure of your answer, if you think about it for too long, you can be sure that, in this case, the answer is usually 'no'.

The questions are divided into eight sections.

Take a pencil and a piece of paper and add up your score as you fill out the test: each question has a negative or positive score. You will start off with a score of 1 000 points and deduct (or add) the results of the eight sections at the end of the test.

- Section 1 -

1 - 1 □ Sex (Gender)		
Male	Deduct 15 points	(-15)
Female	Add 10 points	(+10)
Note : it is well known that women live on average six to seven years longer than men.		

1 - 2 □ Age		
Select the age group in which you belong today.		
0 – 20		(0)
20 – 30	Deduct 25 points	(-25)
30 – 40	Deduct 50 points	(-50)
40 - 50	Deduct 75 points	(-75)
50 - 60	Deduct 100 points	(-100)
60 - 70	Deduct 125 points	(-125)
70 - 80	Deduct 150 points	(-150)
80 et au-delà	Deduct 175 points	(-175)
Note : only select one answer.		

1 - 3 □ Heredity		
One of your parents, or grandparents, has lived older than 80 years old.	If so : Add 10 points	(+10)
Note : if you don't know the answer, skip the question.		

1 - 4 ☐ Family background		
One of your parents, or grandparents, suffered from a stroke or heart attack, BEFORE the age of 50.	If so : Deduct 20 points	(-20)
Note : if you don't know the answer, skip the question.		

1 - 5 ☐ Family history		
One of your ancestors (father, mother, grandparents) suffered from one of the following illnesses before the age of 65–for each illness		
Hypertension	Yes	(-5)
Cancer	Yes	(-5)
Heart disease	Yes	(-5)
Stroke	Yes	(-5)
Diabetes (Type 1 or 2)	Yes	(-5)
Genetic disease	Yes	(-5)
Note : if you don't know the answer, skip the question.		
Add up the answers to question 1- 5 Family history	Min : 0 Max : -30	TOTAL :

SUBTOTAL FOR SECTION 1 (1 - 1 to 1 - 5)	
Negative subtotals :	TOTAL :
Positive subtotals :	
Note : add positive scores together and deduct negative scores (max: +20, min: -240).	

- Section 2 -

2 - 1 ☐ Family income		
Is your yearly income enough to provide for your family's health?	No : Deduct 10 points	(-10)
Note : in certain countries, health costs are out-of-pocket, and studies have shown that low-income individuals tend to neglect their health.		

2 - 2 ☐ Éducation		
No educational background	Deduct 10 points	(-10)
You finished high-school		(0)
You have pursued higher education	Add 10 points	(+10)
Note : it has also been shown that our level of education positively influences our awareness of the importance of health.		

2 - 3 ☐ Occupation		
You do not work, as you are unemployed	Deduct 20 points	(-20)
You do not work, because you are retired		(0)
You do not work, and are older than 65	Add 10 points	(+10)
You mainly work at night	Deduct 20 points	(-20)
Note : only select one answer.		

2 - 4 ☐ Housing		
You live in a large industrial city where pollution spikes are common	Deduct 20 points	(-20)
You live in a large city, with little industrialization		(0)
You live in a quiet suburb or in the countryside	Add 10 points	(+10)
Note : only select one answer.		

2 - 5 ☐ Commuting		
It takes less than 30 minutes for you to get to work		(0)
It takes between 30 and 60 minutes maximum for you to get to work	Deduct 25points	(-5)
It takes at least an hour for you to get to work	Deduct 10 points	(-10)
It takes more than an hour for you to get to work	Deduct 15 points	(-15)
You work at home	Add 5 points	(+5)
Note : only select one answer.		

SUBTOTAL FOR SECTION 2 (2 - 1 à 2 - 5)	
Negative subtotals :	TOTAL :
Positive subtotals :	
Note : add up positive scores and deduct negative scores (max: +35, minimum: -75).	

- Section 3 -

3 - 1 □ Marriage		
You are married or have lived with someone for a long time, and you live in harmony with one another	Add 20 points	(+20)
You are married or live as a couple, but your relationship is unstable	Deduct 20 points	(-20)
You are divorced	Deduct 10 points	(-10)
You live in a different situation		(0)
Note : only select one answer.		

3 - 2 □ Leisure		
You play mentally stimulating games (cards, board games)	Yes : Add 5 points	(+5)
You play a musical instrument	Yes : Add 5 points	(+5)
You speak at least one foreign language	Yes : Add 5 points	(+5)
You are a member of a recreational club or do charity work.	Yes : Add 5 points	(+5)
You have a hobby which relaxes you and which you particularly enjoy	Yes : Add 5 points	(+5)
Note : you may combine these answers.		

3 - 3 ☐ Pets		
You have a dog or cat, or another kind of pet at home	Add 5 points	(+5)

3 - 4 ☐ Children		
You have children	Add 5 points	(+5)
You have grandchildren	Add 5 points	(+5)
Note : you may combine these answers.		

3 - 5 ☐ Friendship		
You have a friend you could trust with anything	Add 10 points	(+10)

SUBTOTAL FOR SECTION 3 (3 - 1 à 3 - 5)	
Negative subtotals :	TOTAL :
Positive subtotals :	
Note : add up positive scores and deduct negative scores (max: +70, minimum: -20).	

- Section 4 -

4 - 1 ☐ Corpulence		
Your BMI is :		
Below 18 kg/m²	Deduct 5 points	(-5)
Between 18 and 25 kg/m²	Add 10 points	(+10)
Between 25 and 30 kg/m²	Deduct 15 points	(-15)
Above 30 kg/m²	Deduct 30 points	(-30)

4 - 2 ☐ Waist		
You are a woman :		
Your waist size is less than 88 cm	Add 10 points	(+10)
Your waist size is between 88 and 95 cm	Deduct 10 points	(-10)
Your waist size is above 95 cm	Deduct 20 points	(-20)
You are a man :		
Your waist size is below 100 cm:	Add 10 points	(+10)
Your waist size is between 100 and 110 cm	Deduct 5 points	(-5)
Your waist size is above 110 cm	Deduct 20 points	(-20)

4 - 3 ☐ Holding your breath		
How long can you hold your breath?		
Less than 30 seconds	Deduct 10 points	(-10)
Between 30 and 60 seconds	Add 5 points	(+5)
Between 60 and 90 seconds	Add 10 points	(+10)
More than 90 seconds	Add 15 points	(+15)

4 - 4 ☐ Flexibility		
Can you touch your toes with your hands without bending your knees?	Yes : Add 5 points	(+5)
Pouvez-vous entrelacer vos doigts dans votre dos ?	Yes : Add 5 points	(+5)
Note : you may combine these answers.		

4 - 5 ☐ Sexual activity		
Do you have sex at least once a week?	Yes : Add 20 points	(+20)

SUBTOTAL FOR SECTION 4 (4 - 1 à 4 - 5)	
Negative subtotals :	TOTAL :
Positive subtotals :	
Note : add up positive scores and deduct negative scores (max: +65, minimum: -60).	

- Section 5 -

5 - 1 ☐ Hypertension		
Do you have high blood pressure (between 140 and 160 mm of Hg systolic and between 90 and 100 mm of Hg diastolic)?	Yes : Deduct 10 points	(-10)
Do you have very high blood pressure (more than 160 mm of Hg systolic and more than 100 mm of Hg diastolic)?	Yes : Deduct 20 points	(-20)
You don't know		(0)

5 - 2 ☐ Cholesterol		
Your total cholesterol is higher than 200	Deduct 5 points	(-5)
Your HDL (good cholesterol) is above 55	Add 10 points	(+10)
Your LDL (bad cholesterol) is above 150	Deduct 10 points	(-10)
You don't know		(0)

5 - 3 ☐ Triglycerides		
You are a man.		
Your blood triglyceride levels are above 150	Deduct 5 points	(-5)
You don't know		(0)

You are a woman.		
Your blood triglyceride levels are above 100	Deduct 5 points	(-5)
You don't know		(0)

Note : triglyceride levels in women are a better predictor of cardiovascular disease than cholesterol levels.

5 - 4 ☐ Diabetes		
You have diabetes (type 2 or type 1)	Deduct 20 points	(-20)

5 - 5 ☐ Cancer		
You have had cancer, but it is in remission		(0)
You have cancer, but it is responding well to treatment	Deduct 10 points	(-10)
You have cancer, but it is responding poorly to treatment	Deduct 30 points	(-30)

SUBTOTAL FOR SECTION 5 (5 - 1 à 5 - 5)	
Negative subtotals :	TOTAL :
Positive subtotals :	

Note : add up positive scores and deduct negative scores (max: +10, minimum: -65).

6 - 1 ☐ Tobacco		
Do you, or have you in the past, smoked more than 5 cigarettes daily :		
For 10 years	Deduct 25 points	(-25)
For 20 years	Deduct 50 points	(-50)
For 30 years	Deduct 75 points	(-75)
For 40 years	Deduct 100 points	(-100)
For 50 years or more	Deduct 125 points	(-125)

6 - 2 ☐ Alcohol		
Do you currently drink MORE THAN the equivalent of three glasses of wine a day?	Yes : Deduct 15 points	(-15)
Are you dependent on alcohol?	Yes : Deduct 20 points	(-20)
Note : only select one answer.		

6 - 3 ☐ Drugs		
Do you regularly consume cannabis?	Yes : Deduct 10 points	(-10)
Do you take any other drugs?	Yes : Deduct 30 points	(-30)
Note : only one answer.		

6 - 4 ☐ Other addictions		
Are you addicted to gambling?	Yes : Deduct 5 points	(-5)

6 - 5 ☐ Medication		
Do you regularly take a lot of medication?	Yes : Deduct 10 points	(-10)

SUBTOTAL FOR SECTION 6 (6 - 1 à 6 - 5)	
Negative subtotals :	TOTAL :
Positive subtotals :	
Note : add up the positive scores and deduct the negative scores (max: +0, minimum: -190).	

7 - 1 ☐ Cardiovascular disease		
Do you have coronary artery disease or do you regularly suffer from angina attacks?	Yes : Deduct 15 points	(-15)
Do you suffer from heart failure?	Yes : Deduct 30 points	(-30)

Note : you may combine these two answers.

7 - 2 ☐ Brain		
Do you suffer from frequent memory loss?	Yes : Deduct 10 points	(-10)
Do you suffer from Alzheimer's disease (or a similar disease)?	Yes : Deduct 25 points	(-25)
Do you suffer from vision impairment, e.g. macular degeneration?	Yes : Deduct 20 points	(-20)

Note : you may combine several answers.

7 - 3 ☐ Auto-immune diseases		
Do you suffer from rheumatoid polyarthritis or a similar disease?	Yes : Deduct 25 points	(-25)

7 - 4 ☐ Stress		
Do you consider that you lead a very stressful life? (Answer quickly and spontaneously!)	Yes : Deduct 25 points	(-25)

7 - 5 ☐ Satisfaction		
Generally speaking, do you think that you lead a happy life?	Yes : Add 10 points	(+10)

SUBTOTAL FOR SECTION 7 (7 - 1 à 7 - 5)	
Negative subtotals :	TOTAL :
Positive subtotals :	
Note : add up positive scores and deduct negative scores (max: +0, minimum: -155).	

- Section 8 -

8 - 1 □ Nutrition		
Do you regularly eat breakfast?	Yes : Add 20 points	(+20)
Do you regularly skip breakfast?	Yes : Deduct 20 points	(-20)
Do you eat at least five servings of fruits and vegetables each day?	Yes : Add 20 points	(+20)
Do you eat red meat more than three times per week?	Yes : Deduct 25 points	(-25)
Do you often feel too full and tired after a large meal?	Yes : Deduct 15 points	(-15)
Do you regularly eat fried foods?	Yes : Deduct 10 points	(-10)
Do you think you eat enough protein each day?	No : Deduct 15 points	(-15)
Do you regularly eat so-called 'whole' foods?	Yes : Add 10 points	(+10)
Do you regularly eat more than three eggs per week?	Yes : Add 10 points	(+10)
Do you regularly eat a lot of sugar?	Yes : Deduct 30 points	(-30)
Do you regularly eat olive oil?	Yes : Add 10 points	(+10)
Do you regularly eat fatty fish?	Yes : Add 10 points	(+10)

SUBTOTAL FOR QUESTION 8 - 1	
Negative subtotals :	TOTAL :
Positive subtotals :	
Note : add up positive scores and deduct negative scores (max: +70, minimum: -145).	

8 - 2 ☐ Dietary supplements		
Do you regularly take multivitamins?	Yes : Add 10 points	(+10)
Do you regularly take vitamin D3?	Yes : Add 10 points	(+10)
Do you regularly take a telomerase activator (TA65)?	Yes : Add 30 points	(+30)
Do you regularly take omega 3?	Yes : Add 20 points	(+20)

SUBTOTAL FOR QUESTION 8 - 2	
Negative subtotals :	TOTAL :
Positive subtotals :	
Note : add up positive scores and deduct negative scores (max: +70, minimum: -0).	

8 - 3 ☐ Physical activity		
Do you exercise less than three hours per week?	Yes : Deduct 20 points	(-20)
Do you exercise vigorously for more than six hours per week?	Yes : Add 20 points	(+20)

8 - 4 ☐ Sleep		
Do you sleep less than five hours per night or more than nine hours per night?	Yes : Deduct 10 points	(-10)
Do you suffer from sleep apnea?	Yes : Deduct 20 points	(-20)
Note : you may combine these two answers.		

8 - 5 ☐ Emotional stress		
Do you think that you are in control of your personal and professional life?	No : Deduct 10 points	(-10)
Do you easily become angry?	Yes : Deduct 5 points	(-5)
Note : you may combine these two answers.		

SUBTOTAL FOR SECTION 8 (8 - 1 à 8 - 5)	
Negative subtotals :	TOTAL :
Positive subtotals :	
Note : add up positive scores and deduct negative scores (max: +160, minimum: -210).	

SCORE

The base score is 1 000 points

Add (or deduct) to 1 000 the scores you received
for each of the eight subsections.

RESULTS FOR SECTIONS 1 TO 8	
Negative subtotals :	TOTAL :
Positive subtotals :	

Note : add up positive scores and deduct negative scores
(max: +360, minimum: -1015).
If your total score is negative (as is most often the case)
deduct this total from the base score (1 000 points.)

Example : total score for sections 1 to 8 = -350,
your score is: 1 000 – 350 = 650 points.

Interprétation

This test, which evaluates your biological age, is a good starting point for further investigation and, most importantly, it will act as a benchmark with which to assess your progress.

Given the subjective variability of most of your answers, we can only provide an approximation of your biological age compared to your chronological age. The important thing is to analyze your answers section by section. Certain sections, which deal with your past and unalterable factors, represent your **genetic** predisposition. Others, which are made of modifiable parameters, represent your **epigenetic** predisposition. These are the parameters which can change your life and your longevity!

- 1 -
Less than 500 points

Your biological age is far higher than your chronological age, in other words: your DNA is aging faster than you are adding on years. We suggest that you perform as many evaluation tests as possible (in particular telomere measurement) and immediately start the lifestyle improvement protocol and taking dietary supplements.

- 2 -
Between 500 and 700 points

You are younger than 60. Your biological age is higher than your chronological age. This demands you take on measures to improve your lifestyle and appropriate dietary supplements. Analyze those sections in which you have many negative numbers and focus on improving those items.

You are older than 60. You are in what would be called the normal range, but you would benefit from following a lifestyle improvement program.

- 3 -
Between 700 and 800 points

Your biological age is between 45 and 60 years old. If you are in the same chronological age range, you appear to be in the norm. If you want to turn this ship around, however, you will have to go the extra mile, especially in those sections where your scores are negative.

If your chronological age is higher than 60, congratulations, you are on the right track.

- 4 -
Between 800 and 900 points

Your biological age is below 50 years old. If your chronological age is above this, you have the cells of a young man or woman. You are on the right track, improve your performance by focusing on every negative number you got in this questionnaire.

- 5 -
Above 900 points

Congratulations, your biological age doesn't exceed 35/40 years of age and you are on the right track. Don't forget that delaying the aging process is a daily battle. Retake this test in 6 months.

Note : this test, which is subjective, is in no way a substitute for a doctor's advice.

Source : **Michael Fossel, Greta Blackburn,** *Dave Woynarowski. The Immortality Edge. Hoboken (New Jersey) : John Wiley & Sons, Inc. ; 2011.*

- Annex 2 -

Dietary profile

The goal of this assessment is to take stock of your CURRENT dietary habits.

This survey is essential as it allows us to understand the relationship you have with food, to discover imbalances as well as nutritional deficiencies. It will bring to light obvious mistakes: no breakfast, skipped meals, harmful dissociations, insufficient fiber intake etc.

- Section 1 -
Dietary balance

A balanced diet is the ultimate goal of any lifestyle modification program. In this case, we do not focus on calories but on the quality and balance of foods and of their components.

Eating a balanced diet is to only eat a little, but a little of everything!

1 ☐ I eat fish	
Very often (e.g. once a day)	(5)
Often (e.g. once every other day)	(4)
Somewhat often (e.g. twice a week)	(3)
Sometimes (e.g. once a week)	(2)
Never (or rarely)	(1)

2 ☐ I eat meat	
Very often (e.g. once a day)	(1)
Often (e.g. once every other day)	(2)
Somewhat often (e.g. twice a week)	(3)
Sometimes (e.g. once a week)	(4)
Never (or rarely)	(5)

3 ☐ I consume milk or dairy products	
Very often (e.g. once a day)	(1)
Often (e.g. once every other day)	(2)
Somewhat often (e.g. twice a week)	(3)
Sometimes (e.g. once a week)	(4)
Never (or rarely)	(5)

4 ☐ I eat eggs	
Very often (e.g. once a day)	(5)
Often (e.g. once every other day)	(4)
Somewhat often (e.g. twice a week)	(3)
Sometimes (e.g. once a week)	(2)
Never (or rarely)	(1)

5 ☐ I go to fast food restaurants	
Very often (e.g. once a day)	(1)
Often (e.g. once every other day)	(2)
Somewhat often (e.g. twice a week)	(3)
Sometimes (e.g. once a week)	(4)
Never (or rarely)	(5)

6 ☐ I eat vegetables	
Very often (e.g. once a day)	(5)

Often (e.g. once every other day)	(4)
Somewhat often (e.g. twice a week)	(3)
Sometimes (e.g. once a week)	(2)
Never (or rarely)	(1)

7 ☐ I eat fruits	
Very often (e.g. once a day)	(5)
Often (e.g. once every other day)	(4)
Somewhat often (e.g. twice a week)	(3)
Sometimes (e.g. once a week)	(2)
Never (or rarely)	(1)

8 ☐ I drink at least 1.5 liters of water or non-sugary drinks every day	
Always	(5)
Very often	(4)
Somewhat often	(3)
Sometimes	(2)
Never or rarely	(1)

TOTAL FOR SECTION 1
TOTAL :

Score and results. Section 1 : dietary balance

30/35

Your dietary balance is very satisfactory, your diet is very varied,
you eat a bit of everything, which is excellent.

24/29

Your dietary balance is satisfactory, your diet is varied,
you eat a bit of everything, which is a good thing.

18/23

Your dietary balance is unsatisfactory,
your diet is not varied enough, it can be improved.

13/17

Your diet is unbalanced and not varied enough,
you should eat only a little, but a little of everything.

7/12

Your diet is completely unbalanced and not varied at all.

- Section 2 -
Excess fat

Excess fat leads to being overweight, but you should remember that fat is often hidden in unexpected foods (cookies, soups, etc.) It is important to evaluate how much fat we consume, knowing that most will be stored.

9 ☐ My meals include processed or cured meats	
Very often (e.g. once a day)	(1)
Often (e.g. once every other day)	(2)
Somewhat often (e.g. twice a week)	(3)
Sometimes (e.g. once a week)	(4)
Never (or rarely)	(5)

10 ☐ I take fat off of meat and / or skin off of chicken	
Always	(5)
Very often	(4)
Somewhat often	(3)
Sometimes	(2)
I eat no meat or chicken	(1)

11 ☐ I eat breaded, fried or battered foods (fish, poultry, vegetables, potatoes)	
Very often (e.g. once a day)	(1)
Often (e.g. once every other day)	(2)
Somewhat often (e.g. twice a week)	(3)
Sometimes (e.g. once a week)	(4)
Never (or rarely)	(5)

TOTAL SECTION 2
TOTAL :

Score and results
Section 2 : excess fat

12/15
Your diet is low in fat.

7/11
Your diet is sometimes high in fat. Try to identify hidden fats.

3/6
Your diet is too high in fat.

- Section 3 -
Excess alcohol

Alcohol contains 7 Kcal per gram, which dissipates as heat, and we do not store alcohol. Theoretically, therefore, alcohol shouldn't make you fat! In practice however, it always leads to excess weight, as it reduces the amount of calories spent on fighting off cold and heat (thermogenesis).

12 ☐ Before lunch and/or dinner, I will gladly have a drink	
Always	(1)
Very often	(2)
Somewhat often	(3)
Sometimes	(4)
I never have a drink before eating	(5)

13 ☐ I drink wine or beer with every main meal	
More than 3 glasses/day	(1)
Often (e.g. 2 to 3 glasses/day)	(2)
Somewhat often (less than 2 glasses/day)	(3)
Sometimes (e.g. 1 glass from time to time)	(4)
Never (or rarely)	(5)

Score and results. Section 3 :
Excess alcohol

8/10
You drink nearly no alcohol.

6/7
You sometimes drink alcohol.

4/5
Your alcohol consumption is relatively high.

2/3
Your alcohol consumption is too high.

- Section 4 -

Excess sugar

Carbohydrates are not only in sweets, but also in starchy foods, bread, pasta, rice, dough, fruit and many others…

Excessive carbohydrate intake will not only lead to excess weight, but also constant hunger.

14 ☐ I eat pizza	
Very often (e.g. once a day)	(1)
Often (e.g. once every other day)	(2)
Somewhat often (e.g. twice a week)	(3)
Sometimes (e.g. once a week)	(4)
Never (or rarely)	(5)

15 ☐ I eat sweets (chocolate, pastries, cookies, ice-cream)	
Very often (e.g. once a day)	(1)
Often (e.g. once every other day)	(2)
Somewhat often (e.g. twice a week)	(3)
Sometimes (e.g. once a week)	(4)
Never (or rarely)	(5)

16 ☐ I sweeten my hot drinks (only count 'real sugar' and not artificial sweeteners)	
Very often (e.g. once a day)	(1)
Often (e.g. once every other day)	(2)
Somewhat often (e.g. twice a week)	(3)
Sometimes (e.g. once a week)	(4)
Never (or rarely)	(5)

17 ☐ I drink sweetened beverages or sodas (Mountain Dew, Sprite, Coca-Cola etc.)	
Always	(1)
Very often	(2)
Somewhat often	(3)
Sometimes	(4)
Never or rarely	(5)

18 ☐ I eat bread, cereal or starches	
Very often (e.g. once a day)	(1)
Often (e.g. once every other day)	(2)
Somewhat often (e.g. twice a week)	(3)
Sometimes (e.g. once a week)	(4)
Never (or rarely)	(5)

19 ☐ I have trouble stopping once I start eating bread, sweets, pasta or pizza	
Always	(1)
Very often	(2)
Somewhat often	(3)
Sometimes	(4)
Never or rarely	(5)

Score and results. Section 4 : Excess sugar

33/40
Your diet is very low in carbohydrates.

27/32
Your diet is low in carbohydrates.

21/26
Your diet is sometimes high in carbohydrates.

14/20
Your diet is often high in carbohydrates.

8/13
Your diet is far too high in sweets and carbohydrates.
We suggest your limit your consumption.

- Section 5 -

Dietary behavior

The rhythm and regularity of your meals are among the key factors for the prevention of excess weight. It is important to know whether your meals are structured and regular or whether you have unstructured meals, leading to constant snacking.

20 ☐ In the evening, I eat while watching TV	
Always	(1)
Very often	(2)
Somewhat often	(3)
Sometimes	(4)
Never or rarely	(5)

21 ☐ I eat between meals	
Very often (e.g. once a day)	(1)
Often (e.g. once every other day)	(2)
Somewhat often (e.g. twice a week)	(3)
Sometimes (e.g. once a week)	(4)
Never (or rarely)	(5)

22 ☐ I know how to read and understand food labels	
Very true	(5)
True	(4)
Somewhat true	(3)
False	(2)
Completely false	(1)

23 ☐ I pay attention to what I eat	
Very true	(5)
True	(4)
Somewhat true	(3)
False	(2)
Completely false	(1)

24 ☐ I know what to eat to have a balanced diet	
Very true	(5)
True	(4)
Somewhat true	(3)
False	(2)
Completely false	(1)

25 ☐ I eat sandwiches	
Always	(1)
Very often	(2)
Somewhat often	(3)
Sometimes	(4)
Never or rarely	(5)

26 ☐ I eat at least three meals a day: breakfast, lunch and dinner	
Always	(5)
Very often	(4)
Somewhat often	(3)
Sometimes	(2)
Never or rarely	(1)

Score and results. Section 5 : Dietary behavior

26/30
Your dietary behavior is very satisfactory.

21/25
Your dietary behavior is satisfactory.

16/20
Your dietary behavior is relatively satisfactory, but could be improved.

11/15
Your dietary behavior is unsatisfactory; it would be advisable to take on a regular rhythm.

6/10
Your dietary behavior is completely out of control and could be the source of unmanageable weight gain.

SCORE

Dietary profile

Total for sections 1 to 5

Total :

110/135
Your answers indicate that your dietary profile is very satisfactory. You only eat a little, but a little of everything.

89/109
Your answers indicate that your dietary profile is satisfactory.

68/88
Your answers indicate a relatively satisfactory dietary profile, but you can do much better.

47/67
Your answers indicate that your diet is unsatisfactory, with irregular rhythms and frequent excesses.

26/46
Your answers indicate that your diet is out of control, with completely irregular rhythms and frequent excesses.

- Annex 3 -

Physical activity profile

Physical activity is the second element of any lifestyle management program. It is just as important as the way you eat, and will be a determining factor of your long-term success. Physical activity does not necessarily mean sports or fitness. Physical activity includes everything which contributes to mobilizing your muscle mass. As you know, every muscle movement (contraction and release of muscle fibers) requires energy.

Improving your physical activity is a key factor. This is why we ask that you fill out a detailed account of your physical activity BEFORE starting the program. We will then show you how to elaborate a physical activity program which is adapted to your needs, your abilities, and especially to your happiness.

1 □ Physical activity at home	
I expend a great deal of energy as I always have something to do (gardening, repairs, cleaning)	(5)
I spend a lot of energy	(4)
I do not spend much energy	(3)
I spend little energy	(2)
I spend nearly no energy	(1)

2 □ Physical activity at work	
My work requires that I expend a great deal of energy	(5)
I spend quite a bit of energy at work	(4)
I spend only some energy at work	(3)
I spend little energy at work	(2)
My job is entirely sedentary	(1)

3 □ Physical activity during leisure time	
I exercise fairly vigorously at least three times a week, and I have done so for several years	(5)
I have exercised moderately for several years	(4)
I have exercised moderately but regularly for several months	(3)
I exercise irregularly, with ups and downs	(2)
I am completely sedentary	(1)

4 ☐ I intend to improve my level of physical activity	
I am absolutely sure of it	(5)
I am sure of it	(4)
Probably	(3)
Maybe	(2)
Certainly not	(1)

Scores and results

17/20
Your lifestyle is very active, you expend a lot of energy, and regularly so.

14/16
You have an active lifestyle, you expend a lot of energy, and regularly so.

11/13
You have a semi-active lifestyle, with some irregularity in your physical activity.

8/10
Your lifestyle is relatively inactive, with irregular physical activity.

4/7
Your lifestyle is completely sedentary, you must urgently improve your level of physical activity.

- Annex 4 -

Assessment of the components of your stress

Stress is a habit, and improving your stress levels therefore requires you to change your habits. Before doing this, however, you should know that, no matter how high your level of stress, your ability to process change manifests itself through physical, psychological, and behavioral reactions. This test will enable you to identify the importance of these three parameters.

It is divided into three sections; answer the questions, then add up the total of each section, your score will indicate which parameter affects you the most, which will allow you to focus on managing that particular parameter.

- Section 1 -

Physical context

1 ☐ I have trouble sleeping (trouble falling asleep or waking up too early)	
Always	(5)
Very often	(4)
often	(3)
Sometimes	(2)
Never	(1)

2 ☐ When faced with an event, even a small one, I tend to have a lump in my throat and sweaty palms, not knowing what to say	
Completely true	(5)
True	(4)
No opinion	(3)
Somewhat false	(2)
Completely false	(1)

3 ☐ I often resort to alcohol or cigarettes (or another drug) in order to relax	
Completely true	(5)
True	(4)
No opinion	(3)

Somewhat false	(2)
Completely false	(1)

4 ☐ I regularly suffer from unpleasant physical manifestations (digestive issues, trouble breathing or heart palpitations)	
Completely true	(5)
True	(4)
No opinion	(3)
Somewhat false	(2)
Completely false	(1)

TOTAL SECTION 1

TOTAL :

Scores and answers. Section 1: Physical context

If your score is higher than 12

Stress mainly affects you physically. There is too much cortisol in your blood, especially when you are upset. By straining your physical reactions to stress in this way, you run the risk of developing cardiovascular disease, diabetes or even cancer later in your life.

- Section 2 -

Psychological and emotional context

5 ☐ I have trouble relaxing during the week-end and forgetting about my work or my hobby	
Always	(5)
Very often	(4)
often	(3)
Sometimes	(2)
Never	(1)

6 ☐ After I have completed a task, I can worry and stay stuck in negative thought patterns	
Always	(5)
Very often	(4)
often	(3)
Sometimes	(2)
Never	(1)

7 ☐ I am happy with myself and always think, I am up to the challenge at my job	
Completely true	(1)
True	(2)

No opinion	(3)
Somewhat false	(4)
Completely false	(5)

8 ☐ I experience less pleasure and interest than before in my professional and leisure activities	
Completely true	(5)
True	(4)
No opinion	(3)
Somewhat false	(2)
Completely false	(1)

TOTAL SECTION 2
TOTAL :

Scores and answers. Section 2 : Psychological and emotional context

If your score is higher than 12

Stress mainly affects you mentally and emotionally. You mull things over too much and tend to have a pessimistic view of things and events you are confronted with. Be careful not to gradually fall into depression or chronic anxiety.

The best way to manage stress in your case is to try to analyze the stressful situations you encounter in a different way. For example, it would certainly be very useful for you to develop more positive lines of reasoning and think in a more optimistic way. In other words, to learn to take a step back and put the importance of things and events into perspective.

- Section 3 -
Behavioral context

9 ☐ I feel annoyed or irritated when things don't go exactly as planned	
Always	(5)
Very often	(4)
often	(3)
Sometimes	(2)
Never	(1)

10 ☐ I interrupt others and try to impose my point of view	
Always	(5)
Very often	(4)
often	(3)
Sometimes	(2)
Never	(1)

11 ☐ I feel as though I rush my work, for lack of time	
Completely true	(5)
True	(4)

No opinion	(3)
Somewhat false	(2)
Completely false	(1)

12 ☐ I sometimes lose my temper with those around me	
Completely true	(5)
True	(4)
No opinion	(3)
Somewhat false	(2)
Completely false	(1)

TOTAL SECTION 3
TOTAL :

Scores and answers. Section 3 : Behavioral context

If your score is higher than 12

Stress mainly affects your behavior. You are a reactive individual, sometimes even hyper-reactive, and you aren't the only one to have noticed. Indeed, those close to you probably suffer from your stress as much as you do. In order to effectively decrease you level of stress, it seems important that you change part of your everyday behavior. In this way you will be able to act less impulsively, and take the time to do things deliberately, as well as be less aggressive and more tolerant of those around you.

Which is the highest score?	
Physical stress score	
Emotional stress score	
Behavioral stress score	
Begin by focusing on the highest score.	
More generally : add up all 3 scores	

- 1 -

Total score: 12 - 23

Apparently stress doesn't affect you. Your body does not react strongly to stress; you can control your emotions. Your behavior is well aligned, you are always calm and peaceful. You have likely managed to place yourself within an environment stripped of any stress.

- 2 -

Total score: 24 - 35

Some stress, yes, but no despair. The situation is under control, and even if stress comes up, you know how to deal with it. Your stress level is low, and it likely allows you to effectively resolve the problems you encounter. You show no physical or emotional reactions.

- 3 -

Total score: 36 - 47

Stress is your thing! As you are often affected by it, it certainly may help you bring your best game to the table, and it stimulates you when faced with constraints and challenges. But careful! Even if stress has not completely overwhelmed you, it is probably in your best interest to try to manage it better in certain situations. At the very least in the interest of your health or your performance.

- 4 -

Total score: 48 – 60

Your level of stress is very high, and even if physical signs are not yet apparent, you can be sure they already exist. Your emotions and your behavior reflect your very high stress levels. There is still time for you to turn things around however, either by changing your environment, or by learning to manage your stress. The help of a specialist will likely be necessary. Do so before burning out completely!

Source : Patrick Légeron. Le stress au travail. Paris : Odile Jacob ; 2001.

Selected bibliography

Works cited

Works in French

☐ De l'ADN moléculaire à l'ADN vibratoire. http://www.spirit-science.fr

☐ Alain Reinberg. Nos horloges biologiques sont-elles à l'heure ? Paris : Le Pommier ; 2004.

☐ Axel Kahn, Fabrice Papillon. Le secret de la salamandre. Paris : Nil Editions ; 2005.

☐ B. Bensaud-Vincent. Les vertiges de la technoscience, façonner le monde atome par atome. Paris : La Découverte ; 2004.

☐ Bruce H. Lipton. Biologie des croyances. Québec : Ariane Editions Inc. ; 2006.

☐ Charles Cungi. Savoir gérer son stress. Paris : Éditions Retz ; 2003.

☐ Christian Drapeau. Le pouvoir insoupçonné des cellules souches. Québec : Les Editions de l'Homme ; 2010.

☐ David Servan-Schreiber. Guérir. Paris : Éditions Robert Laffont ; 2003.

☐ David Servan-Schreiber. Anticancer. Paris : Éditions Robert Laffont ; 2003.

☐ David Servan-Schreiber. Guérir le stress, l'anxiété et la dépression sans médicament ni psychanalyse. Paris : Éditions Robert Laffont ; 2003.

☐ David Servan-Schreiber. On peut se dire au revoir plusieurs fois. Paris : Éditions Robert Laffont ; 2011.

☐ David Servan-Schreiber. Notre corps aime la vérité. Paris : Éditions Robert Laffont ; 2012 (publié à titre posthume).

☐ Dawson Church. Le génie dans vos gènes. Escalquens : Éditions Dangles ; 2013.

☐ Dominique Rueff, Maurice Nahon. Stratégie longue vie. Archamps : Éditions Jouvence ; 2013.

☐ Frédéric Dardel, Renaud Leblond. Main basse sur le génome. Paris : Anne Carrière Éditions ; 2008.

☐ Giorgio Maria Carbone. L'enjeu des cellules souches. Paris : Salvator ; 2006.

☐ Guy Corneau. Revivre. Québec : Les Editions de l'Homme ; 2010.

☐ Helena Baranova. Nos gènes, notre santé, et nous. Paris : Armand Colin ; 2004.

☐ Jean David Ponci. La biologie du vieillissement. Paris : L'Harmattan ; 2008.

☐ Joël de Rosnay, Jean-Louis Servan-Schreiber, François de Closets, Dominique Simonnet. Une vie en plus. Paris : Seuil ; 2005.

☐ Laurent Alexandre. La mort de la mort. Paris : JC Lattes ; 2011.

☐ Liliane Reuter. Votre esprit est votre meilleur médecin. Paris : Robert Laffont ; 1999.

☐ Marie de Hennezel, Bertrand Vergely. Une vie pour se mettre au monde. Paris : Carnets Nord ; 2010.

☐ Miroslav Radman. Au-delà de nos limites biologiques. Paris : Plon ; 2011.

☐ Nathalie Zammatteo. L'impact des émotions sur l'ADN. Aubagne : Éditions Quintessence ; 2014.

☐ Nicole Le Douarin. Les cellules souches. Paris : Odile Jacob ; 2007.

☐ Patrick Légeron. Le stress au travail. Paris : Odile Jacob ; 2001.

☐ Ray Kurzweil, Terry Grossman. Serons-nous immortels ? Paris : Dunod ; 2006.

☐ Thierry Hertoghe, Jules-Jacques Nabet. Comment rester jeune plus longtemps ? Paris : Albin Michel ; 2000.

☐ Walter Wahli, Nathalie Constantin. La nutrigénomique dans votre assiette. Bruxelles : Éditions De Boeck ; 2011.

Works in English

☐ Ann B. Pearson. The Proteus Effect. Washington D.C. : Joseph Henry Press ; 2004.

☐ Aubrey de Grey, Michael Rae. Ending Aging. New-York : St. Martin's Griffin ; 1963.

☐ Andrew Weil. Healthy Aging. New York : Anchor Books ; 2005.

☐ Barry Sears. The Anti-inflammation Zone. New York : HarperCollins ; 2005.

☐ Brandon Colby. Outsmart Your Genes. New York : Perigee Book ; 2010.

☐ David A. Kekich. Smart, Strong and Sexy at 100? New-port Beach, (Californie) : Maximum Life Foundation ; 2012.

☐ David Serban-Schreiber. Anti-Cancer. New-York : Penguin Group ; 2007.

☐ David Stipp. The Youth Pill. New York : Current – Penguin Group ; 2013.

☐ Debra Niehoff. The Language of Life. Washington D.C. : Joseph Henry Press ; 2005.

☐ Eric R. Braverman. Younger You. New York : McGraw Hill ; 2007.

☐ Eric R. Braverman. The Edge Effect. New York : Sterling Publishing Co. Inc. ; 2005.

☐ Frederic J. Vagnini, Dave Bunnell. Count Down your Age. New-York : McGraw-Hill ; 2007.

☐ Ian McDowell, Claire Newell. Measuring Health. New-York : Oxford University Press ; 1996.

☐ James D. Baird. Obesity Genes. Illinois : HWL.Inc. (Naperville) ; 2012.

☐ John M. Emmett. Turning Back the Hands of Time. Baltimore : Abecedarian Books ; 2005.

☐ Joseph C. Maroon. The Longevity Factor. New-York : Atria Books ; 2009.

☐ Joseph C. Maroon, Jeffrey Bost. Fish Oil. Laguna Beach (Californie) : Basic Health Publications ; 2006.

☐ Leonard Hayflick. How and Why We Age. New York : Ballantine books ; 1994.

☐ Marianne J. Legato. Why Men Die First. New York : Palgrave Macmillan ; 2009.

☐ Michael D.West. The Immortal Cell. New York : Doubleday ; 2003.

☐ Michael Roizen, Mehmet Oz. YOU: The Owner's Manual. New York : William Morrow ; 2005.

☐ Michael Fossel, Greta Blackburn, Dave Woynarowski. The Immortality Edge. Hoboken (New Jersey) : John Wiley & Sons, Inc. ; 2011.

☐ Michael Fossel. The Telomerase Revolution. Dallas : Benbella Books Inc. ; 2015.

☐ Myron Wentz. Invisible Miracles. Québec : Medecis, S.C ; 2002.

☐ Oz Garcia. The Balance. New-York : Regan Books ; 2000.

☐ Paul McGlothin & Meredith Averill. The CR Way. New York : Harper-Collins ; 2008.

☐ Paul Yanick Jr, Vincent C. Giampapa. Quantum Longevity. San Diego, CA : ProMotion Publishing ; 1997.

☐ Ray Kurzweil, Terry Grossman. Fantastic Voyage. New York : Plume Book ; 2005.

☐ Ronald Klatz, Robert Goldman. Stopping the Clock. New York : Bantam Books ; 1996.

☐ Ronald Siegel. The Mindfulness Solution. New York : The Guilford Press ; 2010.

☐ Robert A. Freitas Jr. Nanomedicine. Volume I : Basic Capabilities. Austin (Texas) : Landes Biosciences ; 1999.

☐ Stuart J. Olshansky, Bruce A. Carnes. The Quest for Immortality. New York : W.W.Norton & Company ; 2001.

☐ Ted Anton. The Longevity Seekers. Chicago : The University of Chicago Press ; 2013.

☐ Vincent C. Giampapa, Frederick F. Buechel, Ohan Karatoprack. The Gene Makeover. Laguna Beach (Californie) : Basic Health ; 2007.

☐ Vincent C. Giampapa. The Basic Principles and Practice of Anti-aging Medicine & Age Management. Publication universitaire ; 2003.

Websites

Our website : www.Jlife-sciences.com

Useful websites in French

Stem cells :

☐ www.istem.eu

☐ www.inserm.fr

☐ www.eurostemcell.org/fr/

☐ Futura Sciences : www.futura-sciences.com

☐ La Longévité française : www.longevite.fr

☐ Santé : www.maxisciences.com

☐ Allo docteurs : www.allodocteurs.fr/

☐ Health Plexus : www.healthplexus.net

☐ Clés de santé : www.clesdesante.com

☐ Esculape : www.esculape.com

☐ Énergie : www.energie-sante.net

☐ De l'ADN moléculaire à l'ADN vibratoire : www.spirit-science.fr

Dietary supplements :

☐ www.nutranews.org

☐ www. Supermart.com

Useful websites in English

☐ American Aging Association (AGE) : www.americanaging.org

☐ American Academy of Anti-Aging Medicine : www.worldhealth.net

☐ American Federation for Aging Research : www.afar.org

- Alcor Life Extension Foundation (Cryonics) : www.alcor.org
- Anti-Aging Systems : www.anti-agingsytems.com
- Ben Best : www.benbest.com
- The calorie Restriction Society : www.calorierestriction,org
- Dr Dave Woynarowski : www.drdavesbest.com
- Dr Mercola : www.mercola.com
- Fight Aging : www.fightaging.org
- Fitness : www.bodybuilding.com
- Geron Corporation : www.geron.com
- How to meditate : www.how-to-meditate.org
- Immortality Institute : www.imminst.org
- H+Magazine : www.hplusmagazine.com
- Jeunesse : www.jeunesseglobal.com
- Life Enhancement Products : www.lifeenhancement.com
- The Longevity Meme : www.longevitymeme.org
- Manhattan Beach Project to cure aging by 2029 : www.manhattanbeachproject.com
- Maximum Life Foundation : www.MaxLife.org
- Men's fitness : www.mensfitness.com
- My fitness page : www.myfitnesspage.com
- Natural News : www.naturalnews.com
- National Institute on aging : www.nia.nih.gov
- Project LIFE : www.projectlife.org
- Repeat Diagnostics : www.repeatdiagnostics.com
- SENS : www.sens.org
- Sierra Sciences : www.sierrasciences.com
- Spectracell Laboratories : www.spectracell.com
- Stanford Centre on Longevity : www.longevity.stanford.edu
- TA65 : www.tasciences.com
- The Methuselah Foundation : www.methuselafoundation.org
- The Missing Human Manual : www.missinhumanmanual.com
- Third Age : www.thirdage.com
- Women Fitness : www.womenfitness.com
- Yoga today : www.yogatoday.com

Notes

Notes

Notes

Notes

Notes

Notes